PANCE®/PANRE®
Qbook

Sixth Edition

PANCE®/PANRE® Qbook

Sixth Edition

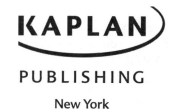

PUBLISHING

New York

© 2016 by Kaplan, Inc.

Published by Kaplan Publishing, a division of Kaplan, Inc.
750 Third Avenue
New York, NY 10017

Printed in the United States of America

10 9 8 7 6 5 4 3 2 1

ISBN-13: 978-1-62523-264-9

Kaplan Publishing books are available at special quantity discounts to use for sales promotions, employee premiums, or educational purposes. For more information or to purchase books, please call the Simon & Schuster special sales department at 866-506-1949.

EDITED BY

James Van Rhee, MS, PA-C

Associate Professor
Program Director
Physician Associate Program
Yale University School of Medicine
New Haven, Connecticut

For Any Test Changes or Late-Breaking Developments

kaptest.com/pages/retail-book-corrections-and-updates

The material in this book is up-to-date at the time of publication; however, the National Commission on Certification of Physician Assistants may have instituted changes in the test after this book was published. Carefully read the materials you receive when you register for the test. If there are any important late-breaking developments—or any changes or corrections to the Kaplan test preparation materials in this book—we will post that information online at kaptest.com/pages/retail-book-corrections-and-updates.

Contents

Part III: Information for Recently Graduated Physician Assistants

Part IV: PANCE/PANRE Practice Tests

Part V: PANCE/PANRE Resources

Preface

Congratulations: By purchasing this book, you're on your way to achieving your highest score possible on the PANCE licensing exam and the PANRE recertification exam.

- Part I: Understanding the Physician Assistant National Certifying Exam (PANCE), opens with Chapter 1, Overview of the PANCE, which discusses the role of the PANCE in obtaining the Physician Assistant–Certified (PA-C) credential. The PANCE examination structure, testing blueprint, and principles of testing are described in detail.

- Chapter 2, Introduction to Computer-Based Testing (CBT), reviews the testing interface and offers the information and strategies you need to be prepared.

- Chapter 3, Registering for the PANCE, is your step-by-step guide through the PANCE registration process.

- Chapters 4 through 6 focus on the study skills and test-taking strategies necessary to be a successful test taker. You will find clear instructions about the areas of study skills that are commonly overlooked, that is, **creating and then executing an effective review plan**. A full discussion of how to create your study plan includes choosing subject versus organ-system review and identifying and correcting patterns of error. The most common test-taker mistakes, strategies, methodologies, and anxiety coping mechanisms are also reviewed.

- Part II: Understanding the Recertification Process, contains Chapter 7, PANRE Recertification. This chapter provides an overview of the PANRE as well as information about registering and reviewing for the test, and what to expect on test day.

- Part III: Information for Recently Graduated Physician Assistants, contains Chapter 8, Transitioning from School to the Workplace. This section gives guidance on navigating the current job market, writing a resume, and establishing a permanent credentials file.

- Two full-length practice tests are provided in Part IV. These practice tests simulate the types of questions you may encounter on the PANCE and PANRE and the length of time each test will take. Each test is broken down into 60-question blocks. Use the first test early in your studies to familiarize yourself with the exam's length and to identify your areas of strength and weakness. Take the second exam closer to the test date to help you practice your timing and incorporate the newly learned test-taking strategies. We recommend that you allot **60 minutes** for each block and allow no more than 45 minutes of total break time between the 5 blocks (total time for the practice test 5 hours and 45 minutes). Using the same timing for the practice tests as for the exam will prepare you for the conditions you'll face on test day. Explanations of both the correct and incorrect answer choices are provided at the end of each exam. These explanations will provide you with the information needed to answer other similar questions on the same topic. A list of standard lab values is found at the back for easy reference (Resource I).

- Finally, PANCE/PANRE Resources (Part V) reference state requirements and laws that you need to take into account when planning your future as a certified physician assistant.

Thank you for choosing Kaplan Medical, the leaders in test preparation of exam review in the medical fields. We wish you the best of luck on the PANCE or PANRE and in your career as a physician assistant!

Kaplan Medical

PART I

Understanding the Physician Assistant National Certifying Exam (PANCE)

Overview of the PANCE

ABOUT THE PANCE

To become certified as a physician assistant, you must first graduate from a training program accredited by the Accreditation Review Commission on Education for the Physician Assistant (ARC-PA). This requirement also applies to those who have earned a medical degree outside the United States. Graduation from an accredited program makes you eligible to take the PANCE, an acronym that stands for **Physician Assistant National Certifying Exam**. The National Commission on the Certification of Physician Assistants (NCCPA) was created to serve as the certifying body for the profession and functions as an independent testing body, autonomous from any particular school or training program.

The PANCE, prepared by the NCCPA, is a test of minimum competency designed to assess whether examinees have the knowledge and skills needed for entry-level practice.

Note

The PANRE, the recertification equivalent of the PANCE, is discussed in greater detail in Part II.

PANCE at a Glance

Examination length: 5 hours and 45 minutes (administered in five 60-minute blocks plus 45 minutes for breaks)

Number of questions: 300 total (approx. 1 minute per question)

Question types: Multiple choice

PANCE CONTENT

Nearly all standardized licensure examinations are constructed around what's called an **exam blueprint**. An examination development group uses a content blueprint to guide the construction of an examination, referring to the blueprint to make decisions about what content to assess and what the emphasis of the exam should be. The NCCPA groups the tasks you will be tested on using seven categories and has set the percent of items in PANCE that will be devoted to each category, as shown in Table 1-1 and explained next.

Table 1-1. PANCE Content by Knowledge/Skill Areas

Percent of Exam Content	Knowledge/Skill Areas
16	History Taking and Performing Physical Examinations
14	Using Laboratory and Diagnostic Studies
18	Formulating the Most Likely Diagnosis
10	Health Maintenance
14	Clinical Intervention
18	Pharmaceutical Therapeutics
10	Applying Basic Science Concepts
Total 100%	

1. History taking and performing physical examinations

These items assess your knowledge of:

- Pertinent history for important medical conditions
- Risk factors for developing important medical conditions
- Signs and symptoms for important medical conditions
- Physical examination techniques
- Physical examination findings associated with important medical conditions
- Appropriate physical examination for important medical conditions
- Differential diagnosis associated with presenting symptoms or physical findings

These items also assess your critical thinking in:

- Conducting comprehensive, focused interviews
- Identifying relevant historical information
- Performing comprehensive, focused physical examinations
- Associating the current complaint with history
- Identifying relevant physical examination information

2. Using laboratory and diagnostic studies

These items assess your knowledge of:

- Indications for initial and subsequent studies (diagnostic or laboratory)
- Cost-effectiveness of diagnostic studies or procedures
- Relevance of common screening tests for selected health conditions
- Normal and abnormal diagnostic ranges
- Risks associated with diagnostic studies or procedures
- Appropriate patient education concerning laboratory or diagnostic studies

These items also assess your critical thinking in:
- Safe and appropriate use of diagnostic equipment
- Choosing appropriate diagnostic or laboratory studies
- Collecting specimens for diagnostic or laboratory studies
- Interpreting the results of diagnostic or laboratory studies

3. Formulating most likely diagnosis

These items assess your knowledge of:
- How to interpret patient history with respect to differential diagnosis
- How to interpret physical findings with respect to diagnosis
- How to interpret diagnostic and laboratory studies with respect to diagnosis

These items also assess your critical thinking in:
- Correlating normal and abnormal diagnostic data
- Establishing the differential diagnosis
- Selecting the most likely diagnosis in with regard to the data presented

4. Health maintenance

These items assess your knowledge of:
- Epidemiology of important medical conditions
- Early detection and prevention of important medical conditions
- Relative merits of common screening tests
- Appropriate patient education regarding preventable conditions or lifestyle modifications
- Healthy lifestyles
- Prevention of communicable diseases
- Immunization schedules and recommendations
- Immunization risks and benefits
- Human growth and development
- Human sexuality
- Occupational and environmental exposure
- Effect of stress on health
- Psychological manifestations of illness and injury
- Effects of aging and changing family roles on health maintenance and disease prevention
- Signs of abuse and neglect
- Barriers to care

These items also assess your critical thinking in:
- Techniques of counseling and patient education
- Effective communication with patients to enhance health maintenance
- Adapting health maintenance to the patient's context
- Use of informational databases

5. Clinical intervention

These items assess your knowledge of:

- Management and treatment of important medical conditions
- Indications, contraindications, complications, risks, benefits, and techniques for selected procedures
- Standard precautions and special isolation conditions
- Sterile technique
- Follow-up and monitoring of therapeutic regimens
- Medical emergencies
- Indications to admit or discharge
- Discharge planning
- Available community resources
- Appropriate community resources
- Appropriate patient education
- Roles of other health professionals
- End-of-life issues
- Risks and benefits of alternative medicine

These items also assess your critical thinking in:

- Formulating and implementing treatment plans
- Recognizing life-threatening emergencies and initiating treatment
- Demonstrating technical expertise related to performing specific procedures
- Communicating effectively
- Using counseling techniques
- Promoting patient adherence and active participation in treatment
- Working effectively in multidisciplinary teams

6. Pharmacological therapies

These items assess your knowledge of:

- Mechanism of action
- Indications for use
- Contraindications
- Side effects
- Adverse reactions
- Follow-up and monitoring of pharmacologic regimens
- Risks for drug interactions
- Clinical presentation of drug interactions
- Treatment of drug interactions
- Drug toxicity
- Methods to reduce medication errors
- Cross-reactivity of similar medications
- Presentation and treatment of allergic reactions

These items also assess your critical thinking in:

- Selecting appropriate pharmacologic therapy for important medical conditions
- Monitoring and adjusting pharmacologic regimens
- Evaluating and reporting adverse drug reactions

7. Applying basic science concepts

These items assess your knowledge of:

- Human anatomy and physiology
- Underlying pathophysiology
- Microbiology and biochemistry

These items also assess your critical thinking in:

- Recognizing normal and abnormal anatomy and physiology
- Relating pathophysiologic principles to specific disease processes
- Correlating abnormal physical examination findings with a given disease process
- Correlating abnormal results of diagnostic tests with a given disease process

The PANCE content also may be understood in terms of the diseases, disorders, and medical assessments that you might encounter during the examination. The percent of questions for various organ systems is shown in Table 1-2.

Table 1-2. PANCE Content by Organ System

Percent of Exam Content	Organ System
16	Cardiovascular System
12	Pulmonary System
10	Gastrointestinal (GI) System/Nutrition
10	Musculoskeletal System
9	Eyes, Ears, Nose, and Throat (EENT)
8	Reproductive System
6	Endocrine System
6	Neurologic System
6	Psychiatry/Behavioral Science
6	Genitourinary System
5	Dermatologic System
3	Hematologic System
3	Infectious Diseases
Total **100%**	

Note

No standardized licensing exam is 100% predictable, and question writers work hard to create questions that require understanding and integration of the material. So the best overall goal in reviewing is to aim for genuine understanding of major concepts, key definitions, and integration of that knowledge across subject areas.

By multiplying the proportional contribution of each disease category by the proportion of the exam dealing with each knowledge/skill area, one can form a matrix that illustrates the relative emphasis for various topics to be tested (Table 1-3). Many students find that this is a rough but helpful way to determine how much study time to invest in reviewing one topic versus another.

The ultimate decision about the amount of time you will need to invest in becoming test-ready for each topic is yours. You must consider your own unique subject strengths and weaknesses. Table 1-3 gives only *approximations* of how the test will distribute content.

Table 1-3. PANCE Content Matrix

Organ System	Knowledge/Skill Areas							
	History and Physical Exam	Labs/ Diagnostic Studies	Formulating a Diagnosis	Clinical Intervention	Clinical Therapeutics	Health Maintenance	Applying Scientific Concepts	Totals ↓
Cardiovascular	8	7	8	7	9	5	4	48
Pulmonary	7	5	6	5	6	3	4	36
GI/Nutrition	5	4	6	4	5	3	3	30
Musculoskeletal	5	4	6	4	5	3	3	30
EENT	4	4	5	4	6	2	2	27
Reproductive	4	4	5	3	4	2	2	24
Endocrine	3	3	3	2	3	2	2	18
Neurologic	3	2	3	3	3	2	2	18
Psych/Beh. Sci.	2	2	3	3	4	2	2	18
Genitourinary	2	3	3	3	3	2	2	18
Dermatologic	2	2	2	2	3	2	2	15
Hematologic	2	1	2	1	1	1	1	9
Infectious Dis.	1	1	2	1	2	1	1	9
Totals:	48	42	54	42	54	30	30	300

Introduction to Computer-Based Testing (CBT)

2

INTRODUCTION

From a testing organization's viewpoint, computer-based testing (CBT) offers many advantages: it can occur year-round at thousands of sites; each test site offers standard testing conditions concerning computer equipment used and rules governing the behavior and monitoring of examinees; and examinees usually receive score reports within 2 to 4 weeks of their test date.

THE COMPUTER-BASED TESTING ENVIRONMENT

The PANCE and PANRE examinations are administered as CBTs at Pearson VUE Test Centers in all 50 U.S. states and at selected locations outside the United States. Typically, within 48 hours of when you receive notification from the NCCPA of your eligibility window, Pearson VUE will also have your eligibility verification, allowing you to go to their website and arrange a test date (see Chapter 3).

Know Where You're Going

Plan to arrive at the test center 30 minutes before your scheduled test appointment to allow time for verification of your credentials and any site-specific introductory information. If you are unfamiliar with the location of the test center, it may be wise to do a scouting run before test day.

Upon Arrival

The NCCPA will inform you what to bring and what to expect on your test day when you are notified of your eligibility window. Make sure you bring 2 forms of identification: a primary identification, which contains a permanently affixed photo of the examinee, along with the examinee's preprinted name and signature (for example: driver's license, passport, military identification, student ID, or state-issued identification), and a secondary identification, which contains the examinee's preprinted name and signature (for example: driver's license, military identification, student ID, employee ID, social security card, or credit card); or 2 forms of primary identification.

Remember

It is recommended that you take breaks only at designated times. The time clock will not be stopped if you leave the testing room during unofficial breaks.

Inside the Testing Area

It is advisable to dress in layers on test day so that you can adjust easily to the testing area temperature. All center locations have storage lockers for personal items; you will be allowed to carry nothing into the examination area.

Food and beverages are not allowed in the testing rooms. You can leave the testing area to get a drink, take medications, or use the restroom, but the time clock does not stop when you are away from your computer, except at designated break times.

Break time is allowed after each 60-minute test block—four breaks overall—but the examinee must decide how long a break to take and must stay within the 45-minute total break time allotted for the whole test day. Examinees are required to scan their finger or palm when leaving or reentering the testing area.

No scratch paper is allowed in the testing rooms. You will be provided with erasable markers and marker boards to use. The testing rooms are monitored, both electronically and by proctors who walk through the test areas periodically. Once you are brought to the test carrel designated for your use, center staff will start your testing software. If there is a hardware or software problem, immediately notify center staff so that they can correct the problem and so that you will not lose valuable test response data or testing time.

Although center policies are designed to provide all examinees with a comfortable test area equipped with functioning equipment and a reasonably quiet environment, do not expect a soundproof cubicle. Other types of exams are being given and other examinees may be taking breaks; therefore, expect some background noise.

☑ *Checklist*

What to Bring

❏ Two forms of photo identification (driver's license, a passport, military identification, or an employee identification card)

❏ Layers of clothing (in case you get too cold or warm)

❏ Snacks for the break (to leave in storage locker)

What Not to Bring

❏ Food and beverages inside the testing room

❏ Scratch paper (erasable marker boards will be provided)

❏ Other personal belongings

Exam Security

To ensure exam security, you will receive one of several versions of the exam, which vary slightly in difficulty. If you receive one of the more difficult versions, then a slightly lower percent correct will be required to pass. If you receive a slightly easier version, then a slightly higher percent correct will be required to pass. Once you complete the examination, results are normally available within 2 weeks of your test date.

Emergency Cancellations

Should an emergency or illness prevent you from keeping your test appointment, you may be allowed to arrange an alternate test appointment either by visiting the Pearson VUE website (www.pearsonvue.com) or, in some cases, by calling the specific center you were scheduled to use. With reasonable advance notice, they will try to accommodate your need for a new appointment time, providing that the date you want falls within the testing eligibility window you received from the NCCPA and that the test site has testing slots available within that eligibility period.

TEST DELIVERY SOFTWARE

Select answers in either of two ways:

1. Position the cursor over the radio button (the circle) for a choice, and then click the mouse, which will darken the radio button for that selection.

or

2. Use the keyboard to press the letter corresponding to your choice, and the radio button will darken.

To change your answer using the mouse, just click on the marked radio button (shaded circle), and the mark will disappear. Then you can select another answer choice. To change an answer using the keyboard, simply type the letter of your new selection and the corresponding radio button will be marked.

Test Items

Test items may contain a variety of material for reference in answering, such as colored photographs, graphs, diagrams, and other reference material.

At all times during a test block, time remaining is shown in the upper right corner of the test screen. By clicking on that area, you can open a window showing the item number of the block you are viewing, as well as the minutes and seconds remaining for all test blocks in your testing session.

The following feature buttons are continually visible onscreen:

NEXT button: lower left corner of the screen

PREVIOUS button: to the right of the NEXT button

ITEM REVIEW button: center, to the right of the PREVIOUS button

HELP button: lower right corner of the screen

MARK box: upper left area of the screen

An example from Kaplan's PANCE Qbank software is shown below.

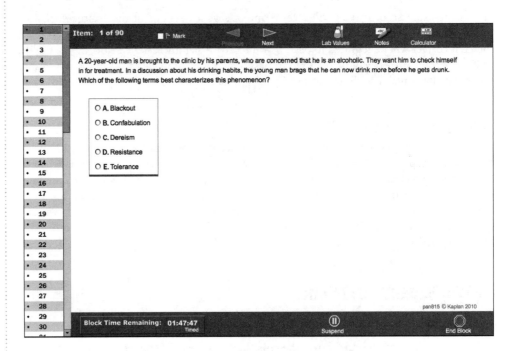

Click the NEXT button to advance to the next item of a block. Click the PREVIOUS button to move to the preceding item. The "Item Review" screen is used in conjunction with the "Mark" feature. For example, you may choose to leave an item blank and return to it for later (although Kaplan does not recommend this), or you may choose to insert a temporary answer and return to it later (much safer). Simply click the MARK box on this item. After you've completed the test block, if time remains, click the ITEM REVIEW button to see a list of your responses to the items in that block. The figure below shows the "Item Review" screen using Kaplan's Qbank software, which is comparable to what you'll see on test day.

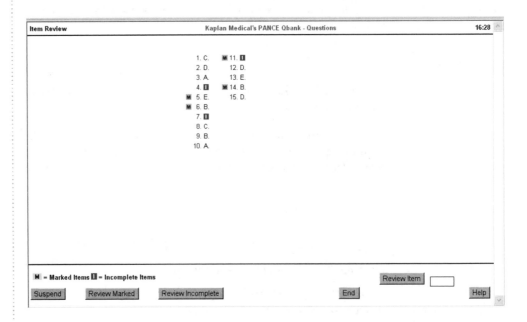

In the "Item Review" screen, all items in the block are listed, along with your response to each item. Items with the letter "I" (incomplete) within a red box were left blank. Items with a black letter "M" (marked) inside a yellow box were marked for later review. The "Item Review" screen appears automatically once you answer the last question, ensuring that you will see any skipped items. This screen also provides easy navigation to return to items by simply entering the number of an item you wish to review.

The SUSPEND button shown in the screen illustration above is *not* an option provided on the actual test screen. There are navigation buttons at the bottom of the "Item Review" screen that allow you to successively look at all items you have marked (next to the REVIEW MARKED button), and a similar button (REVIEW INCOMPLETE) to successively look at all unanswered, or incomplete, items. To navigate directly to specific items, you can double-click inside the REVIEW ITEM entry box, located at the lower right section of the screen, and then enter the number of any item that you wish to review.

If you are within an item screen when time runs out, you can still answer that item; doing so immediately ends the testing session. If you are not within an item when time expires, then the session ends immediately. To end a session early, click the ITEM REVIEW button, then click the END button to exit the session.

At the end of the testing day, you will receive a certificate for your records indicating that you appeared for the testing appointment.

Score Reporting

PANCE testing sessions are scored immediately, and results are normally posted to your online personal certification record within 2 weeks of your test appointment. The NCCPA no longer publishes the percentage correct required to pass the exam.

Testing Center Policies

Before beginning your examination, you will be asked to read and sign a statement of test center regulations, which lays out behaviors that violate testing policies. Within this statement is a promise that you will not share or discuss questions with anyone else, talk to other examinees, or bring any unauthorized items into the testing area. Violation of any of the policies and regulations will cause the violator's examinations to be invalidated. Testing areas are continuously monitored by center staff, and your testing session may be recorded on video.

Registering for the PANCE

3

To register to take the PANCE, you first must be certified as eligible by the NCCPA. After graduating from an accredited physician assistant program, or after completing the requirements for graduation from an accredited program, you must submit proof to the NCCPA and then be verified as eligible. This initial eligibility lasts for 6 years, and the exam may be taken up to six times during that initial 6-year period.

Access the PANCE online registration application here:

https://www.nccpa.net/n0/Account/FirstTime

To sign on to the site, enter your birth year and NCCPA ID number. This will allow you to access your personal certification record. You will be asked for your credit card information to pay the $475 examination fee. During the registration/exam application process, you will choose one of four 90-day exam windows. There are several factors to bear in mind before selecting your exam window.

The NCCPA must verify your graduation date with the director of your accredited program. If you are graduating soon, check with your program director before applying for the exam and follow your school's recommendations about when to register. If the program director does not verify within 72 hours of the NCCPA's request, you will be withdrawn automatically from your requested exam window.

The NCCPA needs time for the verification process, and it may require additional time to obtain a test date at your chosen test site. *Choose a testing window with at least 4 weeks remaining after your expected graduation date.* If you will graduate close to the end of your initially preferred testing window, choose the next testing window so that there is time for your school to verify your graduation, for the NCCPA to verify your exam eligibility, and to secure an acceptable test date at the test center you have chosen.

Once you have registered for the PANCE examination and the NCCPA has processed your application, you will receive an email telling you how to access, download, and print your permit from your personal certification record at the NCCPA website. The permit will be accessible until your examination window has expired. Your exam-scheduling permit will specify the exact beginning and end dates during which you are eligible to test.

Once you have the permit, wait at least 3 days to allow the NCCPA to notify Pearson VUE Test Centers of your eligibility. Then go online to www1.pearsonvue.com/testtaker/signin/SignInPage/NCCPA to schedule your exam date at the center of your choice.

Stay flexible and plan ahead. Before scheduling your test date, visit the website and make a note of one or two specific centers that are convenient to you. Sometimes you can schedule a test almost immediately; other times you may have to wait 6 to 7 weeks.

Have necessary information on hand when you schedule your test date. You will be asked for your name as you would like it to appear on your certification document, your Social Security number, a phone number at which you can be contacted if the test center needs to reach you, the mailing address to which you would like your certificate mailed, the exam eligibility information that you received from the NCCPA, your email address, and your credit card information.

Preparing for the PANCE

WHY DEVELOP A REVIEW PLAN?

PANCE is not just another test. It is comprehensive, assessing the basic science and clinical science knowledge acquired from many different courses and clinical experiences. PANCE questions are designed to require critical thinking in order to apply knowledge in a wide variety of contexts and patient-care situations. PANCE questions are likely to be quite different from the questions you saw on examinations in your physician assistant program. PANCE assesses everything you are supposed to have learned, which is analogous to compressing all of the final exams you took into one.

In order to be able to walk into the testing center on test day with confidence, you need a plan. Your PANCE study plan will enable you to manage your review time, sequence the subjects, determine how and when you practice with questions, and help you judge when you are test-ready.

CREATING A GOOD REVIEW PLAN

An effective study plan involves the following key factors:

1. Determining how much time you need for each area
2. Setting a sequence of topics
3. Establishing a good study process
4. Retaining your review
5. Monitoring your performance
6. Determining when you are test-ready

Assess your strengths and weaknesses. If you aren't sure, use practice questions to measure your current level of knowledge. Take 20 to 25 questions per subject area, and score the items. Calculate your percent correct for each area. This initial performance profile will help you determine where to focus more time. Also, faculty members probably mentioned some topics that they know are heavily tested; these topics need attention. Finally, the ultimate source of information about the number of items used to test topics is the PANCE blueprint, which you can find at the NCCPA website (www.nccpa.net). Your personal mix of current recall and topics that faculty emphasized, combined with the exam blueprint, will help you determine how much time you will need to devote to reviewing each area. By thinking carefully about what needs more time and what needs less, you will derive the maximum benefit from your review.

At this point, you are ready to sequence the subjects in your study plan. Because the PANCE tests even basic science information in clinical contexts, one way to sequence your review is to move through the content by organ systems.

Note

Studying everything equally wastes limited review time by investing the same amount in every subject, whether you need it or not.

Organ System Reviewing

Systemic pathology provides the ideal organizer for organ system reviewing. The initial part of your review in this method is general principles, which includes preliminary material, such as physiology, cell biology, general pathology, pharmacokinetics, pharmacodynamics, and genetics.

Once you have finished general principles, begin reviewing each organ system by starting with the embryologic development of that organ, its gross anatomy, the physiology of the organ, the pathology associated with the organ, and finally, the drugs used to treat problems with that organ system. Repeat this process for each of these organ systems:

Note

Study the aspects of each organ system in the following order:

1. Embryology

2. Gross anatomy

3. Physiology

4. Pathology

5. Pharmacology

- Special senses
- Skin and breast
- Cardiovascular
- Pulmonary
- Renal
- Endocrine
- Hepatobiliary
- Gastrointestinal
- Musculoskeletal
- Female reproductive
- Male reproductive
- Blood and lymph
- Immunology
- Nervous system

Once you have finished reviewing all of the systemic topics, move on to the remaining subjects:

- Microbiology
- Biochemistry
- Behavioral Sciences

Advantages of reviewing by organ system

One of the advantages of organ system–based review is that practicing clinicians organize their knowledge this way: It allows them to interpret patient signs and symptoms, arrive at a differential diagnosis, and form a treatment plan efficiently. You are thus getting a head start on thinking like a clinician.

Another benefit is that this sequence of reviewing helps you integrate subjects that you learned separately. What integration really means is that instead of studying anatomic structures independently from their functions and how they malfunction in disease processes, you will tie all these perspectives together, forming a working understanding of the human body's dynamics in both the healthy and diseased states. People who review this way often report that they can reason their way to correct answers far more easily and don't need to memorize as much.

Subject-Based Reviewing

If your school uses a problem-based or integrated curriculum, then you might want to review by subject instead of by organ system. Changing the path that you take through the material helps you fill gaps and provides some novelty in that you are moving through the material in a different manner. If you decide that a subject-based method is right for you, then sequence your review as follows:

1. Behavioral Sciences
2. Physiology
3. Immunology
4. Genetics
5. Anatomy
6. Pathology
7. Pharmacology
8. Microbiology
9. Biochemistry

This sequence works well for most people because it allows them to begin by studying material that involves lots of concepts, mechanisms, and processes, which tend to remain in memory longer. The plan then moves on to the content material that involves more memorization as the exam date gets closer. This keeps any forgetting to a minimum, which is an advantage when there is so much material to cover.

ESTABLISHING A GOOD STUDY PROCESS

Merely going through the material does not enable you to successfully apply the learned material to test items. Use your time strategically, and systematically work to address what you don't know, using practice questions to test how well you can apply what you are studying rather than simply studying in isolation from application.

Begin test preparation by scanning lecture notes and then the text. Think about what the lecturers emphasized. Make a list of key study objectives—primary topics—and aim to know them extremely well, a secondary group of topics and aim to know them pretty well, and a third group and aim to be familiar with but not obsess about if time runs short. Then study your notes and review sections that you highlighted or pulled out of the textbook when you read it initially. After completing your review of a topic on your study objectives list, quiz yourself with questions related to that topic, analyze your mistakes, and review aspects you don't understand. And then move down your list to the next topic. Take a practice test similar in length to the real exam and allow the same amount of time to complete it as you will have on test day. After scoring the practice test, analyze your errors and clarify any still-problematic aspects.

Actively Engage with the Material

Effective studying requires that you stay mentally engaged with the content. But how can you learn to stay engaged? You have to *do* something with what you are reading. Here are some methods:

- Transform the material by extracting key aspects into a briefer, personally meaningful version.
- Use arrows and boxes to diagram a process.

Note

Passive study methods are deceptive in that you tend to assume that you know, when in reality, you merely followed along and recognized the material as familiar. If what you do when you study results in frequent nodding off or mind wandering, then you need to change your methods.

- Stop after reviewing a topic and summarize it out loud.
- Do practice questions that relate to what you just read, and clarify any misunderstandings or forgotten elements by searching your notes or the textbook.
- If you must know features of various viruses, bacteria, or drugs, make flash cards with the name on one side and brief lists of key features on the flip side. Look at the name side of the card, and try to recite the features. Highlight or make a checkmark by features you failed to recall. Do card sorts by posing a Task, such as "Find all the bacteria that can cause respiratory infections." Next, scan the features side of the cards to see if you can accurately recall the names associated with each list of features. Again, make a mark by the names of those you have trouble with.

Study methods that require you to make judgments about the material, express it in your own words, show linkages between things, or mimic the demands of actual test items are all effective techniques for actively engaging with the material.

Methods of Remembering

Everyone must deal with the forgetting problem because there is so much to review that whatever you study first is going to fade away to some degree by the time you finish studying everything else. To combat this problem, create a greatly condensed summary of notes that you can use to refresh your memory during the final weeks or days before the examination. Tackling practice questions on a regular basis that cover *all previously reviewed material* is another tried and true method of keeping material fresh in memory. If you don't address the forgetting issue, your performance will reflect how recently you studied each area, with earlier topics yielding a lower performance than the topics you studied closer to test day.

Note

Test taking is a performing art. To perform well, you must practice the skills, get feedback, and try again until the whole thing becomes internalized and finely tuned, and every aspect of the process has been rehearsed in advance.

Practice What You Learn

If you are serious about doing well on the PANCE (and future examinations), adopt the "questions all along" approach, that is, use practice questions regularly to determine what you know versus what you need to work on. Saving the use of practice questions to the very end (or even worse, never doing any at all) is analogous to preparing to run in a marathon by reading about marathon running, perhaps watching people running marathons, talking with your friends about how you plan to run, but never actually hitting the pavement.

Knowing When You're Ready

The final aspect of a solid study plan is determining if you are test-ready. The most reliable way to do this is to take a practice test that is as similar as possible to the testing conditions you will face on test day. This means that if the items are all mixed together, then your simulation test should also mix up the items among subjects. If you have 5 hours to complete 300 items on test day, then your simulation test should also be taken at that same pace. And, obviously, the items in the simulation must be as similar as possible to those you will see on test day (how you do on the simulation will be a reliable indicator of how you might score on the actual examination).

As mentioned before, you should take this "readiness" simulation exam earlier than the last day or two before your test date, so that you will have time to analyze your errors and clarify any misunderstandings or forgotten elements.

Test-Taking Skills 5

IDENTIFYING ERROR PATTERNS

Several times in the preceding chapter we mentioned the need to analyze your errors. Do this routinely throughout your preparation process. Most people look at two things after they take a test: their overall performance and which items they answered incorrectly. Looking at just these two aspects wastes a lot of potentially valuable information.

Overall performance tells you how you did on a mixture of items covering various aspects of the material. If your practice test covered an entire subject, first compare this score with your initial score on the subject profile testing you used to determine strengths and weaknesses.

Second, take time to sort out where you made your mistakes. Did errors load up on a particular type of question, such as items involving calculations or use of graphs and data sets? If so, you may have discovered a type of material that you tend to understudy or avoid. Continue looking for patterns among the items that you missed.

Test anxiety

If many of your errors occurred on items early in the exam, this may reflect the fact that difficult content happened to be asked early in the test. Or, more likely, it may be an indicator of test anxiety, which is often felt most strongly during the early stages of taking an exam.

Pacing/fatigue setbacks

If many errors occurred on the final pages of the exam and you answered the items in numerical order, then pacing or mental fatigue may be a problem for you. How much sleep did you get the night before the exam? Did you run short of time near the end of the exam, causing you to rush through answering the final items? Was the most difficult material covered mainly in the final portion of the exam?

Misreading

Reading mistakes are common during exams. People feel nervous, rushed, or simply tired toward the end and may easily misread a word or key phrase. They may even answer the question that they expected to be asked, rather than one actually asked. How can you tell if an error was due to a reading mistake? Read the item and note the correct answer, as well as the answer you selected. If your choice makes no sense, given what was asked, then it is highly likely that you misread the question at the time.

Note

Negatively phrased items (e.g., "What is the least likely diagnosis?") commonly cause confusion.

Note

Beware of misreading. Only a few letters in a prefix or suffix can change the entire meaning of a question (e.g., *hyper* versus *hypo*).

Anger management

Were there any items on the exam that, at the time, made you very upset or frustrated? Students often describe such questions as tricky or picky, if not downright unfair. Test takers frequently make silly mistakes on items following the ones that made them upset. Their strong emotions interfered with their concentration on subsequent items.

Directionality

When a test question asks about information from an unexpected direction, performance on the item tends to decrease. For example, a physiology question might ask what effect living at high elevation might have on variables of the respiratory system. If, while studying, the test taker reviewed notes that presented such unusual conditions (e.g., high altitude, deep sea diving) followed by a discussion of the effects such environments have on the lung, then the item would not cause much trouble. However, if the test writer instead created a description of a patient with pulmonary function test results, chief complaint, and results of history and physical exam, then asked what might account for the patient's respiratory findings, then simply changing the task of the item from "state cause → ask about effects" to "describe effects → ask about cause" may affect the test taker's performance.

Another problem test takers sometimes struggle with during exams is determining what the item writer is actually asking when the question involves a series of steps. For example, if a certain mechanism proceeds A → B → C → D → E, a test question might ask what causes E but list answer choices that include both A and D. Which answer is correct? With exam questions of this type, test takers should choose the response that is the most immediate cause of E, not the initial cause. Thus, in this example, the correct answer to the question of what causes E would be D. The best way to deal with this is to be sure you know *exactly* what the question is asking by reading carefully and not making quick assumptions. Be on the alert.

Delineation

A question may require knowing how a specific member of a group with shared features is different from the other group members. These questions are commonly asked in subjects such as pharmacology, microbiology, and disease groups, such as the anemias. Questions may ask what is unique to a member of one of these groups or may require the test taker to know the shared or common features in that group.

Answer-changing

Before you insist that when you change answers you invariably change from correct to incorrect, do the math. Make a mark (e.g., a delta—Δ—in the margin) so that you will be able to spot all items where you changed your initial answer. Now tally the three possibilities:

- Column 1: Wrong to wrong
- Column 2: Wrong to right
- Column 3: Right to wrong

You may discover that most changed answers end up in Column 1. These reflect knowledge gaps. If the sum of Column 2 is greater than that of Column 3, then you are using good judgment and should change answers as you see fit. Only in relatively rare cases in which the sum of Column 3 is greater than that of Column 2 is there evidence of an answer-changing problem, and the solution is simple: Adopt a rule, based on the data you've collected and analyzed, that you will *never* change an answer.

Knowledge gaps

Are many of the errors you make referring to a common topic or similar kind of material? For example, you might notice that test after test, you tend to miss items that ask you to calculate an answer. This pattern clearly signals its own solution—if you want to improve, you must spend more time working with calculations and memorize a few formulas. Perhaps you notice that you often miss items that present an image, such as a photomicrograph, and require you to recognize structures within the image. This signals that you need more visual review. Failing to note how rare or common diseases are, what lab tests are appropriate, and how to interpret lab results all are common problems when students study material without thinking about *how* they might be asked about what they're studying. The obvious solution is to adjust your study efforts accordingly, putting more time into and practicing more dynamically with the problematic aspects identified in your error analysis.

Other obstacles

The potential patterns identified in error analyses can't all be described here. Some will be unique to an individual, whereas others might be related to which professor taught a particular topic. Not every test error will fall into a pattern. But if you have adopted active, sound study strategies, you are trying to anticipate what you might be asked, and your test performance is still not improving, then scanning your performance for patterns is a worthwhile exercise.

DEVELOPING A STANDARD APPROACH TO QUESTIONS

Habits are very comforting. We all establish personal rituals, and we tend to do these things in the same order repeatedly. Routines free us to think about other things; our actions are running in the background, sort of on automatic pilot. Many people remark that they sometimes drive between two places they know very well without really remembering the drive or any specifics of how they got there.

In common, habitual behaviors, our brains are constantly trying to reduce the demands and complexity of situations by storing the sequence of steps, much as a computer program does. Because all that stored, habitual information is running in the background, our minds free up more processing power to deal with new or unexpected challenges. This "back burner/front burner" strategy that the brain uses to deal efficiently with numerous demands is evident in what we experience while learning a new behavior pattern or set of skills. Think back to when you first learned to drive a car. Remember how difficult it was for you to listen to the instructor, change lanes in traffic, depress the accelerator and brake pedals smoothly, check your mirrors, and remember to signal the lane change? It likely felt overwhelming, even scary, because none of these separate actions had been linked together into a smoothly automated behavioral set.

STRATEGIES FOR MASTERING EXAM QUESTIONS

What are the steps you should aim to incorporate into your approach to dealing with questions? They need to be generic enough to work with different kinds of questions. Using our driving analogy again, these steps also need to protect you from making mistakes that could hurt you, much like defensive driving habits such as checking your mirrors. Let's look at the approach to questions used by many good test takers and focus on why it works.

Note

Test taking is a complex behavioral pattern and, like driving proficiently, one that can be improved with practice until what needs to be done becomes smooth and automatic.

Note

Often there is more than one right answer, but the question is asking for the *best* answer. Read *all* answer choices before jumping to a conclusion.

The Basic Steps

1. Read the question carefully to locate the important clues.

2. Make sure you fully understand what's being asked.

3. Before looking at any answer choices, put the clues together with what you are being asked and allow your mind to form an answer.

4. Look at the choices offered, and if one of them fits your anticipated answer, mark it.

5. If no choice is a good fit, use general knowledge, larger concepts, and logic to eliminate as many choices as you can.

6. Select an answer from the remaining choices.

Not all of these steps will necessarily be used with every question. For example, if a question asked which bacterial organism is most commonly responsible for neonatal pneumonia and you remembered it, then the process would stop at Step 4. However, in most standardized examinations, many questions will ask you to assess specifics that you won't be able to recall. It is in dealing with these questions that good test takers have a real advantage over those who are less adept. So, just what methods are used to get more correct answers?

The Methods

The arsenal of test strategies is hinted at in Step 5 above, which directs the use of general knowledge, larger concepts, and logic. Unconfident test takers are prone to an either/ or mindset when they encounter questions. If, after reading the question, they aren't sure of an answer based on what they recall, they quickly give up and guess. Good test takers use information presented in the question itself or more of their general knowledge to chip away at the question. By persevering and exploiting whatever they can to eliminate choices, they more frequently end up with correct answers. But frankly, just talking about what's involved in abstract terms isn't likely to make you a better test taker. To accomplish that goal, you will have to see test strategies in action.

Strategies really can't be taught out of context. To give you a sense of how to use strategies, we are going to illustrate them with examples, followed by a discussion of how applying a strategy narrows the possible answers and, in many cases, allows a test taker to obtain correct answers by knowing something about the topic of the question but not enough to mark an answer using only recalled information.

Eliminate distractors by applying basic principles

An 8-year-old boy is seen for a routine checkup. His vaccinations are current, and he has been healthy. The child is at the fifth percentile for height and at the 20th percentile for weight. His thumbs are disproportionately small compared with his other digits. There are several round, smooth, flat, light-brown areas ranging in size from 3 to 5 cm on his trunk and extremities. Which of the following genetic disorders is this child most likely at risk for?

A.   Down syndrome

B.   Fanconi syndrome

C.   Fetal alcohol syndrome

D.   Trisomy 18

E.   Cri du chat syndrome

Strategy: The most basic knowledge of the symptoms of Down syndrome, fetal alcohol syndrome, trisomy 18, and cri du chat syndrome reveals that these severe disorders would have become evident and been diagnosed long before this child reached age 8. By exclusion, then, if not through any direct knowledge of Fanconi syndrome, this would be the best answer (choice B).

A 62-year-old man is complaining of fatigue of 4 months' duration. He was recently seen by another physician for nephrolithiasis. He takes no medications and is otherwise healthy, except for mild hypertension controlled with diet. CBC is normal. Which of the following lab values would suggest primary hyperparathyroidism?

A.   Decreased calcium, decreased phosphorus, and increased parathyroid hormone

B.   Decreased calcium, increased phosphorus, and increased parathyroid hormone

C.   Increased calcium, decreased phosphorus, and increased parathyroid hormone

D.   Increased calcium, increased phosphorus, and increased parathyroid hormone

E.   Increased calcium, decreased phosphorus, and decreased parathyroid hormone

Strategy: This item illustrates how basic science questions can still be asked on a licensure examination. This item is an endocrine physiology question, but it looks clinical because the test writers attached a vignette introduction. But none of the clinical vignette information is necessary to answer the question. (The correct answer is C.)

A neonate has a flat, dark-pigmented area of skin over the sacral region. The area is roughly oval, has a clearly defined border, and differs from surrounding skin only in color. Which of the following is the most likely diagnosis?

A. Diastematomyelia

B. Mongolian spot

C. Nevus flammeus

D. Pilonidal cyst

E. Spina bifida

Strategy: The use of strategies never guarantees a correct answer; however, they allow you to extrapolate from what you do recall and relate that knowledge to the specifics of a given question. In this item, if you didn't know the answer (choice B), you could still eliminate choice E because the patient's findings would be more severe for spina bifida. You might also reason that it wouldn't be a cyst (choice D) because the stem of the question states that the area differs only in color, whereas with a cyst, you would expect a palpable mass. Knowing some word etymology might help you eliminate choice C ("flammeus" [flame] suggests either redness or heat, which is not mentioned in the description). This leaves choices A or B to choose from. Now you have a 50%—instead of a 20%—chance of getting the question right.

A 55-year-old woman with no significant medical history complains of difficulty with keeping her balance. Cranial nerve, motor, and mental status examination results are all within normal limits. There is diminished proprioception in the joints of all four extremities, with a greater deficit on the right side. She is able to stand with a narrow base and with her arms extended and eyes open. However, when she stands in a similar manner with her eyes closed, she immediately begins to fall. Which of the following is the most likely site of the lesion?

A. Cerebellum

B. Cerebral cortex

C. Peripheral nerve

D. Pons

E. Posterior column

Strategy: Even if you are not that knowledgeable in neuroanatomy, you could still figure out the correct answer to this item. This patient has a problem with balance, so for that reason, the answer isn't likely to be choice C because peripheral nerves aren't part of the central nervous system. It also isn't likely to be choice B because the cortical functions involve higher-order thought, and this question deals with balance, not thought disruption. The correct answer is choice E, and this could also have been chosen because of a mnemonic which says, "The body, like a temple, stands because of its *columns*."

A 20-year-old football player is sent to the campus health clinic by his coach after complaining of neck pain following a hard tackle during practice. He has a normal neurologic exam, but his posterior neck is tender. Which of the following would be the best initial step in management?

A. Administer nonsteroidal anti-inflammatory (NSAID) agents

B. Apply a hard cervical collar and immobilize his spinal cord

C. Apply a soft cervical collar and order bed rest

D. Send him to the hospital for a cervical spine x-ray

E. Apply ice directly to the affected area

Strategy: This question illustrates the principle of recognizing potentially serious findings and dealing with them first. The test writer has masked the seriousness by making the situation a campus clinic rather than an emergency room. Use a systematic decision-making process: Ask first, "What do I know? In this case, do I really know the extent of the young man's injuries? No? Then it is wisest to act cautiously by applying a hard cervical collar (choice B) until his injuries can be further explored at a hospital."

A 4-year-old boy with a displaced supracondylar fracture of the humerus without neurovascular complication is placed in skeletal traction. Six hours later, he has severe pain in the forearm and increased pain on passive extension of the wrist and fingers. Which of the following is the most appropriate next step in management?

A. Increased weight on the traction apparatus

B. Administration of analgesic medication

C. Exploration of the fracture and fasciotomy of the flexor compartment of the forearm

D. Closed reduction with the patient under anesthesia

E. Open reduction and internal fixation of the fracture

Strategy: Once again, this item can be worked through with a systematic, logical series of questions. Ask yourself, "What do I actually know about this boy's injuries? If the treatment given so far was appropriate but now the symptoms are worsening, what do I need at this point?" If you need more information about the true nature of the fracture damage, it makes sense to look for an answer that would provide more information (choice C).

> A 16-year-old boy is brought to the emergency room after the sudden onset of severe abdominal and scrotal pain. There is severe tenderness in the region of the inguinal canal on the right, and the right side of the scrotum is empty. Urinalysis is normal. Which of the following is the most effective management?
>
> A. Administration of analgesics and observation
>
> B. Administration of gonadotropic hormones
>
> C. Insertion of a nasogastric tube
>
> D. Cystoscopy
>
> E. Immediate operation

Strategy: You can often rely on the information given in question stems, along with logical reasoning from basic principles and concepts in biology, to arrive at a correct answer. In this item, using the concepts of acute and chronic, you can reason that the "sudden onset" of these symptoms indicates that something has recently changed to create the problem. So it's logical that some action needs to be taken. This rules out choices A and B because neither of these immediately resolves anything. It's difficult to see how inserting a nasogastric tube will help manage this patient's problem, so choice C also can be eliminated. Choice D would provide more information about what cells are lurking in the affected area, but it sounds as though the scrotum's contents have gone elsewhere. Therefore, you could reason that it would most likely require a surgical procedure to put the contents back in place. The correct answer is choice E, which is the only choice that offers immediate restorative action for an acute condition.

> A 2-year-old boy with several episodes of rectal bleeding is brought to the clinic by his mother. Evaluation with a technetium-99m perfusion scan reveals a 3-cm ileal outpouching located 60 cm from the ileocecal valve. This structure most likely contains which of the following types of ectopic tissue?
>
> A. Duodenal
>
> B. Esophageal
>
> C. Gastric
>
> D. Hepatic
>
> E. Jejunal

Strategy: A vital clue here is that the boy has been bleeding rectally. This suggests that tissue somewhere in the gastrointestinal tract has been damaged, rupturing blood vessels in the area. It's then most logical that gastric tissue (choice C) is correct because gastric tissue produces acid, which is capable of eroding the surrounding tissue and producing bleeding at some point in the process.

A 65-year-old man was diagnosed with carcinoma of the colon 7 months ago. An operation was successful, but he continues to receive adjunctive chemotherapy with methotrexate. Over the past several months, he has developed insomnia, fatigue, crying spells, feelings of guilt, and anhedonia. Which of the following is the most likely cause of this patient's behavior?

A. Normal adjustment

B. Metastatic cancer

C. Reaction to methotrexate

D. Personality disorder

E. Major depressive disorder

Strategy: If you recognize that this man's depression developed long after he was put on medication, then it is logical to rule out choice C. And because colon cancer doesn't easily spread to the brain, it isn't choice B either. This is a psychiatry question, and so the correct answer is likely to be either choice D or E. His symptoms and their duration seem to fit those of depression (choice E) more than a personality disorder, so this would be the best guess.

In the two oxygen-hemoglobin dissociation curves shown below, normal findings are represented by the solid line and abnormal findings are represented by the dotted line, indicating a situation in which the curve has been shifted. Shifts such as this can occur under which of the following circumstances?

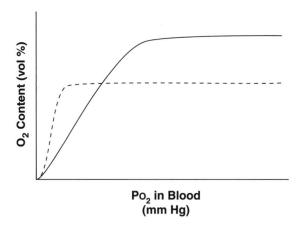

A. Carbon monoxide poisoning

B. Decreased pH

C. Increased 2,3-diphosphoglycerate (2,3-DPG)

D. Increased pCO_2

E. Increased temperature

Strategy: If you recall that a left shift causes oxygen to load and a right shift causes oxygen to unload, then you can figure out the answer to this item without strategies. If you don't recall, however, you can analyze the choices, seeking interrelationships. Look at choices B, C, D, and E, which would all occur when a person exercises. With exercise, more oxygen is needed, so you would want the body to react with a right shift. By elimination, the factor causing a left shift must be choice A, carbon monoxide poisoning, because it is the only effect not likely resulting from the oxygen demands being increased due to vigorous exercise.

A 60-year-old man with heart disease is brought to the emergency department by paramedics because he is short of breath. Cardiovascular evaluation reveals a resting O_2 consumption of 200 mL/min, a peripheral arterial O_2 content of 0.20 mL O_2/mL of blood, and a mixed venous O_2 content of 0.15 $O2$/mL of blood. What is his cardiac output?

A. 2.5 L/min

B. 4 L/min

C. 10 L/min

D. 25 L/min

E. 100 L/min

Strategy: It is stated that this elderly man has heart disease; therefore, it is unlikely that his heart is working efficiently. Even if you can't recall the formula for calculating cardiac output, if a normal heart pumps about 5 L/min, then this man's cardiac output is going to be decreased. So choices A and B are the most likely, giving you a 50% chance of getting the item correct. Choices C, D, and E would both mean that his diseased heart is actually pumping more blood than normal, so these answers can't be correct. (The correct answer is B.)

As part of an exercise tolerance test, a healthy 27-year-old man has just jogged 2 miles on a treadmill. As a result, his mean arterial blood pressure has increased (95 to 130 mm Hg). Similarly, his cardiac output has doubled. Which of the following would most accurately describe what has happened to his total peripheral resistance?

A. It is one-half the resistance at rest.

B. It is the same as the resistance at rest.

C. It is twice as great as the resistance at rest.

D. It is between 50 and 100% of the resistance at rest.

E. It is between 100 and 150% of the resistance at rest.

Strategy: Try thinking like a biologic engineer who is creating the body. You would want the resistance to the increased blood flow this healthy man's heart is pumping to decrease in order to supply those hardworking muscles. So this narrows the possibilities to choices A or D. A second tactic is to select choice D because it is more consistent with the fact that physiologic variables normally fluctuate within a range. Therefore, choice D is better than choice A, which indicates that it decreases to half of normal. In short, choice D fits the general pattern of variables in physiology.

Recognizing a question in disguise

What Is Really Being Asked?

A 16-year-old girl comes from a very religious family and denies any sexual activity. She has severe acne unresponsive to previous treatment of conventional therapy. Which of the following laboratory studies should be performed prior to prescribing isotretinoin?

A. Lipid profile

B. Liver function studies

C. Measurement of serum urea nitrogen (BUN)

D. Complete blood count (CBC)

E. Measurement of urine β-hCG

Strategy: First, make sure you understand what is actually being asked. You're dealing with someone who is potentially sexually active (any young woman of reproductive age should be assessed for pregnancy); therefore, it is always necessary to check for pregnancy before prescribing a drug that could affect a developing embryo. Knowing this, you could correctly answer this item (choice E) without knowing much, if anything, about the properties of the specific drug isotretinoin.

A 4-year-old boy is admitted with respiratory difficulty. He has had several previous admissions for pneumonia. History is significant for the failure to pass meconium at birth. Temperature is 101.1°F, and respirations are 35/min. Physical examination reveals a thin, malnourished boy <5th percentile for height and weight. Rales are heard over the left lower lobe, and percussion over the region is dull. Sputum culture grows *Pseudomonas aeruginosa*. Which test would confirm the diagnosis?

A. Bronchoscopy

B. Chloride sweat test

C. CT scan of the thorax

D. D-xylose absorption test

E. Pulmonary function tests

Strategy: This item illustrates the policy of portraying diseases in their most classic presentations on entry-level licensure examinations. The boy's history and symptoms are textbook indications of cystic fibrosis, so the correct answer is B. Notice that examinees don't receive credit for knowing what disease the boy has, only for reaching a correct diagnosis and then using that knowledge to answer the question posed (i.e., which test would confirm that diagnosis).

A 30-year-old woman with no significant past medical history presents with serosanguinous discharge from one of her breasts. She is not lactating and has no family history of breast disease. Physical examination reveals a moderate amount of serosanguinous discharge expressed from the left nipple. Cytologic exam of the fluid is negative. What is the most appropriate next step in management?

A. Advise the patient to return in 6 months for re-evaluation

B. Obtain a mammogram

C. Perform a chest x-ray

D. Perform an excisional biopsy of the retroareolar area

E. Perform a needle biopsy of the retroareolar area

Strategy: This item illustrates one of the common themes in clinical items—assessing whether examinees know the proper sequence in which to order lab tests. Here, although a mammogram (choice B) may not provide definitive diagnostic information about this patient's problem, it is standard procedure to order a mammogram before ordering more invasive or expensive tests. The trap is to opt for the test that would yield information allowing you to confirm the diagnosis, which isn't what is being asked.

Red Herrings

A 52-year-old physician whom you know socially has taken secobarbital, 2 g daily, for 7 years, despite several attempts to stop using the drug. He has been abstinent from alcohol for 10 years. The patient weighs 72 kg (158 lb). Examination shows no abnormalities. Which of the following is the most appropriate next course of action?

A. Detoxification as an outpatient and referral for group treatment

B. Discontinuation of secobarbital and prescription for a benzodiazepine in equivalent doses

C. Hospitalization for detoxification

D. Psychotherapy

E. Suggest that he gradually reduce the dosage of secobarbital

Strategy: Watch out for the item-writing tactic displayed in this question. The stem clearly states that this man has a history of addictive behavior (alcohol, drugs). But by making the patient a physician, the test writer is trying to confuse the strength of your convictions. Are you willing to hospitalize him, even though this might be a difficult step for you to take? Because the patient has responsibility for the well-being of others, it is even more important to take the tough but appropriate action so that his addiction won't negatively affect patients' welfare. Therefore, he should be hospitalized for detoxification (choice C).

A patient in chronic renal failure has five relatives as potential donors. A one-way mixed lymphocyte reaction is performed, isolating lymphocytes from each relative and treating the cells with mitomycin-C to prevent DNA replication. The cells are incubated with the patient's untreated lymphocytes in the presence of titrated thymidine for 2 days. The DNA is isolated, and the radioactive counts (CPM) are measured. Based on the assays, who is the best potential donor?

A. Father   (lymphocytes 24,000 CPM)

B. Mother   (lymphocytes 18,000 CPM)

C. Grandfather   (lymphocytes 30,000 CPM)

D. Brother   (lymphocytes 1,500 CPM)

E. Sister   (lymphocytes 6,000 CPM)

Strategy: Item writers love to make questions look complex! A question like this becomes straightforward when you realize that rejection is the big worry in all transplants. When potential donor and recipient cells are mixed together, you would want the smallest number of lymphocytes, as it would indicate the least interaction between the cells. Therefore, the correct choice is D.

A 20-year-old pregnant woman (para 1, gravida 0) comes to your office at 23 weeks' gestation complaining of polyuria. Because of the concern for gestational diabetes, a glucose tolerance test is ordered. The following values are obtained:

Time	Glucose (mg/dL)	Normal (mg/dL)
0	115	<105
1 hour	180	<175
2 hours	144	<145
3 hours	133	<140

What is the polyuria this patient is experiencing most likely due to?

A. The baseline value

B. The 3-hour value

C. The average of all values

D. Increased GFR and plasma volume

Strategy: This is an example of what could be called the *myopia trap* because the way the stem is written can cause you to focus too closely on the data and therefore lose sight of the bigger picture. (In other words, the presentation of unnecessary specific data could sway the test taker into thinking that the answer lies in correctly analyzing the data.) The correct answer is choice D because it's the only choice that relates to her pregnancy, in that her GFR and plasma volume will increase to support the developing child. When items present data, be sure to keep perspective on the overall patient presented in the question stem.

Visualize the correct situation

A convenience store clerk is hit in the face multiple times with a baseball bat during a robbery. Upon arrival at the emergency department, the patient is cyanotic and stridulous, with copious amounts of blood in his mouth. He has a markedly displaced mandible and midface, and clear fluid is draining from his nose. Two attempts at orotracheal intubation fail. Which of the following is the most appropriate next step in management?

A. Administer a high concentration of oxygen delivered through a tight-fitting face mask

B. Administer humidified oxygen and bronchodilator treatment

C. Intubate with a fiberoptic scope

D. Perform an emergency cricothyroidotomy

E. Perform a nasotracheal intubation

Strategy: Visualization of stem information is critically important to getting more items correct. If you picture what this patient's face must look like and what's already been tried, then choices A, B, C, and even E all seem unlikely to be successful. The only way to establish an airway with any certainty of success, thus keeping your patient alive for his other injuries to be treated, is choice D, which is the correct answer.

A 27-year-old man is brought to the emergency department by paramedics after being thrown from the back of a pickup truck at high speed. He received 2 liters of intravenous (IV) fluid in transit. His pulse on arrival is 120/min and BP is 60/40 mm Hg. He is awake and without focal neurologic signs. He has a distended tender abdomen and a stable pelvis, with no deformities of the lower extremities. Portable chest x-ray results are normal. Which of the following is the most appropriate next step in management?

A. CT scan of the abdomen and head

B. Diagnostic peritoneal lavage and fluid administration while awaiting cell counts on lavage fluid

C. Dopamine infusion to improve BP, followed by observation

D. Exploratory laparotomy and administration of blood products

E. Spine films to rule out vertebral fracture

Strategy: If you visualize this patient's injuries, it should be rather obvious that he is bleeding into the abdominal area because his blood pressure is still low (despite the IV) and his abdomen is tender and distended. This must be dealt with immediately or a rupture could kill him; there is no time for scheduling diagnostic tests (which rules out choices A and E). Choice C is clearly wrong because waiting and observing won't stop his bleeding. You would then guess either choice B or D. In considering these final two, it would probably be smarter to pick choice D (the correct answer) because choice B also mentions waiting for cell counts.

A 33-year-old man complains that recently his chest hurts when he eats, especially when he eats meat. An x-ray shows a dilated esophagus, and achalasia is suspected. Esophageal manometry is used to confirm the diagnosis. Swallowing-induced relaxation is most likely to have been reduced at which anatomic location in this patient?

A.   Lower esophageal sphincter

B.   Lower esophagus

C.   Middle esophagus

D.   Pharynx

E.   Upper esophageal sphincter

F.   Upper esophagus

Strategy: The problem depicted here seems to be that food gets into the upper gastrointestinal tract, but then is blocked in such a way that it becomes trapped in the esophagus. Picturing this, it seems logical that the lower esophageal sphincter (choice A) would be the problem; this would allow food to get into the esophagus, but then trap it there if the lower esophageal sphincter won't allow it to move out. The upper sphincter (choice E) is less likely because it would be felt high in the back of the throat, not in the chest area. Picturing what's happening in a clear, concrete way is often a big help in answering multiple-choice questions.

Don't let sharp turns confuse you

In recent years, most HMOs have instituted plans involving patient copayments. A local HMO has just raised copayments by $15 in an attempt to reduce costs. Studies have shown that the effect of increasing patient copayments in the United States has been which of the following?

A.   Decreased utilization in direct proportion to the required copayment

B.   Decreased utilization of unnecessary services only

C.   Decreased use of tertiary services, but increased use of primary services

D.   Increased utilization in a nonlinear fashion

E.   Increased utilization in a linear fashion

Strategy: This is a good example of what might be called a bait-and-switch question. The item writer is hoping that you'll assume the medical professionals' viewpoint so that you'll get slightly thrown off when the focus of the question is switched to the impact, not the intent, of increasing copayments. The correct answer is choice A, not choice B, because the typical citizen lacks the medical knowledge to know what is necessary and what isn't necessary. So he or she will tend to use less of all kinds of services.

> Malpractice insurance rates have continued to soar in recent years, adding to the overall cost of healthcare in the United States. It is recommended that physicians become more knowledgeable about this issue to exert peer influence on their medical colleagues. In this context, which of the following cases represents the best grounds for malpractice?
>
> A. A 19-year-old model undergoes breast augmentation and is left with breasts of slightly unequal size.
>
> B. A 27-year-old man dies from penicillin allergy after he receives a shot for strep throat in the emergency room.
>
> C. A 51-year-old woman is diagnosed with breast cancer metastatic to her lungs. One month earlier, her mammogram was read as normal.
>
> D. A 55-year-old businessman suffers peritonitis when operative sponges were not removed during his appendectomy.
>
> E. A 77-year-old woman falls out of bed in the hospital and suffers a hip fracture.

Strategy: This is another example of the bait-and-switch in the point of view. It tries to trap the test taker into evaluating the choices from the medical practitioner's viewpoint when in actuality, the question is asked from a malpractice attorney's viewpoint. Choice D is the correct answer because it's the only one that mentions any concrete physical evidence for the attorney to show a jury (the sponge). This makes it the easiest case to prove legally. Recognizing the point of view saves time and leads to fewer incorrect answers in questions like these.

When in doubt, be open and empathetic

> A 13-year-old boy with poor impulse control is brought to the office for an evaluation. During the interview, the boy expresses concern at his inability to control his temper, but he subsequently becomes enraged. With clenched fists and in a trembling voice, he tells the physician to "Stop bugging me or I'll hit you!" Which of the following would be the physician's best response?
>
> A. "You should never hit people."
>
> B. "Do you think you are really going to hit me?"
>
> C. "It must be frightening to be that angry."
>
> D. "I don't believe that you really want to hit me."
>
> E. Sit quietly, watching the patient attentively but doing nothing.

Strategy: Only choice C shows empathy with the boy's feelings. By not judging his behavior, the clinician encourages the boy to confide more information and avoids provoking him into further negative emotions. When encountering questions dealing with communication skills, always search for the answer that is most likely to lead to the patient saying more. This will usually be the most open-ended, nonjudgmental question or statement on the part of the clinician. Similarly, if the question deals with an ethical situation, it makes sense to search for the choice that is most relevant or consistent with the ethical principle involved in the situation, such as patient confidentiality or patient autonomy.

Be wary of suspicion

A 52-year-old man with a 10-year history of hypertension complains of abdominal and back pain for the past 6 months, a 10-lb weight loss, and greasy, foul-smelling stools. He smokes 2 packs of cigarettes and drinks a pint of whiskey/day. On physical examination, he is afebrile with mild epigastric tenderness but no guarding, rigidity, or distension. Bowel sounds are present, and rectal exam is normal. Laboratory tests reveal the following:

Hematocrit	48%
Sodium	141 mEq/L
Potassium	3.9 mEq/L
Glucose	148 mg/dL
ALT, AST	16, 24, respectively
Albumin	4.7 g/dL
Prothrombin time	11 sec

Chest x-ray is normal, and abdominal plain film shows pancreatic calcifications. Which of the following is most likely responsible for his weight loss?

A. Alcoholic hepatitis

B. Duodenal ulcer

C. Gastric ulcer

D. Pancreatic insufficiency

E. Thiamin deficiency

Strategy: People who have struggled to do well on multiple-choice exams often carry around strong negative emotions about having to take these kinds of tests. Sometimes they feel that the items are expressly designed to trick them into choosing wrong answers. Such feelings in this case could easily lead the examinee toward avoiding answer D. The question stem lists "pancreatic calcifications"; therefore, a suspicious test taker might reason that the pancreatic calcifications clue was just to lure him or her into making a mistake. Wary test takers therefore choose another answer, the wrong one.

Notice also how the wrong answers each agree with at least part of the patient's findings. The patient drinks heavily, so choices A and E relate to this fact. The patient has abdominal symptoms, so choices B and C relate to those symptoms. In a well-written test, nearly every incorrect choice fits at least some part of the stem information, but only the correct answer fits all of the clues given in the stem.

Strategy Summary

- Rely more on general recall and concepts.

- Familiarity and life experience have validity.

- Consider what's common versus what's rare.

- Visualize what question stems describe.

- Use homeostasis as a guide to what the body would try to do to keep a healthy balance.

- Know important definitions.

- Rule out extreme or unrelated choices.

- Use decision rules to manage time use.

- In items with tables, seek patterns.

- In items with graphs, seek trends and anchor points.

- Always seek relationships.

- Use the whiteboard and marker to sketch or calculate.

- Use logical analysis based on concepts and information given in the question.

- Watch for hinge words in questions.

- Develop a mindset to reject choices.

- Look for the best fit with clues in the stem and with what you feel is the point of the question.

Advice for Test Day

6

As test day approaches, many test takers become increasingly anxious. This is a natural reaction, but it is wise to recognize the symptoms of pre-exam anxiety and to take steps to manage it. You don't want your anxious feelings to lead to counterproductive behaviors that can decrease your examination performance.

MENTAL TURMOIL

One of the most common symptoms of test anxiety is to lose focus and concentration. Rather than thinking about the material they are studying, people's minds race with thoughts about the material they haven't mastered, questions about whether they should stop studying this topic and review another topic instead, or worry about what they will do if they fail the examination. Their regimen of studying, taking breaks, and practice testing become harder to adhere to; many abandon their study plans and begin to flit from one thing to another. Others decide to do only practice questions, believing that the more items they see in the final days, the more likely it is that they will encounter similar items on the actual exam. Still others poll their classmates and colleagues, believing that whatever their friends are doing in these final days must be the right thing for them to do as well.

All of these behaviors are symptomatic of test anxiety and often result in feeling less and less in control at the worst of times. *Remember:* Your goal is to adhere firmly to your study plan and to allow the structure it provides to help you rein in the pre-exam jitters.

BIORHYTHMS

When you routinely study late into the night, your body becomes habituated to operate at peak efficiency nearly 12 hours later than what you will need on examination day. This calls for a readjustment period, beginning at least a week before the exam. After months or weeks of sleeping late because you didn't turn in before 3 A.M., you will not miraculously be able to awaken early on test day feeling alert and ready to tackle a long exam.

To readjust your biorhythms, begin setting the alarm clock to wake you an hour earlier each day so that by the night before the examination, you'll be able to fall asleep and awaken the morning of the exam feeling rested and ready for the mental tasks ahead.

NUTRITION

Eating habits affect everyone's ability to deal with life's challenges. All of us are affected by fluctuations in blood-sugar levels and excessive intake of junk foods. As stated earlier, test-taking is a performing art and as such requires that you eat a variety of foods and avoid certain substances, such as caffeine and alcohol, that can disrupt metabolism and leave you feeling short of energy or overstimulated.

Taking a long exam burns many calories, so think of the kinds of high-energy snacks and fluids and energy-sustaining foods that you'll want to bring to the testing center. Avoid heavy foods or a large lunch, which can leave you suffering from postprandial drop, resulting in grogginess or abdominal discomfort. Finally, be sure to bring fluids, such as bottled water or fruit juice. Dehydration is a potential cause of fatigue, headache, and general feelings of listlessness.

INSOMNIA

Note

Two factors can influence one's ability to fall asleep:

- Avoid consuming caffeine after dinnertime.

- Carefully choose the personal level of stimulation required for you to fall asleep the night before (e.g., a tiring workout but not too close to turning in).

People's personalities vary greatly. Some react to increased stress by seeking out favorite activities that help them mentally regroup and feel physically tired, allowing them to fall asleep and regain their equanimity. Other people turn to drugs or alcohol, self-medicating to bring on sleep. Nearly everyone occasionally finds sleep elusive when they are worried about something. Although many adults can function perfectly well on a good six hours of sleep, some require eight or nine hours to feel fully rested and alert.

Sedatives, stimulants, and medications

Prescribed medications can alter sleep requirements, making it difficult to fall asleep or to wake without grogginess. Avoid foods or beverages containing caffeine later than dinnertime the evening before the test. Some people find that drinking milk before bedtime also helps make them sleepy.

Side stroke, anyone?

The second factor preventing sleep is the general level of stimulation prior to retiring. Strenuous physical activities before bedtime can be a double-edged sword. Exercise may tire you out; however, if done too soon before retiring, it can overstimulate you. In short, if you do a physical activity that tends to wear you out so that you feel generally limp, such as swimming, then it is wise to engage in this activity early enough on the day before the exam that you have time to settle down before bedtime.

Hide the books

Finally, late on the day before your exam, *avoid studying*. Whatever content you madly race through that evening is not going to settle into your long-term memory. Bits and pieces of it will still be spinning around in working memory the following morning, and this can directly interfere with recall of the far larger body of information that you spent the last few months and weeks working with. This phenomenon is so well researched that it has a label, *retroactive interference*. Resist the temptation to look at anything related to tomorrow's exam the night before.

FIVE TIPS FOR CONCENTRATION, PACING, AND TEST ANXIETY MANAGEMENT

Tip 1

Several weeks before the exam, list on an index card several of your greatest personal strengths and attributes, such as, "I'm an intelligent person who reacts well under pressure," or, "I know I'm going to be a great physician assistant." Keep this card handy so that whenever negative thoughts intrude while you are studying or practicing with questions, you can pull the card out, read the statements, and reflect on their truth. Luxuriate in the calm, positive feelings you associate with each of these statements. Fairly soon, you won't even need the card because you will know all the statements by heart and will be able to mentally review them as an antidote to negative thoughts and self-doubt.

Tip 2

Keep a master tally sheet nearby each time you sit down to study. Make a mark each time you find yourself engaging in negative thinking, daydreaming, or otherwise mentally escaping from the study situation. For many, the very act of counting the frequency of mind-wandering or lapses in concentration actually reduces the frequency of these behaviors, and they find that their daily tallies decrease over time. This is a mild form of behavior modification that you can apply to your own study behavior.

Tip 3

Months (or at least a few weeks) before the exam, spend some quiet time thinking back over your life experiences to select one event in which you were the "hero" of the situation. Perhaps you walked in on a serious fight between two friends and were able to bring about a peaceful resolution. Perhaps you administered CPR successfully to someone or orchestrated a successful fund-raising event for a charitable cause during college. Whatever life event you select, it must be a situation in which your abilities and actions solved a problem or redeemed a bad situation.

Spend at least 10 minutes each day in a quiet place reliving this event, trying to bring back the memory in as much detail as possible. What time of year/day was it? What were you wearing? What was the setting like? As you practice this, it will take less and less time for you to retrieve the memory in graphic detail. The purpose of this exercise is to allow you to mentally revisit the event quickly, because stored with this remembered event are all of the associated psychological feelings of being in control, a successful problem solver, confident, and, in general, winning over adversity. When anxious feelings arise during the exam and you take a brief time-out to retrieve this memory, these positive emotions serve to counteract the negative emotions associated with the test-taking process.

Tip 4

Pacing problems will be far less likely if you work through lots of sample tests during your preparation. With practice, you will sense the right pace and will be able to walk in on test day confident in the knowledge that you can handle it. The test setting will feel less strange—and the more familiar it feels, the less anxious you will feel.

During the actual test, use the same pacing plan that you used in practice testing in the final week or two. Before you begin, determine the items that correspond with 1/4, 1/2, and 3/4 points. When you take the test and reach a time-marker item, check your time. For example, in a 60-item test, you might write numbers 16, 31, and 46 on the marker board. When you reach Question 16, you should have used roughly a quarter of the total time; by Question 31 half of the time; and so on. Worrying about running out of time contributes to anxiety and often leads to time-wasting behaviors, such as checking the clock every couple of minutes—a nervous habit that continually interrupts your thought process and often results in the need to re-read once you return to the question.

If you do run short of time toward the end of a session, use question "triage," that is, scan the remaining items to find the ones that are easiest and mark the answers to these first. Return to the remaining items and mark some answer for *all* of them. Remember that giving no answer is an automatic error, so *never* leave items blank. The item-review option allows you to easily check to see what you have done with all items in the section, so always use this feature before exiting the test session.

Tip 5

If you feel anxiety during the exam that is interfering with your ability to concentrate on the questions, take a brief mental "time-out." Shut your eyes, lean back, and slowly rotate your neck and roll your shoulders to relax them. Take several slow, cleansing, deep breaths and exhale each breath slowly. This time-out helps break the cycle of anxiety and will usually help you focus with a greater sense of calm and improved concentration.

Signs of Anxiety That May Require Professional Help

If you experience significant anxiety symptoms, such as muscle twitching, chronic insomnia, nausea, hyperventilation episodes, or chest tightness when you think about taking exams or while taking them, then self-help tactics may not be enough. If you experience several of these symptoms and they are severe, *seek professional help* from either a psychiatrist or a cognitive psychologist who is experienced in helping people overcome situational anxiety. Therapies may include antianxiety medications, behavioral retraining, or a variety of other interventions. Do not delay making an appointment—each of these treatment modalities requires time to become effective.

MANAGING TIME DURING THE EXAMINATION

Don't skip around frantically searching for easier items. Doing this can result in missing items and will leave you feeling out of control in the test situation—something you definitely want to avoid. Also, because you won't easily be able to estimate how many items you have left to answer at any given point, skipping around makes following any pacing plan very difficult.

Decision Rules

Rule One

Use decision rules to make the most of your testing time. Everyone needs at least two decision rules. Rule One is used when you are able to narrow the possible answers to two options. At this point, self-honesty is paramount. If you have already used recall and any strategies appropriate to such a question, it's time to choose and move on. Rule One prevents you from ineffectually reading and re-reading the item. Mark the *upper* of the final two choices and move to the next question. The second half of Rule One says that the next time you are faced with the same "final two choices" dilemma, you should mark the *lower* of the final two choices and then move on. This is actually a time-management rule, designed to prevent you from obsessing between those two options.

Note

Remember to answer all questions on the PANCE. Every blank item counts as an error, so you might as well take a guess.

Note

Throughout the exam, change an answer *only* if you realize that you initially misread the question or because new and specific recall occurs that now allows you to answer the question correctly.

Rule Two

The second time-management rule pertains to questions about material that you've never come across before. You are unlikely to encounter many of these "clueless" items. Most test takers report that on standardized examinations, they encounter only a handful of items that they truly have no idea how to answer. If you encounter a question dealing with totally unknown content, then have a favorite letter between A and E in mind, mark the choice that corresponds to the favorite letter, and move on. There is little to be gained from re-reading the item multiple times.

Note

Decision rules save time, and adequate time results in more correctly answered items.

☑ *Checklist*

Concentration, Anxiety Prevention, and Pacing Routine Checklist

❏ Have you created self-affirming index cards?

❏ Have you identified, monitored, and changed your mind-wandering behaviors?

❏ Have you mastered a memory that provokes self-confidence during anxious moments?

❏ Have you implemented the practice of marking time junctures during exams?

❏ Have you found a quick relaxation routine (e.g., deep breaths, shoulder rolling) that works for you during high-stress moments?

❏ Have you established and mastered "decision rules" to save time in answering questions that you don't know?

PART II

Understanding the Recertification Process

PANRE Recertification

7

OVERVIEW OF THE PANRE

Physician assistants who currently hold NCCPA certification must pass a recertification exam, the Physician Assistant National Recertifying Examination (PANRE), before the expiration of their certificates, which occurs at the end of the tenth year of the certification maintenance cycle. The exam may be taken as early as year 9.

The PANRE is a timed, 240-item, multiple-choice examination covering a wide range of clinical topics. The content distribution and format are the same as that of the PANCE, but the PANRE is 60 items shorter than the PANCE. Examinees have 4 hours to complete the 240 items on the PANRE.

REGISTERING FOR THE PANRE

Physician assistants holding a valid NCCPA certificate who are in the ninth or tenth year of the certification cycle are eligible to take the PANRE. Registration is online at the NCCPA website (www.nccpa.net/panre). Registrants sign into their personal certification record to submit their application information. A valid credit card is required to pay the $350 examination fee. Examinees can choose to have 40% of the test directed toward one of the following three topics: adult medicine, surgery, or primary care. The test is offered year round, except in the last week and a half of December. The PANRE may be taken at any of the Pearson VUE Testing Centers. Locations of test centers can be accessed by visiting the Pearson VUE website (www.pearsonvue.com/nccpa/).

TEST-PREP REFRESHER FOR THOSE PREPARING FOR THE PANRE

To Know Yet Not to Know

One can know the material and yet still have problems applying that knowledge to test questions. It is possible that knowledge may be stored rigidly in memory, so that only certain cues will trigger recall. In clinical practice, knowledge is usually triggered by seeing a real patient, an x-ray, or some other concrete visual stimulus. On an examination, however, questions appear mainly as written vignettes, occasionally with visual cues, such as photographs.

To prepare for this type of examination, you need to consider the kinds of cues likely to occur in questions as you review content, so that the information stored in memory is linked to those cues. In other words, organize information using categories of information deemed likely to be presented in questions. For example, rather than memorizing bacterial names and a list of features associated with each, organize the bacteria using features such as their Gram stain results, drug sensitivity, or production of low-grade fever. These organisms are more likely to appear in questions, triggering recall.

More Sources Are *Not* Necessarily Better

Using too many review sources will hurt your review process, making it less effective and leaving you feeling overwhelmed. If you use too many sources, at some point you will realize that there is no way to complete your review because you spent time reviewing multiple versions of the same material and consequently fell way behind. **Choose your review resources wisely and use only one source for any given topic.**

Capture the Essence

As a busy professional, you have limited time to spend preparing for the PANRE. You probably don't plan to take time off for your preparation. This means that you will be using briefer review sessions, which may be spread out over several weeks or months. Consequently, there's a fairly good chance that you will forget what you learned early on, when you first began to study. To minimize this problem, each time you review, **try to capture the key elements of what you reviewed in condensed personal notes**. This aids concentration during study and gives you a way to refresh highlights of much of the material in the final days before your test appointment.

Study What You Don't Often Work With

Because job demands differ and because few positions are likely to involve using all of the clinical knowledge you studied during PA school, preparing for the recertifying exam requires you to **focus your review efforts on the aspects of clinical medicine that you don't routinely deal with at work.** What's not used is rapidly forgotten. For example, if your practice seldom involves seeing pediatric patients, you will want to spend more time reviewing pediatrics rather than adult medicine.

Solid Frameworks Support More Material

Just as the framework of a building supports all of the other materials that will be added to form the final structure, a solid mental framework provides a useful way to organize and store what you review. **Major categories within that mental framework can then function during the exam to help you sort out the kind of problem you are dealing with.** Examples of these major categories include:

- Acute versus chronic
- Benign versus malignant
- Laboratory tests that confirm versus laboratory tests that help monitor treatment
- Patient variables, such as age, sex, or risk groups more prone to suffer certain diseases

Fit the Task to the Time Available

Many people feel that it isn't worth using small periods of time to review, but busy professionals must grab those many small opportunities because they rarely have longer periods of time available. If you capture key aspects in brief notes, **even a half-hour spent reviewing moves you closer to being test-ready**.

As the Exam Date Nears

When your PANRE date is only a week or so away, it's time to review your personally con- densed notes to refresh your recall of key aspects of all the material you have reviewed over the preceding weeks or months. At this time, you might find it helpful **to take a longer, timed practice test, and then let the errors you make on this practice test guide what you still need to clarify.** Give yourself the day before the exam off to let things settle in your mind. Reviewing right before the exam leaves disconnected bits floating around in working memory that interfere with earlier studied material. Relax and treat yourself to a mindless, pleasant activity the day before your test.

ON PANRE TEST DAY

When the correct answer isn't immediately apparent, focus your efforts on eliminating choices. In general, rule out choices that:

- Are too aggressive
- Are too extreme
- Are totally unfamiliar
- Don't fit one or more facts presented in the question stem
- Overlap too much with other choices for that question
- Don't really answer what is being asked

Manage Your Testing Time Wisely

With 240 items to complete and 4 hours of testing time, you must average answering one question per minute to finish all of the items. To set up a pacing plan that will make sure this happens, follow this simple procedure:

1. Divide the time allowed for a test session into fourths.
2. Divide the number of items you must complete in that session by 4.
3. Check your time use when you come to these quarterly "checkpoint" item numbers, and adjust your pace accordingly.

Another time-management tactic that works for many people is to **adopt a decision rule** for the frequent occasions when you have narrowed the likely answer choices down to two. If you have used all possible recall and reasoning and still can't decide between the final two options, alternate between marking the upper and the lower of the final two. Keep track of which (upper/lower) you used last by jotting "U" and "L" or ↓↑ on the marker board each time you invoke the rule. This doesn't change the odds of making correct choices, but it will ensure that you don't waste testing time with useless vacillation over which of the final two to mark. If you waste time in such a manner, you'll have to rush through final items in each test session, thereby missing relatively easy items.

PART III

Information for Recently Graduated Physician Assistants

Transitioning from School to the Workplace

8

If you will be graduating from physician assistant school soon or just recently graduated, you are moving into a challenging transition period—from full-time student to full-time employment as a physician assistant. This is a busy time and will require that you think about a new and wider range of issues as you prepare your credentials, look at locations and settings where you might want to work, and, most likely, adjust from living on student loans to earning a professional salary.

This section discusses various aspects of the job-seeking process, as well as a few things you need to prepare for to do a great job of presenting yourself to prospective employers.

ESTABLISHING A PERMANENT CREDENTIALS FILE

Documentation of your professional education, your PA certification, and eventually records of the continuing medical education credits you earn will be maintained by the National Commission on Certification of Physician Assistants (NCCPA). However, for purposes of applying for a position, you will need to create your own credentials file, both on paper and electronically.

Applying for positions involves not only completing applications and writing cover letters but also preparing and sending your professional resume to prospective employers. Other documents you'll want to keep handy for the applications include:

- School transcripts
- Copies of letters of recommendation
- A list of references and their contact information
- Any other certifications related to clinical practice, such as basic or advanced life support training, certifications of proficiency on medical apparatus, or EMT certification

As time passes, update your resume to keep it current.

Obtaining an NPI number

In order to work as a physician assistant in the United States, you must obtain an NPI number and a DEA number.

The Administrative Simplification provisions of the Health Insurance Portability and Accountability Act of 1996 (HIPAA) requires each U.S. health care provider and health plan to use a National Provider Identifier, or NPI number. Using these standard, unique identifiers is meant to facilitate electronic transmission of health information.

To obtain an NIP number, apply online with the National Plan and Provider Enumeration System (NPPES) at https://nppes.cms.hhs.gov/NPPES/Welcome.do. After setting up a login, estimated time to complete the NPI application form is 20 minutes.

Obtaining a DEA number

The U.S. Department of Justice's Drug Enforcement Administration (DEA) is responsible for suppressing illegal drug distribution and use in the United States. To this end, the DEA's Office of Diversion Control issues DEA numbers to legitimate prescribers. This unique prescriber number is used to track distribution from authorized prescribers, thus assuring adequate distribution of drugs for legitimate medical, commercial, and scientific needs while avoiding diversion of controlled pharmaceuticals and their precursors for illicit use.

You can apply for a DEA number online at http://www.deadiversion.usdoj.gov. Begin by clicking on "Registration," then select "Mid-Level Practitioner" to locate the appropriate form.

WRITING YOUR PROFESSIONAL RESUME

A good resume is essential, so draft it carefully and then share it with experienced reviewers for feedback. There are commercial services that will help you prepare a resume, but the cost tends to be high, so try to spend the time to develop your own.

Scrutinize a sample version

There are guides to writing resumes that contain examples of good formatting. If you are still in school, ask Student Affairs staff or a faculty advisor if they have some good examples you can see.

Once you have looked at some well-done examples, note how they are organized using headings such as Educational Experience, Work Experience, Honors, Research Experience, Publications & Presentations, and Other Interests. Within each category, list each entry from most recent to least recent (i.e., in reverse chronology).

Piece together your information

Begin jotting down information about your own educational experiences, previous job history, and other medically related activities, such as certifications and volunteer activities. Once you have listed what you might want to include under the major headings, list starting and ending dates and institution names and locations for each educational experience, work history, and activity you want to include. Once you have drafted the document, scrutinize it to be sure that it contains no typographic or spelling errors. Then check to ensure that all time intervals are accounted for. Unaccounted for gaps in time always raise questions in the minds of prospective employers.

RESEARCHING THE JOB MARKET

If you haven't already decided exactly which factors you want most from a position, spend some time thinking about what is essential and what is optional to you. Some factors to consider include:

Note

The more sample resumes you look at, the more ideas you have when creating your own.

Note

Show a few trusted people the latest draft of your resume for comment. You'll be surprised at how many good pointers people have to offer.

- The diversity of the patient mix you want
- The type of clinical setting you prefer (rural or urban, clinic or hospital)
- Whether you prefer to be relatively closely supervised or function more autonomously
- Whether the position offers the opportunity to further specialize in specific areas, such as critical care, family medicine, pediatrics, nephrology, geriatrics, or women's health

This written "wish list" is a valuable tool. With it, you'll have an easier time identifying the job elements you feel are "must-haves" versus those you can be flexible about. This will help you select positions you'd like to apply for, and, once the job offers come in, decide which to accept.

Determine which state(s) you might want to work in, and then do research to learn about the specific state laws and temporary licensure requirements for newly graduated or about-to-graduate PAs. The 50 states vary considerably in terms of whether they offer a temporary license so that you can begin work before your PA certification is finalized, how long it will take for that state to process your temporary license, and what documentation you must submit to that state to secure temporary licensing.

All states give PAs prescriptive authority, but some prohibit them from writing prescriptions for certain controlled substances. To find out what laws apply in states where you are considering working:

- Contact the licensing agency for the states of your choice (see Resource III at the back of this book); or
- Check the summary of all the state laws on the AAPA's website (http://www.aapa.org/threeColumnLanding.aspx?id=328); or
- Visit the U.S. Drug Enforcement Administration website (http://www.deadiversion.usdoj.gov). You can also get a DEA number at this site by clicking on registration and selecting "Mid-Level Practitioner."

Begin exploring job opportunities through your PA school's placement or alumni office, state PA chapters, professional organization websites and newsletters, PA journal classifieds, local classifieds, general internet searches, and specific hospital or clinic websites. Medical clinics and hospitals where you did clinical rotations are also good places to inquire about job opportunities.

Do research on employment aspects that will come up repeatedly during job interviews so that you will understand what job benefits are typically offered and what's included in a standard job contract. Have relevant questions ready to ask potential employers, such as PA hospital privileges, whether you will be allowed to write prescriptions, any fees you will be required to pay, and how malpractice coverage works.

Financial Planning

Schedule a meeting with your PA school's financial aid office to review your loans and gain an accurate picture of the repayment schedule. You also might want to ask if they have any suggestions or information about loan forgiveness programs or any advice about loan consolidation plans should you need to consider them.

Note

See Resource III at the back of this book for a listing of all State/U.S. Territory Licensing Authorities.

Interview Preparation

Contact your school's alumni or placement office to ask if they have materials on interviewing skills or if they have compiled a list of the types of questions you should be prepared to answer at a job interview. Many schools also sponsor or participate in job fairs, which bring together graduating students and prospective employers. If your school doesn't offer these services, ask your student PA organization to organize a job fair or bring in a speaker from a local healthcare institution to discuss their interviewing and hiring process. At a minimum, find a good book on interviewing skills. If you want to present yourself well at a job interview, you have to prepare in advance.

Once you have been offered an interview, find out as much as you can about the hiring organization. Their website may tell you a great deal about the clinical services they provide, the patient mix they serve, and any new areas of health research or community outreach that they are involved in. Knowing this kind of information about a prospective employer is extremely useful during the interview; it enables you to appear knowledgeable and to ask questions specific to their institution's goals and mission. This wins points for any job applicant—and it increases the chances that you will be offered a position.

PART IV

PANCE/PANRE Practice Tests

Test 1

Block 1

1. Which of the following produces the first heart sound?

   A. Closing of the mitral and tricuspid valves

   B. Closing of the aortic and tricuspid valves

   C. Closing of the aortic and pulmonic valves

   D. Closing of the mitral and pulmonic valves

   E. Closing of the aortic and mitral valves

2. Which of the following provides the most sensitive test for primary hypothyroidism?

   A. Triiodothyronine

   B. Thyroid-stimulating hormone (TSH)

   C. Thyroxine

   D. Triiodothyronine uptake

   E. Thyroxine-binding globulin

3. A peripheral blood smear shows a microcytic anemia with basophilic stippling. Which of the following is the most likely cause of this patient's anemia?

   A. Anemia of chronic disease

   B. Folate deficiency

   C. Hereditary spherocytosis

   D. Iron-deficiency anemia

   E. Lead poisoning

4. Which of the following describes periods of deep breathing alternating with periods of no breathing and can be caused by heart failure?

   A. Kussmaul breathing

   B. Obstructive breathing

   C. Ataxic breathing

   D. Cheyne-Stokes respiration

   E. Tachypnea

5. Which of the following describes a papule?

   A. A small, discolored spot on the skin that lacks depression or elevation

   B. A palpable, solid lesion smaller than 0.5 cm in diameter

   C. An elevated, fluid-filled, circumscribed lesion smaller than 0.5 cm in diameter

   D. A well-demarcated, plateau-like, elevated lesion larger than 0.5 cm in diameter

   E. An elevated, fluid-filled, circumscribed lesion larger than 0.5 cm in diameter

6. An 82-year-old woman with a history of a previous myocardial infarction and hypertension arrives at the emergency department complaining of severe abdominal pain. The pain started suddenly with her last meal and has progressively worsened since its onset one hour earlier. She had a single episode of bloody diarrhea prior to arrival and is currently afebrile. The abdominal examination is significant for mild, diffuse tenderness. Which of the following is the most likely diagnosis?

   A. Acute cholecystitis

   B. Diverticulitis

   C. Acute pancreatitis

   D. Mesenteric ischemia

   E. Pyelonephritis

7. A 25-year-old man reports he went hiking a week ago. At the end of the day, his friend noticed a tick on him and removed it. The patient now reports fever, chills, and body aches and has a skin lesion where the tick bit him. The lesion has a red border with central clearing. Which of the following is the most appropriate intervention?

   A. Acetaminophen

   B. Ceftriaxone

   C. Doxycycline

   D. Erythromycin

   E. Rifampin

8. A woman is 35 weeks pregnant; a routine vaginal culture is positive for group B streptococci. Which of the following is the most appropriate therapeutic intervention?

   A. Antibiotic treatment at the time of diagnosis

   B. Antibiotic treatment during labor

   C. Antibiotic treatment for the newborn postdelivery

   D. No treatment is needed if the newborn is asymptomatic

   E. No treatment is needed if the pregnant woman is asymptomatic

9. A 43-year-old woman is diagnosed with a condition that causes excruciating pain near her nose and mouth. The involved nerve is derived from which of the following branchial arches?

   A. First

   B. Second

   C. Third

   D. Fourth

   E. Sixth

10. All of the following are common signs and symptoms of withdrawal that an opiate abuser might experience **EXCEPT**?

   A. Bradypnea

   B. Diarrhea

   C. Piloerection

   D. Rhinorrhea

   E. Sweating

11. Which of the following is a disadvantage of using acetaminophen over aspirin?

   A. There is a decreased effect on uric acid excretion.

   B. There is a decreased anti-inflammatory effect.

   C. There is less gastric irritation.

   D. There is less of a risk for occult blood loss.

   E. There is no alteration of bleeding time.

12. All of the following are characteristics of tetralogy of Fallot **EXCEPT**?

   A. Large, nonrestrictive ventricular septal defect

   B. Severe right ventricular outflow obstruction

   C. Right ventricular hypertrophy

   D. Overriding of the aortic root over the ventricular septum

   E. A left-to-right cardiac shunt

13. A 46-year-old obese man is at the clinic for an annual examination. He reports no complaints, and the physical exam is unremarkable. Laboratory results show a fasting plasma glucose of 142 mg/dL. A repeat fasting plasma glucose is performed the next day, and the result is 150 mg/dL. Which of the following is the most appropriate conclusion?

   A. The patient is classified as having diabetes mellitus.

   B. The patient is classified as hyperglycemic.

   C. No conclusions can be made.

   D. No treatment is currently needed.

   E. The patient is hypoglycemic.

14. Which of the following best describes the laboratory evaluation of a patient diagnosed with acute myeloid leukemia?

   A. Elevated white blood cell count greater than 100,000/μL, detection of the Philadelphia chromosome, and a markedly decreased leukocyte alkaline phosphatase

   B. Isolated lymphocytosis; lymphocytes appear mature and small

   C. Pancytopenia and "hairy cells"

   D. Pancytopenia with circulating blasts and the presence of Auer rods

   E. Paraprotein on serum protein electrophoresis

15. A patient has respiratory acidosis. Which of the following blood gas findings match the patient's condition?

   A. pH 7.52, P_{CO_2} 45 mm Hg, P_{O_2} 93 mm Hg, HCO_3^- 37 mEq/L

   B. pH 7.30, P_{CO_2} 50 mm Hg, P_{O_2} 75 mm Hg, HCO_3^- 25 mEq/L

   C. pH 7.65, P_{CO_2} 20 mm Hg, P_{O_2} 70 mm Hg, HCO_3^- 28 mEq/L

   D. pH 7.42, P_{CO_2} 38 mm Hg, P_{O_2} 98 mm Hg, HCO_3^- 24 mEq/L

   E. pH 7.33, P_{CO_2} 34 mm Hg, P_{O_2} 85 mm Hg, HCO_3^- 16 mEq/L

16. A 60-year-old man has a lesion on his chest that is well-demarcated, raised, round-shaped, and brown in color. It has a 3-cm diameter and a greasy, stuck-on appearance. Which of the following is most consistent with these findings?

   A. Actinic keratosis

   B. Basal cell carcinoma

   C. Rosacea

   D. Seborrheic keratosis

   E. Vitiligo

17. Which of the following is a clinical feature of esophageal achalasia?

   A. Fever

   B. Regurgitation of predigested food

   C. Epigastric pain

   D. Dysphagia to solids and liquids

   E. Hematemesis

18. Which of the following can cause Rocky Mountain spotted fever?

   A. *Bordetella pertussis*

   B. *Borrelia burgdorferi*

   C. *Corynebacterium striatum*

   D. *Rickettsia prowazekii*

   E. *Rickettsia rickettsii*

19. A diagnosis of menometrorrhagia is made when a patient has

   A. absence of menses

   B. difficult and painful menstruation

   C. excessive menstrual bleeding

   D. excessive or irregular menstrual bleeding during and between periods

   E. irregular menstrual bleeding between periods

20. An injury to a patient's right orbit results in entrapment of the inferior rectus muscle in the orbital floor. The patient will have double vision upon

    A. converging the eyes to view a near object.
    B. diverging the eyes to view a distant object.
    C. gazing to the left.
    D. looking downward.
    E. looking upward.

21. A 54-year-old man with chronic renal failure receives a kidney transplant and is given immunosuppressive therapy with cyclosporine. Over the next 6 months the patient's creatinine levels progressively rise, and a needle biopsy of the kidney is performed. What is the biopsy most likely to show?

    A. Intimal fibrosis, interstitial fibrosis, and tubular atrophy
    B. Linear deposition of immunoglobulin and complement in glomeruli
    C. Neutrophils, immunoglobulin, and complement in blood vessel walls
    D. T cell interstitial infiltrate and edema
    E. Thickening of the blood vessel intima due to cellular proliferation

22. Which of the following is the drug of choice for anti-hypertension therapy during pregnancy?

    A. Benazepril
    B. Methyldopa
    C. Amlodipine
    D. Atenolol
    E. Losartan

23. Which of the following is a characteristic of the Somogyi effect?

    A. Occurs in insulin-dependent and non-insulin-dependent diabetics
    B. Reduced tissue sensitivity to insulin between 5 and 7 AM
    C. Hyperglycemia in the evening
    D. Occurs following an episode of nighttime hyperglycemia
    E. Hyperglycemia in the morning

24. An adult is diagnosed with idiopathic thrombocytopenic purpura. Which of the following is the most appropriate first step in management?

    A. Heparin
    B. Infusion of factor VIII
    C. Plasmapheresis
    D. Prednisone
    E. Splenectomy

25. A patient has a history of eczema and seasonal allergies. Which of the following is the patient most likely to develop?

    A. Emphysema
    B. Chronic bronchitis
    C. Asthma
    D. Bronchiectasis
    E. Bronchogenic cancer

26. A young, sexually active woman complains of painless bumps around her groin and genital region. The bumps are skin-colored, umbilicated, 2-mm papules. Which of the following is the most likely diagnosis?

    A. Condylomata acuminata
    B. Folliculitis
    C. Herpes simplex
    D. Hidradenitis suppurativa
    E. Molluscum contagiosum

27. A 52-year-old man presents with burning epigastric pain brought on by eating, abdominal bloating, early satiety, and weight loss of 8 lb over the past month. The only significant physical examination finding is well-localized epigastric tenderness. Stools are negative for occult blood. Serum lipase is normal. What is the most likely diagnosis?

    A. Gastroesophageal reflux disease
    B. Acute pancreatitis
    C. Gastric ulcer
    D. Esophageal spasm
    E. Duodenal ulcer

28. A 25-year-old man presents to your office complaining of a painless lesion on his penis. He reports no penile discharge. Physical examination reveals inguinal adenopathy and a 1-cm ulcer on the distal shaft of the penis. The ulcer has a clean base with indurated borders. Which of the following is the most likely diagnosis?

    A. Chancroid

    B. Genital warts

    C. Gonorrhea

    D. Herpes simplex

    E. Syphilis

29. A woman has two children. Her first child was born premature. She has also had one abortion. Which of the following describes the woman's reproductive history?

    A. G3P2111

    B. G3P1112

    C. G2P3121

    D. G2P1113

    E. G1P3112

30. A 29-year-old woman diagnosed with AIDS has had a progressive blurring of vision in her right eye. On funduscopic examination, a small white opaque lesion is noted on the retina of her right eye. Which of the following is the most appropriate therapy for this patient?

    A. Acyclovir

    B. Amantadine

    C. Flucytosine

    D. Ganciclovir

    E. Zidovudine

31. Which of the following groups of viruses is most likely to be the etiology of viral meningitis?

    A. Adenoviruses

    B. Enteroviruses

    C. Human papillomaviruses

    D. Poxviruses

    E. Reoviruses

32. A 46-year-old man presents with a four-week history of recurrent headaches. He states the headaches awaken him at night and last approximately one hour. The pain is described as deep burning, centered behind the left eye. The pain is rated as 10 out of 10. Associated symptoms include watery eyes, sensation of warmth on the face, and nasal discharge. The patient denies any recent life changes or major stressors. Physical examination is normal. Which of the following is the most likely diagnosis?

    A. Tension headache

    B. Cluster headache

    C. Migraine headache

    D. Subdural hematoma

    E. Subarachnoid bleed

33. Which of the following diuretic agents is most likely to cause hyperkalemia?

    A. Acetazolamide

    B. Furosemide

    C. Hydrochlorothiazide

    D. Metolazone

    E. Triamterene

34. A teenager presents to the office for a school physical. He has no complaints. Blood pressure in the left arm is 150/90 mm Hg and in the right arm is 152/94 mm Hg. His femoral pulses are weak bilaterally. There is a harsh systolic murmur heard best at the back. Which of the following is the most likely diagnosis?

    A. Patent ductus arteriosus

    B. Atrial septal defect

    C. Transposition of the great arteries

    D. Ventricular septal defect

    E. Coarctation of the aorta

35. Laboratory results show a prolonged partial thromboplastin time, a normal prothrombin time, a normal bleeding time, normal fibrinogen levels, and normal factor VIII:R antigen levels. Which of the following is the most likely diagnosis?

    A. Disseminated intravascular coagulation

    B. Hemophilia A

    C. Idiopathic thrombocytopenic purpura

    D. Thrombotic thrombocytopenic purpura

    E. von Willebrand disease

36. Which of the following conditions is likely to present with cor pulmonale, severe hypoxia, and edema of the legs?

    A. Bronchiolitis obliterans

    B. Pneumonia

    C. Lung abscess

    D. Chronic bronchitis

    E. Bronchiectasis

37. Which of the following laboratory examinations is consistent with a herpes simplex infection?

    A. Elevated serum IgE levels

    B. A giant, multinucleated keratinocyte on a Giemsa-stained smear

    C. Large pseudohyphae forms and budding yeasts on 10% KOH

    D. Microscopic demonstration of a mite from skin scraping

    E. Septal panniculitis histologic findings

38. A 25-year-old woman presents with complaints of abdominal distension and bloating; intermittent, crampy, abdominal pain relieved by defecation; and more frequent and loose stools when she has pain. She has not had any weight loss. She has had diarrhea on some occasions and constipation at other times. Her physical and laboratory examinations are unremarkable. What is the most likely diagnosis?

    A. Ulcerative colitis

    B. Crohn's disease

    C. Viral gastroenteritis

    D. Irritable bowel syndrome

    E. Diverticulitis

39. A sexually active female is seen for her annual Pap smear and examination. She reports no problems. Speculum examination reveals a fish-like odor and grayish discharge. A wet mount shows clue cells. Which of the following is the most appropriate treatment?

    A. Ceftriaxone

    B. Clotrimazole

    C. Acyclovir

    D. Metronidazole

    E. Podophyllum resin

40. A patient is 26 weeks pregnant. Her pregnancy has been uneventful until today. She presents with painless vaginal bleeding. Which of the following is the most likely diagnosis?

    A. Abruptio placentae

    B. Uterine atony

    C. Placenta previa

    D. Preeclampsia

    E. Premature rupture of membranes

41. An otherwise healthy patient who wears contact lenses develops a small ulceration of the eye. Which of the following organisms is most likely involved?

    A. *Acanthamoeba*

    B. Cytomegalovirus

    C. Herpes simplex

    D. *Toxocara*

    E. *Toxoplasma*

42. A 35-year-old man is brought to the emergency department following an accident. He was walking across the street when he was struck by a man on a motorcycle. He complains of severe leg pain. Physical examination shows a foot drop and weakness of foot eversion. Radiographic studies do not reveal any abnormalities. Which of the following is the most likely location of this patient's injury?

    A. At the inguinal ligament

    B. At the neck of the fibula

    C. Near the medial malleolus

    D. Near the sciatic notch

    E. Proximal to the inguinal ligament

43. A 16-year-old girl confesses that she started smoking cigarettes when she was 14 years old. "I've heard about how bad this is for me and I want to stop smoking," she says, "but I just can't seem to stop." She asks the physician to prescribe "this patch thing I've heard about." Physical examination shows the girl is below normal body weight for her height. Both of the girl's parents are smokers as well. At this point, what would be the best thing to say?

    A. "I'm going to give you something called bupropion which has helped a lot of people to quit smoking."

    B. "I'm going to sign you up with a program for people your own age who are trying to quit smoking."

    C. "Let's schedule a time that you, I, and your parents can all talk about this issue together."

    D. "Quitting smoking sure is tough, but you just have to keep trying."

    E. "Tell me a bit more about what happened when you tried to quit smoking in the past."

44. A 64-year-old man complains of increasing shortness of breath, especially when he tries to sleep. Physical examination reveals a blowing pansystolic murmur best heard at the apex. The murmur radiates to the axilla. What is the most likely diagnosis?

    A. Tricuspid regurgitation

    B. Aortic stenosis

    C. Mitral regurgitation

    D. Aortic regurgitation

    E. Tricuspid stenosis

45. A 46-year-old obese man visits the clinic for his annual examination. He reports no complaints, and his physical examination is unremarkable. Laboratory results show a fasting plasma glucose of 142 mg/dL. A repeat fasting plasma glucose is performed, and the result is 150 mg/dL. Which of the following is the most appropriate treatment?

    A. Start metformin

    B. Follow up in 3 months and evaluate for symptoms

    C. Start glipizide

    D. Recommend diet and exercise

    E. Start pioglitazone

46. A 50-year-old is diagnosed with polycythemia vera. Which of the following is the most appropriate treatment for this patient?

    A. Heparin

    B. Phlebotomy

    C. Plasmapheresis

    D. Prednisone

    E. Splenectomy

47. A 60-year-old obese, otherwise healthy, woman presents with progressive swelling and pain in the left knee over the past 18 months. She states the symptoms worsen after activity and late in the day. She notes little to no pain or swelling early in the day. She denies any other joint involvement. Which of the following is the most likely diagnosis?

    A. Gout

    B. Osteoarthritis

    C. Reiter's syndrome

    D. Rheumatoid arthritis

    E. Calcium pyrophosphate deposition disease

48. An 18-year-old woman living in Florida notices areas of hypopigmented patches on her arms and neck. Examination with a Wood's lamp reveals yellow-green fluorescence. Which of the following is the most appropriate pharmacotherapy for this patient?

    A. Mupirocin ointment

    B. Oral acyclovir

    C. Oral corticosteroid

    D. Selenium sulfide lotion

    E. Topical retinoid application

49. A patient presents with right upper quadrant pain that is described as sharp but subsides in an hour. She has had several occurrences, usually after eating fatty foods. Which diagnostic study would you recommend first to confirm your diagnosis?

    A. Ultrasound of the gallbladder

    B. Oral cholecystography

    C. Endoscopic retrograde cholangiopancreatography (ERCP)

    D. Exploratory surgery

    E. Complete blood cell count

50. A 6-month-old child has an eye surgically enucleated because it contains a retinoblastoma. To which of the following structures should the pathologist pay particular attention when evaluating the specimen?

    A. Anterior chamber

    B. Cornea

    C. Lens

    D. Optic nerve

    E. Vitreous

51. A 50-year-old woman is seen for an annual examination. She has no complaints, and her physical examination is unremarkable. Laboratory testing reveals an elevated TSH; normal free T_4 level, T_4 level, and T_3 level; and detectable antithyroid antibodies. Which of the following is the most appropriate intervention?

    A. Radioactive iodine

    B. Monitor for symptoms

    C. Levothyroxine

    D. Propylthiouracil

    E. Recheck free T_4 levels in 3 months

52. A patient has right-sided sensorineural hearing loss. Which of the following would you expect to find?

    A. Bone conduction greater than air conduction on the right side during the Rinne test

    B. An abnormality visualized during otoscopy

    C. The sound lateralizes to the left side during the Weber test

    D. When the patient is placed in a noisy room the patient reports hearing has improved

    E. Air-fluid level behind the tympanic membrane

53. Which of the following is a common EKG finding noted in a patient with COPD?

    A. A large S wave in lead I and a Q wave and an inverted T wave in lead III

    B. Left ventricular hypertrophy

    C. Sinus bradycardia

    D. Atrial fibrillation

    E. Right axis deviation

54. A 4-year-old boy is brought in by his mother for fever, cough, sore throat, and conjunctivitis. Physical examination shows generalized lymphadenopathy, pharyngeal erythema, and Koplik spots. Which of the following is the most likely diagnosis?

    A. Erythema infectiosum

    B. Mumps

    C. Roseola

    D. Rubella

    E. Rubeola

55. Which of the following is used to treat hypoxemia in COPD patients?

    A. Oxygen

    B. Cromolyn sulfate

    C. Ipratropium bromide

    D. Albuterol

    E. Oral corticosteroids

56. Which of the following antihypertensives causes hyperglycemia?

    A. Propranolol

    B. Hydrochlorothiazide

    C. Benazepril

    D. Clonidine

    E. Terazosin

57. A 21-year-old man is competing in a weight-lifting competition. He lifts 325 lb over his head and holds it there for 5 seconds. Suddenly, his arms give way, and he drops the weight to the floor. Which of the following receptors is responsible for this sudden muscle relaxation?

    A. Free nerve ending

    B. Golgi tendon organ

    C. Merkel disk

    D. Muscle spindle

    E. Pacinian corpuscle

58. Which of the following best describes the primary mechanism of action of biguanides?

   A. Inhibits hepatic gluconeogenesis

   B. Stimulates pancreatic insulin release

   C. Increases insulin sensitivity

   D. Delays digestion of carbohydrates

   E. Promotes liver gluconeogenesis

59. Which of the following is considered an absolute contraindication to intrauterine device (IUD) use?

   A. Abnormal shape of uterus

   B. History of pelvic inflammatory disease (PID)

   C. Menorrhagia

   D. Multiple sexual partners

   E. Purulent cervicitis

60. A 12-year-old girl has been known to have cystic fibrosis since age 3. A chest x-ray film demonstrates tubular, air-filled structures that extend to near the edges of the lung fields. The intervening lung tissue appears normal. Which of the following is the most likely diagnosis?

   A. Asthma

   B. Bronchiectasis

   C. Chronic bronchitis

   D. Emphysema

   E. Pneumonia

End of Block 1

Block 2

1. A 24-year-old man comes in with a history of a sore on his glans penis. Physical examination reveals a non-tender indurated ulcer over the glans, and nontender inguinal lymphadenopathy. The organism causing this disease can best be visualized in the lesion using which of the following?

   A. Fluorescent treponemal antibody-absorption test (FTA-ABS)

   B. Gram stain

   C. Giemsa stain

   D. *Treponema pallidum* enzyme immunoassay (TP-EIA)

   E. Dark field microscopy

2. A patient experiences episodes of sharp stabbing pain that radiates over the mandible and extends around the temporomandibular joint and then deep into the ear. These episodes are triggered by smiling and by touching his face. Which of the following cranial nerves is involved?

   A. CN I

   B. CN II

   C. CN IV

   D. CN V

   E. CN VII

3. Which of the following differentiate into osteoblasts that form bone for remodeling and repair?

   A. Interstitial lamellae

   B. Osteoclasts

   C. Osteocytes

   D. Osteogenic cells

   E. Osteons

4. Which of the following hypertensive medications should be used cautiously in a diabetic patient?

   A. Clonidine

   B. Atenolol

   C. Nifedipine

   D. Benazepril

   E. Terazosin

5. An 18-year-old male athlete presents to your office for a physical. He has no complaints and presents a form from his college requesting medical clearance to participate in track and field. The medical clearance requires a urinalysis, an EKG, and a CBC. The urinalysis and CBC are pending. EKG is noted below. Which of the following is the most likely diagnosis?

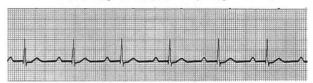

   A. The patient has first-degree heart block

   B. The EKG is normal

   C. The patient needs permanent pacing

   D. The patient needs to be treated prophylactically with warfarin

   E. The patient has Mobitz type I heart block

6. Which of the following physical examination findings is consistent with a diagnosis of acromegaly?

   A. Double vision and exophthalmos

   B. Enlarged hands and a doughy, soft, sweaty handshake

   C. Moon-shaped facies, buffalo hump, and central obesity

   D. Abdominal tenderness, hypotension, skin hyper-pigmentation, and confusion

   E. Clitoromegaly, deepening of voice, and increased muscularity

7. A 25-year-old man comes to the clinic for evaluation of a painless lump just above the collarbone. The lump is nontender, rubbery, round, 1 cm in diameter, has smooth edges, and is in the supraclavicular region. Which of the following is most consistent with the history and physical findings?

   A. Hairy cell leukemia

   B. Hodgkin disease

   C. Multiple myeloma

   D. Polycythemia vera

   E. von Willebrand disease

8. Which of the following is most likely to cause a lung abscess?

   A. *Chlamydia pneumoniae*

   B. *Mycoplasma pneumoniae*

   C. *Haemophilus influenzae*

   D. *Staphylococcus aureus*

   E. *Streptococcus pneumoniae*

9. Which of the following is the most appropriate treatment for severe cystic acne?

   A. Benzoyl peroxide topical gel

   B. Clindamycin lotion

   C. Comedone removal with comedo extractor

   D. Oral isotretinoin

   E. Oral tetracycline

10. A 76-year-old man with mild dementia chokes and coughs when he eats. His wife says the problem is worse with liquids than with solids. On examination, the patient begins coughing immediately after drinking water. The quality of his voice is then altered. Which of the following is the most likely diagnosis?

    A. Diffuse esophageal spasm

    B. Esophageal cancer

    C. Oropharyngeal dysphagia

    D. Schatzki ring

    E. Achalasia

11. Which of the following is a contraindication to a varicella vaccination?

    A. A child between 12 and 18 months of age

    B. A history of a serious allergic reaction to eggs

    C. A history of mild, intermittent asthma

    D. Pregnancy

    E. A 25-year-old with no prior history of chickenpox

12. Which of the following history and physical examination findings is consistent with fibrocystic disease?

    A. Bilateral milky discharge from multiple ducts in a nonlactating 35-year-old woman

    B. A firm, nontender mass with ill-defined margins in a 45-year-old woman

    C. Premenstrual, tender, rope-like changes of both breasts in a 30-year-old woman

    D. Redness, tenderness, increased warmth, and induration of a breast of a lactating woman

    E. A round, rubbery, movable, nontender, 1-cm mass in a 25-year-old woman

13. A 36-year-old Caucasian male archeologist who had lived in Egypt for several years complains of a history of painful urination and some blood in his urine. Ultrasound and intravenous pyelography confirm the presence of a filling defect in the urinary bladder. How did the patient most likely acquire his infection?

    A. Ingestion of eggs in water

    B. Ingestion of larvae in meat

    C. Ingestion of oocysts from fecal contamination

    D. Skin penetration by cercariae

    E. Mosquito transmission of microfilariae

14. A patient presents with a spastic left hemiparesis and an extensor plantar reflex on the left. The right side of the patient's face is numb, and the jaw deviates to the left upon protrusion. Where is the most likely location of a lesion?

    A. Cervical spinal cord on the left

    B. Right cerebellopontine angle

    C. Right cerebral hemisphere

    D. Right midbrain

    E. Right rostral pons

15. A 25-year-old woman comes to the office because of palpitations. She states that she thinks she has a "thyroid condition," based on research from medical websites. She drinks 4 cups of coffee a day, drinks a "moderate" amount of alcohol, and smokes a pack of cigarettes a day. She does not take any medications, and she denies feeling unusually sad or anxious lately. Physical examination and laboratory test results are all normal. The physician explains to her that the palpitations are probably not due to a medical condition, but most likely precipitated by the caffeine, alcohol, and cigarettes. The patient remains convinced that she has a "thyroid condition," and returns to the same physician many times over the next few months, requesting treatment. Which of the following is the most likely diagnosis?

    A. Body dysmorphic disorder
    B. Malingering
    C. Conversion disorder
    D. Hypochondriasis
    E. Somatization disorder

16. Which of the following will accentuate a mitral stenosis murmur during cardiac auscultation?

    A. Ask the patient to roll partly onto the left side and you place the bell of your stethoscope on the apical impulse.
    B. Ask the patient to sit up, lean forward, and exhale completely, and you place the diaphragm of your stethoscope along the left sternal border.
    C. Ask the patient to roll partly onto the left side and you place the bell of your stethoscope on the left sternal border.
    D. Ask the patient to sit up, lean forward, and exhale completely, and you place the bell of your stethoscope on the apical impulse.
    E. Ask the patient to sit up, lean forward, and inhale completely, and you place the diaphragm of your stethoscope on the apical impulse.

17. A patient complains of nausea, abdominal pain, fatigue, and weakness. The patient is hypotensive, is mildly confused, and has hyperpigmentation of the skin. Laboratory findings note hyponatremia, hyperkalemia, and hypoglycemia. Which of the following is the most appropriate test to confirm the possible diagnosis?

    A. Dexamethasone suppression test
    B. Antidiuretic hormone level
    C. Schilling test
    D. Direct Coombs test
    E. Cosyntropin stimulation test

18. Which of the following patients would benefit most from a pneumococcal vaccine?

    A. Patient with folic acid deficiency
    B. Patient with G6PD deficiency
    C. Patient with iron deficiency
    D. Patient with sickle cell anemia
    E. Patient with vitamin B_{12} deficiency

19. Which of the following is the most likely complication of a pneumonia caused by *Mycoplasma pneumoniae*?

    A. Pleural effusion
    B. Pneumothorax
    C. Endocarditis
    D. Bullous myringitis
    E. Cavitation

20. An 18-year-old African woman notices a thick, raised, smooth area on her shoulder, where a previous surgical incision healed. Which of the following is the most appropriate next step in management?

    A. Antibiotics
    B. Curettage
    C. Excision
    D. Intralesional injection of triamcinolone acetonide
    E. Topical corticosteroid

21. A 60-year-old man has constant epigastric pain with radiation to the back. He has lost 20 lb in the past 4 months. Physical examination reveals jaundice and a positive Courvoisier sign. Which of the following is the most likely diagnosis?

    A. Chronic cholecystitis

    B. Gastric ulcer

    C. Hepatic abscess

    D. Pancreatic carcinoma

    E. Acute cholecystitis

22. A sexually active woman reports genital itching and vaginal irritation. Inspection of the vulva and speculum examination reveal a malodorous, frothy, greenish discharge with diffuse vaginal erythema. Microscopic examination of a wet mount shows flagellated motile organisms. Which of the following is the treatment of choice?

    A. Ceftriaxone

    B. Doxycycline

    C. Metronidazole

    D. Miconazole

    E. Penicillin

23. Rheumatic fever is most frequently associated with which of the following cardiac lesions?

    A. Tricuspid regurgitation

    B. Mitral stenosis

    C. Aortic stenosis

    D. Aortic regurgitation

    E. Pulmonic stenosis

24. During cardiac auscultation, you listen to the patient's heart while the patient is in the squatting position and again in the standing position to help distinguish between mitral valve prolapse and aortic stenosis. Which of the following statements is true?

    A. Standing increases the prolapse of the mitral valve

    B. Standing increases the murmur intensity of aortic stenosis

    C. Standing decreases the prolapse of the mitral valve

    D. Squatting decreases the murmur intensity of aortic stenosis

    E. Squatting increases the prolapse of the mitral valve

25. During pregnancy at 20 weeks, where should the uterine fundus be palpable?

    A. The midpoint between the pubic symphysis and the umbilicus

    B. The midpoint between the umbilicus and the xiphisternum

    C. The pubic symphysis

    D. The umbilicus

    E. The xiphisternum

26. A 35-year-old man complains of his heart racing. It typically lasts 3 hours and then resolves spontaneously. Shortness of breath is noted only when his heart races. The patient's past medical history is unremarkable. Objective findings show a pulse of 180 beats per minute. An EKG shows a regular narrow complex tachycardia. A Valsalva maneuver was unable to interrupt the attack. What is the first-line drug therapy?

    A. Lidocaine

    B. Adenosine

    C. Verapamil

    D. Propranolol

    E. Amiodarone

27. Which of the following signs and symptoms is sufficient to make a diagnosis of chronic bronchitis?

    A. An increase of mucous secretions, which leads to chronic cough and infection

    B. Sputum production for longer than 3 months of the year for more than 2 successive years

    C. An increase in AP diameter of the chest

    D. Wheezing, productive cough, and decreased Pa_{O_2} and increased Pa_{CO_2}

    E. A decreased FEV_1:FVC ratio

28. Which of the following diagnostic tests is most useful in assessing a chronic obstructive pulmonary disease (COPD) patient's disease state?

    A. Chest radiograph

    B. Sputum culture

    C. FEV_1:FVC ratio

    D. EKG

    E. Arterial blood gases

29. Folate supplements during pregnancy have been shown to reduce the risk of which of the following fetal abnormalities?

    A. Arnold-Chiari malformations

    B. Germinal matrix hemorrhage

    C. Holoprosencephaly

    D. Neural tube defects

    E. Syringomyelia

30. A 30-year-old woman has chronic, silver-white, scaly patches on the skin of her knees and elbows. Which of the following is the most likely etiology of this condition?

    A. Autoimmune disease

    B. Bacterial disease

    C. Fungal disease

    D. Granulomatous disease

    E. Large vessel vasculitis

31. Which of the following FDA pregnancy categories denotes a drug that has demonstrated fetal risk in human studies and greater risk than benefit?

    A. A

    B. B

    C. C

    D. N

    E. X

32. A bronchial biopsy from a long-term smoker demonstrates focal areas where the normal respiratory epithelium is replaced by keratinizing squamous epithelium. The same change may occur as a pathologic response to deficiency of which of the following vitamins?

    A. Vitamin A

    B. Vitamin B_{12}

    C. Vitamin C

    D. Vitamin D

    E. Vitamin E

33. A 53-year-old married man is diagnosed with essential hypertension. Family history reveals a history of hypertension in males. After a discussion, the physician and patient agree on a course of treatment that includes exercise and daily medication. Knowing that adherence rates with antihypertension medications are low, what additional course of action is most likely to increase the chance of this patient's adherence?

    A. Ask for a joint consultation with the patient and his wife to explain the details of the treatment to the patient's spouse

    B. Describe the potential side effects of the medication in detail and ask the patient to call if any of them appear

    C. Provide an informative pamphlet describing the dangers of untreated hypertension

    D. Remind the patient of how his father and grandfather died of hypertension, as revealed in his family history

    E. Send the patient a reminder postcard in 1 week and schedule him for a follow-up visit in 2 weeks

34. Which of the following antihistamines would be the most appropriate treatment for an airline pilot with hay fever?

    A. Chlorpheniramine

    B. Diphenhydramine

    C. Meclizine

    D. Pyrilamine

    E. Terfenadine

35. A patient with severe systemic lupus erythematosus is receiving long-term glucocorticoid therapy. She should consequently receive supplemental therapy with which of the following?

    A. Calcium

    B. Carotene

    C. Folate

    D. Iron

    E. Vitamin B_{12}

36. A 45-year-old man complains of intermittent chest pain since yesterday. The pain is substernal and crushing in nature. EKG is noted below. Which type of myocardial infarction does the EKG show?

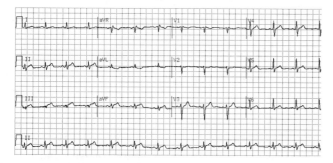

   A. Posterior infarction
   B. Lateral infarction
   C. Anterior infarction
   D. Inferior infarction
   E. Subendocardial infarction

37. Which of the following is considered first-line treatment for acute exacerbations of COPD?

   A. Ipratropium bromide and theophylline
   B. Albuterol
   C. Theophylline
   D. Methylprednisolone sodium succinate (Solu-Medrol)
   E. Ipratropium bromide and albuterol sulfate (Combivent)

38. Ten days ago, the spouse of a patient noticed a bright red, oval lesion of approximately 3 cm on her husband's back. Now, the patient presents with a generalized rash. There are multiple discrete, dull pink, fine-scaling papules and plaques in a Christmas tree distribution on the patient's back. Which of the following is the most likely diagnosis?

   A. Lichen simplex chronicus
   B. Nummular eczema
   C. Pityriasis rosea
   D. Pityriasis versicolor
   E. Shingles

39. A 60-year-old man with a long history of alcohol abuse presents with painless hematemesis. The patient states he was vomiting and then vomited up a large amount blood. Which of the following is the most likely diagnosis?

   A. Gastric cancer
   B. Duodenal ulcer
   C. Gastric ulcer
   D. Mallory-Weiss tear
   E. Gastroesophageal reflux disease

40. A 55-year-old Pennsylvania coal miner consults his physician about increasing respiratory distress. He is also experiencing troubling bouts of arthritis. A chest x-ray film demonstrates massive fibrosis of his lungs. Biopsy of a 2-cm lump on his arm demonstrates a rheumatoid nodule. Which of the following is the most likely diagnosis?

   A. Caplan syndrome
   B. Goodpasture syndrome
   C. Plumbism
   D. von Gierke disease
   E. WAGR syndrome

41. A homosexual man develops small, purplish nodules on his legs and chest. Biopsy of one of these nodules demonstrates a malignant vascular neoplasm. Which of the following viruses has been implicated in the pathogenesis of this type of tumor?

   A. Epstein-Barr virus
   B. Herpes simplex I
   C. Herpes simplex II
   D. Herpesvirus 8 (HHV8)
   E. Human papilloma virus

42. A pregnant woman is diagnosed with hyperthyroidism. Which of the following is the most appropriate treatment?

    A. Propylthiouracil

    B. Methimazole

    C. Radioactive iodine

    D. Thyroid surgery

    E. Propranolol

43. A patient is hospitalized for a deep vein thrombosis of the left lower extremity. Which of the following is the most appropriate next step?

    A. Warfarin therapy

    B. Insertion of a vena cava filter

    C. Heparin therapy

    D. Simultaneous heparin and warfarin therapy

    E. Streptokinase

44. Which of the following is the most common etiology of chronic bronchitis?

    A. Smoking

    B. Air pollution

    C. Pneumonia

    D. Alpha-1-antitrypsin deficiency

    E. Allergy

45. At the conclusion of his annual physical examination, a 65-year-old man confides that he has had some difficulty with his sexual functioning lately. Further questioning reveals the problem to be one of the orgasm disorders. Which of the following is the most likely diagnosis?

    A. Anorgasmia

    B. Dyspareunia

    C. Premature ejaculation

    D. Retarded ejaculation

    E. Secondary impotence

46. The area of auscultation for the aortic valve in the heart is performed at which of the following anatomic positions?

    A. Inferior border of the heart

    B. Left second intercostal space

    C. Left fifth intercostal space

    D. Right second intercostal space

    E. Xiphisternal junction

47. A patient reports a new onset of palpitations over the last month. When further questioned, the patient states this happens every couple of days and usually lasts less than an hour. An EKG performed in the office shows a normal sinus rhythm. What is the most appropriate next step?

    A. Holter monitor

    B. Stress exercise test

    C. Echocardiogram

    D. Prescribe a low-dose beta-blocker

    E. Radioablation therapy

48. A known drug user has been taking large doses of a drug for the past few days. He is excited, has persecutory ideas, and demonstrates stereotypic, nondirective behavior. On physical examination, he has warm, moist skin. His mouth is dry and his eyes are sunken. Fresh "tracks" are visible on his forearms. Which of the following drugs has he most likely been injecting?

    A. Butabarbital

    B. Diazepam

    C. Heroin

    D. Methamphetamine

    E. Phencyclidine

49. A 53-year-old man with a known gastric ulcer on upper gastrointestinal imaging is given ranitidine for 12 weeks. On follow-up examination, he reports that his epigastric pain persists. What is the next step in his management?

   A. Continue ranitidine for another 4 weeks.

   B. Increase the dose of ranitidine until the patient responds.

   C. Repeat the upper gastrointestinal imaging.

   D. Refer for endoscopic evaluation.

   E. Refer for vagotomy.

50. A couple trying to get pregnant recently purchased a home ovulation urine test kit. The increase in which of the following would indicate a higher probability of fertilization?

   A. Follicle-stimulating hormone (FSH) levels

   B. Human chorionic gonadotropin (HCG) levels

   C. Luteinizing hormone (LH) levels

   D. Progesterone levels

   E. Prolactin levels

51. A 25-year-old woman comes to the emergency room complaining of tachycardia, palpitations, neck pain, and insomnia that has progressed over the past 8 days. Further questioning reveals noticeable weight loss and heat intolerance. She denies methamphetamine use, and a urine screen supports her claim. Physical examination notes generalized nervousness, mild tremor, exophthalmos, and an enlarged thyroid. She has an elevated free T4 and decreased thyroid-stimulating hormone. Which of the following would *NOT* be an acceptable treatment option for this patient?

   A. Propylthiouracil (PTU)

   B. Methylcellulose eye drops

   C. Levothyroxine

   D. Radioactive iodine

   E. Propanolol

52. A patient reports that earlier in the day she had a brief episode of unilateral blindness. She describes the episode as a vertical curtain passing across her visual field with subsequent unilateral blindness that lasted approximately 2 minutes. She describes a similar vertical curtain passing over her visual field as her vision returned. Currently, she has no visual deficits, and funduscopic examination is normal. Which of the following is the most likely diagnosis?

   A. Central retinal vein occlusion

   B. Central retinal artery occlusion

   C. Retinal detachment

   D. Open angle glaucoma

   E. Amaurosis fugax

53. A patient presents to the emergency room with shortness of breath. Objective findings show muffled heart sounds and tachycardia. In addition, there is a >10 mm Hg decline in systolic blood pressure during inspiration. Which of the following is the most likely diagnosis?

   A. Aortic dissection

   B. Pericarditis

   C. Cardiac tamponade

   D. Myocardial infarction

   E. Congestive heart failure

54. An alcoholic man is diagnosed with Wernicke triad and Korsakoff syndrome. Which of the following would be the most appropriate treatment for this patient?

   A. Biotin

   B. Niacin

   C. Pyridoxine

   D. Riboflavin

   E. Thiamine

55. Which of the following is the most common etiology of acute pharyngitis?

   A. Group A beta-hemolytic *Streptococcus*

   B. *Mycoplasma pneumoniae*

   C. *Chlamydia pneumoniae*

   D. Viral

   E. *Neisseria gonorrhoeae*

56. A 32-year-old woman has a history of abnormal menstruation and infertility. She and her husband want to have a child and went to a fertility specialist. The woman was started on an oral medication for ovarian stimulation. A few months later, she presents to the ER with sharp pelvic pain and light, persistent vaginal bleeding. On physical examination a right adnexal mass is palpated. Which of the following is the most likely diagnosis?

    A. Ectopic pregnancy

    B. Endometrial cancer

    C. Endometriosis

    D. Pelvic inflammatory disease

    E. Uterine prolapse

57. Which of the following conditions is associated with a human papillomavirus infection?

    A. Actinic keratosis

    B. Dyshidrosis

    C. Seborrheic dermatitis

    D. Seborrheic keratosis

    E. Squamous cell carcinoma

58. A pregnant woman is possibly exposed to rubella. Which of the following is the most appropriate next step?

    A. Administer live attenuated rubella virus vaccine

    B. Advise therapeutic abortion

    C. Obtain hemagglutination-inhibiting rubella antibody level

    D. Provide counseling

    E. Recommend acetaminophen for symptomatic relief

59. A 40-year-old, overweight woman complains of bilateral lower extremity discomfort. She describes the discomfort as an achy heaviness that is worse with prolonged periods of standing. Physical examination reveals bilateral, dilated, tortuous veins beneath the thighs and legs. Which of the following diagnoses do you suspect?

    A. Chronic venous insufficiency

    B. Thrombophlebitis of the deep veins

    C. Varicose veins

    D. Livedo reticularis

    E. Acute arterial occlusion

60. Which of the following viruses produces disease or sequela that is more severe if the infection occurs at a very young age?

    A. Epstein-Barr virus

    B. Hepatitis B virus

    C. Measles virus

    D. Poliovirus

    E. Varicella-zoster virus

End of Block 2

Block 3

1. A patient has chronic atrial fibrillation. He is currently on warfarin anticoagulation therapy. He presents to the office for his monthly PT and INR blood draws. All of the following will affect the coagulation status **EXCEPT?**

   A. Recent diagnosis with a platelet disorder

   B. Ingestion of excessive green, leafy vegetables

   C. Chronic diarrhea

   D. Alcoholism

   E. Biliary obstruction

2. Which of the following is the most common cause of urge incontinence in females?

   A. Detrusor overactivity

   B. Urinary tract infection

   C. Beta-adrenergic agents

   D. External urethral sphincter spasm

   E. Menopause

3. A 62-year-old man is prescribed a pharmaceutical agent that inhibits the activity of the enzyme HMG-CoA reductase. This patient most likely has which of the following conditions?

   A. Chronic inflammation

   B. Familial hypercholesterolemia

   C. Hypertension

   D. Hyperuricemia

   E. Type 2 diabetes

4. A 7-year-old girl is brought to the emergency department by her parents with a complaint of severe polyuria and polydipsia. Laboratory examination reveals ketones in her urine. Which of the following is the most likely source of the ketones?

   A. Free fatty acid breakdown

   B. Gluconeogenesis

   C. Glycogenolysis

   D. Protein breakdown

   E. Triglyceride breakdown

5. A newborn presents with a possible cyanotic, congenital heart disease. Which of the following is in the differential diagnosis?

   A. Patent ductus arteriosus

   B. Coarctation of the aorta

   C. Complete transposition of the great arteries

   D. Atrial septal defect

   E. Aortic stenosis

6. A 55-year-old man complains of fever, headaches, and scalp tenderness. The headache is severe, throbbing, and localized over the frontotemporal region. The right temporal artery is tender and has a diminished pulse. Which of the following is the most appropriate initial step in management?

   A. Refer patient for an arterial biopsy

   B. Order an elevated sedimentation rate (ESR)

   C. Order a complete blood count (CBC)

   D. Start prednisone therapy

   E. Obtain a chest radiograph

7. A patient complains of a dramatic increase of thirst and going to the bathroom frequently. He states that he drinks approximately 10 L of water daily and feels like he urinates the same amount. He denies dysuria. An initial battery of labs is performed and shows hyperuricemia and a low urine specific gravity. Which of the following is the most appropriate test to confirm the diagnosis?

   A. Urine culture

   B. Oral glucose tolerance test

   C. Vasopressin challenge test

   D. Dexamethasone suppression test

   E. Plasma growth hormone levels

8. A 6-year-old boy is brought in by his father for evaluation of a facial rash. The boy had stayed home from school in the past 2 days because he generally didn't feel well and had a mild fever. He presents with intensely erythematous cheeks and circumoral pallor. Which of the following is the most appropriate intervention?

    A. Antibiotics
    B. Antiviral therapy
    C. Immunoglobulin
    D. Racemic epinephrine
    E. Symptomatic treatment

9. A 72-year-old man has a 6-month history of dysphagia, mainly for solids. It has been getting progressively worse, and he has noted a 15-lb weight loss over that same time period. He is a heavy smoker and a recovering alcoholic. What is the most likely diagnosis?

    A. Esophageal carcinoma
    B. Gastric carcinoma
    C. Achalasia
    D. Esophageal stricture
    E. Barrett's esophagus

10. Last year's influenza A vaccine is unlikely to be effective today because influenza A

    A. has a heavy polysaccharide coat
    B. immunosuppresses the patient
    C. kills lymphocytes
    D. resists inactivation by complement
    E. undergoes genetic reassortment

11. Which of the following laboratory results is suggestive of a postmenopausal woman?

    A. A decreased serum alkaline phosphatase level
    B. A decreased serum luteinizing hormone level
    C. A decreased urine estradiol level
    D. An increased serum follicle-stimulating hormone level
    E. An increased serum total testosterone level

12. An elderly woman reports episodes of dizziness upon standing. She has no other medical problems. She is diagnosed with orthostatic hypotension. You make recommendations for her continued care. Which of the following would you NOT recommend?

    A. Wearing waist-high elastic hosiery
    B. Daily use of an alpha blocker
    C. Adding potassium supplementation
    D. Getting up quickly from sitting to standing
    E. Prolonged recumbency

13. A 41-year-old obese woman with a history of biliary colic presents with right upper quadrant discomfort and pain in her right shoulder after eating a fatty meal. Physical examination is significant for marked right upper quadrant tenderness during inspiration. Which of the following structures is most likely involved in producing her shoulder pain?

    A. Expiratory motor neuron
    B. Inspiratory motor neuron
    C. Intercostal nerve
    D. Phrenic nerve
    E. Vagus nerve

14. A 45-year-old man stops his exercise program and begins to gain weight. When asked why he stopped he states, "It just made me feel too uncomfortable." The mechanism causing this man to stop exercising would best be described as which of the following?

    A. Extinction of a classically conditioned response
    B. Extinction of a positive operant response
    C. Negative reinforcement
    D. Punishment of an instrumental response
    E. Withdrawal of secondary reinforcement

15. A 24-year-old woman is taken to the emergency department because of severe pelvic pain. The attending physician suspects a rupturing ovarian cyst and wants to take a sample of the contents of the pouch of Douglas. This structure is found between the uterus and which of the following structures?

    A. Bladder

    B. Cervix

    C. Fallopian tube

    D. Ovary

    E. Rectum

Items 16–17: The response options for the next two items are the same. You'll be required to select one answer for each item in the set.

For the following neoplasms, select the most commonly associated chemical carcinogen (choices A–E).

    A. Aflatoxin

    B. Arsenic

    C. Asbestos

    D. Nitrosamines

    E. Vinyl chloride

16. Hepatocellular carcinoma

17. Mesothelioma

18. After recovering from a recent thyroidectomy, a patient reports muscle aches, increased moodiness, and tingling around the mouth and hands and feet. Objective findings reveal a positive Chvostek sign. Which of the following is among the differential diagnoses?

    A. Hyperthyroidism

    B. Myxedema

    C. Diabetes insipidus

    D. Hypoparathyroidism

    E. Addison disease

19. A patient with a history of intravenous (IV) drug use complains of abrupt onset of fever, cough, and joint pain. Physical exam shows painless erythematous lesions on the palms and petechiae beneath several fingernails. Lungs are clear to auscultation and a diastolic murmur is newly discovered. Which of the following diagnoses is consistent with the history and physical?

    A. Polymyalgia rheumatica

    B. Infectious mononucleosis

    C. Infective endocarditis

    D. Scarlet fever

    E. Dermatomyositis

20. A 4-year-old boy presents with fever, a strawberry tongue, reddening of the palms and soles, and bilateral conjunctival inflammation. Which of the following is the most appropriate treatment?

    A. Acetaminophen

    B. Amoxicillin

    C. Oral hydration

    D. Aspirin

    E. Ibuprofen

21. A 35-year-old man presents 2 months after treatment for a gastric ulcer discovered on endoscopy. At the time of endoscopy, *Helicobacter pylori* infection was identified. Which of the following is the most appropriate therapeutic management for eradication of *H. pylori*?

    A. Bismuth subsalicylate, two tablets QID for 14 days

    B. PPI BID and ranitidine 400 mg BID for 14 days

    C. PPI BID, clarithromycin 500 mg BID, and amoxicillin 1 gram BID for 14 days

    D. PPI BID and bismuth subsalicylate, two tablets QID, and amoxicillin 1 mg BID for 14 days

    E. Ofloxacin 400 mg PO BID for 14 days

22. Which of the following is the most common type of lung cancer in *non*smokers?

    A. Bronchioloalveolar carcinoma

    B. Bronchogenic adenocarcinoma

    C. Large cell (anaplastic) carcinoma

    D. Small cell (oat cell) carcinoma

    E. Squamous cell carcinoma

23. An accident in a dry cleaning facility exposes an employee to massive amounts of carbon tetrachloride, both on the skin and by inhalation. Severe damage to which of the following organs is most likely to occur?

    A. Heart

    B. Intestine

    C. Kidney

    D. Liver

    E. Stomach

24. A 50-year-old man is evaluated by a physician after developing recurrent bouts of bilateral pneumonitis with nodular and cavitary pulmonary infiltrates. The man also has a long history of sinusitis. Nasal biopsy demonstrates a necrotizing vasculitis with granulomas. This man is also particularly vulnerable to serious disease of which of the following organs?

    A. Heart

    B. Kidneys

    C. Liver

    D. Testes

    E. Thyroid

25. A postmenopausal woman reports vaginal soreness and painful intercourse. Pelvic examination reveals thin, pale vaginal walls. No malodorous discharge, cervical motion tenderness, or vulvar lesions are noted. A wet prep is unremarkable. Which of the following is the most likely diagnosis?

    A. Atrophic vaginitis

    B. Bacterial vaginosis

    C. Cervicitis

    D. Endometrial cancer

    E. Uterine prolapse

26. A 4-year-old is referred to a pediatrician for evaluation after a Head Start program teacher notices that the child seems to have stopped developing mentally and has developed behavior problems. The pediatrician notes that the child is lethargic and that there is a dark line near the teeth in the patient's gingiva. Which of the following is the most likely diagnosis?

    A. Acetaminophen poisoning

    B. Arsenic poisoning

    C. Carbon monoxide poisoning

    D. Lead poisoning

    E. Mushroom poisoning

27. After receiving a heart transplant and immunosuppressive therapy, a 56-year-old Vietnam War veteran develops fever and pulmonary infiltrates. Microscopic examination of bronchoalveolar lavage fluid reveals a 1-mm worm. Which of the following is the most likely means by which this infection was acquired?

    A. Ingestion of eggs in contaminated water

    B. Ingestion of infected feces

    C. Ingestion of larvae in infected meat

    D. Mosquito inoculation of larvae

    E. Skin penetration by larvae

28. A 35-year-old woman complains of vomiting dark, greenish material approximately 1 hour after eating. She is scheduled for a barium meal to evaluate the upper portion of the gastrointestinal tract. She denies pain and is anicteric. Which of the following is the most likely cause of this woman's condition?

    A. Annular pancreas

    B. Esophageal atresia

    C. Gallstones

    D. Meckel diverticulum

    E. Pyloric stenosis

29. A 20-year-old woman complains of easy fatigability. Physical examination reveals a grade II/VI systolic ejection murmur best heard over the pulmonic region and a fixed split second heart sound. Which of the following is the most likely diagnosis?

    A. Aortic stenosis

    B. Ventricular septal defect

    C. Atrial septal defect

    D. Mitral regurgitation

    E. Tricuspid regurgitation

30. A 13-year-old boy with known sickle cell anemia presents with increased fatigue. Physical examination is unremarkable. Complete blood count reveals a white blood cell count of 2.0×10^3/mL, hemoglobin 6 mg/dL, hematocrit 18%, and platelet count 90×10^9/L. Urinalysis is negative for blood. The patient's condition is most likely related to infection with which of the following?

    A. Cytomegalovirus (CMV)

    B. Epstein-Barr virus (EBV)

    C. Herpes simplex I

    D. Human papillomavirus (HPV)

    E. Parvovirus B19

31. A pregnant woman is diagnosed with eclampsia. Two weeks later she presents to the emergency room convulsing. Which of the following is the most appropriate next step?

    A. Calcium gluconate

    B. Diazepam

    C. Magnesium sulfate

    D. Obstetric consult

    E. Phenytoin

32. Which of the following is the recommended antidote for an overdose of heparin?

    A. *N*-acetylcysteine

    B. Platelets

    C. Vitamin K

    D. Protamine sulfate

    E. Flumazenil

33. A 35-year-old pregnant woman is in her tenth week. She presents with nausea, vomiting, and uterine bleeding. Objective findings note a larger uterus than expected for the weeks of gestation. An ultrasound reveals a snowstorm appearance, an enlarged uterus, and a lack of a fetus. Which of the following is the most likely diagnosis?

    A. Ectopic pregnancy

    B. Hemorrhage

    C. Hydatidiform mole

    D. Intrauterine infection

    E. Spontaneous abortion

34. An elderly patient presents with attacks of dizziness. Objective findings note a slow pulse. What is the appropriate treatment?

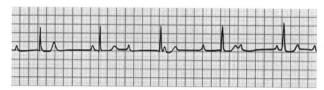

    A. Pacemaker

    B. Thrombolytic treatment

    C. Cardioversion

    D. Adenosine

    E. Propranolol

35. A patient with acute lymphocytic leukemia is treated appropriately with antineoplastic therapy. Inhibition of which of the following enzymes will help prevent side effects of this therapy?

    A. Alpha-glucosidase

    B. Angiotensin-converting enzyme

    C. Beta-lactamase

    D. Cyclooxygenase

    E. Xanthine oxidase

36. After eating a dinner of leftovers that included rewarmed vegetable fried rice, a 17-year-old boy develops diarrhea and stomach pain. Which of the following is the most likely pathogen?

    A. *Bacillus cereus*

    B. *Campylobacter jejuni*

    C. *Clostridium botulinum*

    D. *Clostridium difficile*

    E. *Escherichia coli*

37. A 57-year-old alcoholic man is brought to the emergency department in a state of global confusion, psychosis, and ataxia. On examination, ophthalmoplegia and polyneuropathy are also noted. Administration of which of the following would be the most appropriate treatment for this patient?

    A. Biotin

    B. Niacin

    C. Pyridoxine

    D. Riboflavin

    E. Thiamine

38. You suspect a patient has coarctation of the aorta. Which of the following blood tests would help confirm your diagnosis?

    A. CBC

    B. Partial thromboplastin time

    C. Renin levels

    D. Prothrombin time

    E. Total metanephrine

39. A patient complains of discomfort around the intravenous site. Findings show induration, redness, and tenderness that is localized. What is the most appropriate treatment?

    A. Heparin

    B. Warm soaks and NSAIDs

    C. Warfarin

    D. Cephalexin

    E. Excision of vein

40. A pregnant woman is in her 30th week and presents for a checkup. She reports no problems. Her blood pressure is 140/90 mm Hg, and she has 2+ albuminemia. Which of the following is part of your recommendations?

    A. Decrease water intake.

    B. Increase salt intake.

    C. Instruct patient to lie on her right side while sleeping.

    D. Monitor urine output.

    E. Strict bed rest.

41. A 6-month-old male infant is brought in by his mother for feeding poorly and appearing lethargic for 1 day. In an attempt to make the bottle feedings easier, she put a dab of honey on the nipple of the bottle to tempt her son. Now, her son will not feed at all. Physical examination reveals decreased muscle tone and a weak cry. Which of the following is most consistent with the history and physical examination?

    A. Adenovirus infection

    B. Botulism

    C. Congenital hypothyroidism

    D. Congenital myasthenia gravis

    E. Reye syndrome

42. A young woman complains of an itchy, red, bumpy rash. The lesions are erythematous, perifollicular lesions with some pustules. Upon questioning, the patient reports that 2 nights ago, she came back from a spa retreat where she spent a lot of time in a hot tub. Which of the following organisms is the most likely cause of her skin condition?

    A. *Escherichia coli*

    B. *Malassezia furfur*

    C. *Pseudomonas aeruginosa*

    D. *Staphylococcus aureus*

    E. *Streptococcus pyogenes*

43. A routine hepatitis screen performed on a unit of donated blood reveals the following:

    HB$_c$Ab negative

    HB$_s$Ag negative

    HB$_s$Ab positive

    HB$_e$Ag negative

    HB$_e$Ab negative

    Which of the following is the correct interpretation of the status of the blood donor?

    A. Successfully vaccinated

    B. Resolved acute infection

    C. Chronic carrier

    D. Acutely infected

    E. Infectious to others

44. A 25-year-old woman complains of palpations when she exercises. Physical exam reveals a high-pitched late systolic crescendo-decrescendo murmur best heard at the apex. An echocardiogram is performed and reveals mitral valve prolapse without regurgitation. Which of the following is the most appropriate treatment?

    A. Valve repair

    B. Beta-blocker

    C. Aspirin

    D. Reassurance

    E. Digitalis therapy

45. Which of the following is not a risk factor for hyaline membrane disease?

    A. Premature infant

    B. An L/S ratio of 2:1

    C. Maternal diabetes

    D. Being a second twin

    E. Male sex

46. What is the treatment of choice for patients with non–small cell carcinoma?

    A. Chemotherapy

    B. Chemotherapy and radiation

    C. Corticosteroids and chemotherapy

    D. Surgical resection

    E. Radiation

47. A 50-year-old man presents with sudden onset of severe chest pain that radiates to the back. A chest radiograph shows widening of the mediastinum. Which of the following is the most likely diagnosis?

    A. Myocardial infarction

    B. Pulmonary embolism

    C. Aortic dissection

    D. Cor pulmonale

    E. Constrictive pericarditis

48. A patient is diagnosed with Prinzmetal angina. Which of the following is the prophylactic treatment of choice?

    A. Propranolol

    B. Aspirin

    C. Amlodipine

    D. Streptokinase

    E. Heparin

49. Which of the following is an absolute contraindication to fibrolytic therapy in acute myocardial infarction?

    A. Known bleeding diathesis

    B. Active peptic ulcer disease

    C. History of chronic severe hypertension

    D. History of hemorrhagic stroke

    E. Pregnancy

50. How is secondary hypertension different from essential hypertension?

    A. Blood pressure is refractory to antihypertensives

    B. Systolic blood pressure does not exceed 200 mm Hg

    C. The onset is in the patient's late 20s

    D. There is a positive family history of hypertension

    E. In the majority of cases, no cause can be established

51. Which of the following medications should a hypertensive diabetic patient be prescribed?

    A. Hydrochlorothiazide

    B. Benazepril

    C. Propranolol

    D. Atorvastatin

    E. Furosemide

52. A 25-year-old woman has a hot-potato voice, high fever, dysphagia, and a sore throat. Objective findings note that the uvula is swollen and displaced to the left, the soft palate is edematous and erythematous, and a peritonsillar abscess displaces the right tonsil medially. Which of the following is the most appropriate intervention?

    A. Referral to ENT for incision and drainage

    B. Tonsillectomy

    C. Penicillin

    D. Viscous lidocaine

    E. Aspirin

53. A nonsmoking woman complains of bilateral calf achiness when walking. The pain is relieved by rest. The skin of the lower extremities is atrophic, cool, and hairless. There are weak pedal pulses. Which of the following is the most likely diagnosis?

    A. Venous insufficiency

    B. Varicose veins

    C. Thrombophlebitis

    D. Thromboangiitis obliterans

    E. Arterial insufficiency

54. A formula-fed, 1-month-old boy is exposed to his sister, who has chickenpox. His mother had the infection 5 years ago. Which class of immunoglobulins did he acquire from his mother in utero that protected him from this virus?

    A. IgA

    B. IgD

    C. IgE

    D. IgG

    E. IgM

55. A 33-year-old man with diabetes has not been monitoring his blood sugar on a regular basis. His glycolated hemoglobin (HbA_{1c}) is 11.4, and random blood glucose is 513 mg/dL. What would be the best agent to lower his blood glucose level right now?

    A. Glucagon

    B. Metformin

    C. Insulin glargine

    D. Insulin lispro

    E. Exercise and weight loss

56. Which of the following is recommended for the reduction of morbidity in a patient with rosacea?

    A. Avoid swimming pools

    B. Avoid rubbing and scratching

    C. Avoid suspected allergen

    D. Eliminate hot beverages

    E. Frequently wash the face

57. A 60-year-old woman with a history of congestive heart failure presents to the emergency room. She complains of abdominal pain, nausea, and fatigue. An EKG shows frequent premature ventricular contractions. A laboratory result shows hypokalemia. During the history-taking, which of the following questions aids the most in obtaining the diagnosis?

    A. "Do you smoke?"

    B. "What medications do you take?"

    C. "Do you have a history of heart disease?"

    D. "Do you have a history of abdominal pain?"

    E. "Do you drink alcohol?"

58. A G3P3 40-year-old woman complains of constipation and difficulty with evacuation. She states that her vagina bulges when she strains to have a bowel movement. At times, she even needs to press against the vaginal bulge to help her have a bowel movement. The history is most consistent with which of the following diagnoses?

    A. Cystocele

    B. Enterocele

    C. Incompetent cervix

    D. Rectocele

    E. Uterine prolapse

59. A patient reports a week ago he had an acute onset of a runny nose with nasal congestion, sneezing, and malaise. He took acetaminophen and used an oxymetazoline nasal spray. He states the medicine helped his symptoms for 4 days. Now he reports that he feels fine but can't get rid of his nasal stuffiness, which is worse than when it first started. Which of the following diagnoses is most consistent with the history?

    A. Allergic rhinitis

    B. Viral rhinitis

    C. Nasal polyps

    D. Rhinitis medicamentosa

    E. Nasal vestibulitis

60. A patient is admitted to critical care and confined to bed. Which of the following is used in the prevention of venous thromboembolism?

    A. Heparin

    B. Warfarin

    C. Streptokinase

    D. Intermittent pneumatic compression

    E. Early ambulation

End of Block 3

Block 4

1. A 35-year-old male farmer complains that his right eye has a nonpainful, unsightly lesion on it. He states that he has had it for many years; however, it seems to get a little bigger each year. Objective findings notes a fleshy, white tissue with blood vessels in a triangular shape that extends from the conjunctiva on the right nasal side of the eye over the cornea toward the pupil. Which of the following is most consistent with the history and physical examination?

    A. Hordeolum
    B. Pterygium
    C. Chalazion
    D. Conjunctivitis
    E. Cataract

2. Which of the following objective findings is consistent with right unilateral blindness with normal sympathetic and parasympathetic innervations to both irises?

    A. A light directed in the left eye produces a consensual reaction in the right eye
    B. A light directed in the right eye produces a direct reaction in the right eye
    C. A light directed in the right eye produces a consensual reaction in the left eye
    D. A light directed in the left eye produces a sluggish direct reaction
    E. A light directed in the left eye fails to produce a direct reaction

3. A 23-year-old woman with a history of sickle cell disease presents with fever and severe bone pain localized to her left tibia. A bone culture grows gram-negative rods. Which of the following is the most likely infecting organism?

    A. *Vibrio*
    B. *Legionella*
    C. *Salmonella*
    D. *Pseudomonas*
    E. *Shigella*

4. All of the following are lifestyle modifications recommended for prevention and management of hypertension **EXCEPT?**

    A. Losing weight, if overweight
    B. Increasing aerobic physical activity to 30 to 45 minutes for most days of the week
    C. Stopping smoking
    D. Maintaining adequate intake of dietary potassium, approximately 90 mmol/day
    E. Reducing sodium intake to no more than 6 g of sodium per day

5. A 65-year-old woman with an 8-year history of type 2 diabetes dies in the hospital. She had no other significant medical history. Which of the following was the *MOST* likely cause of death?

    A. Diabetic ketoacidosis (DKA)
    B. Infection
    C. Myocardial infarction
    D. Renal failure
    E. Stroke

6. Which of the following periconceptional supplementations can lower the risk of a neural tube defect?

    A. Calcium
    B. Folate
    C. Iron
    D. Vitamin A
    E. Vitamin B_{12}

7. A 3-year-old boy is brought in by his mother for an infection around the mouth and nose. The lesions are honey-crusted and weeping and have a stuck-on appearance. Which of the following is the most appropriate treatment?

    A. Amoxicillin
    B. Benzoyl peroxide wash
    C. Ketoconazole cream
    D. Mupirocin ointment
    E. Topical glucocorticoids

8. A 4-year-old was playing with Legos and suddenly started wheezing. The mother states that her child previously seemed well. Objective findings note labored breathing, wheezing, and absent right breath sounds. Which of the following is the most likely diagnosis?

    A. Croup

    B. Pertussis

    C. Foreign body aspiration

    D. Acute epiglottitis

    E. Bronchiolitis

9. A patient has atrial fibrillation. Which of the following physical examination findings confirms the diagnosis?

    A. Palpation of an irregularly irregular rhythm

    B. Palpation of a regular irregular rhythm

    C. Auscultation of an S_3

    D. Auscultation of an S_4

    E. Auscultation of a systolic ejection murmur

10. A 65-year-old man undergoes coronary artery bypass surgery that entails grafting the left internal mammary artery to the left main coronary artery to form an alternative conduit for blood flow. This patient received a(n)

    A. allograft

    B. autograft

    C. homograft

    D. isograft

    E. xenograft

11. A 27-year-old, HIV-positive patient complains of visual disturbances. The patient is referred to an ophthalmologist, who notes perivascular hemorrhage and bilateral retinal exudates. The virus responsible for this patient's retinitis belongs to which of the following viral families?

    A. Adenovirus

    B. Herpesvirus

    C. Orthomyxovirus

    D. Paramyxovirus

    E. Retrovirus

12. A patient is diagnosed with a disease in which autoantibodies "inactivate" receptors at the neuromuscular junction. This patient would most likely derive benefit from an agent that inhibits which of the following enzymes?

    A. Acetylcholinesterase

    B. Angiotensin-converting enzyme

    C. Cyclooxygenase

    D. DOPA decarboxylase

    E. Phenylalanine hydroxylase

13. If a patient is diagnosed with a condition that is caused by a deficiency of aldolase B, which of the following findings would be most prominent?

    A. Cataracts

    B. Hemolytic anemia

    C. Hepatomegaly

    D. Hypoglycemia

    E. Mental retardation

14. Before a 36-year-old man can go to bed each night, he must turn around three times and touch each of the four corners of his bed. Should he fail to do this, he is extremely restless and unable to sleep. Even after these actions, he reports that he often has trouble falling asleep, and that he lies awake thinking about all the bad things that could happen to his family during the night. PET scans of the activity in his brain will most likely show increased activity at which of the following locations?

    A. Amygdala

    B. Caudate nucleus

    C. Cerebellum

    D. Hippocampus

    E. Pons

15. A 55-year-old chronic alcoholic man is found wandering on the street and brought to the emergency department by paramedics. The patient has a high fever, a cough productive of gelatinous red sputum, and difficulty breathing. Examination of the chest reveals wheezes and rales over the left lower zone and a chest x-ray film confirms pneumonia. Gram stain of the sputum reveals rather large gram-negative bacteria and many white blood cells. Which of the following is the most likely pathogen?

    A. *Candida albicans*

    B. *Klebsiella pneumoniae*

    C. *Legionella pneumophila*

    D. *Mycoplasma pneumoniae*

    E. *Streptococcus pneumoniae*

16. Which of the following is the leading cause of blindness for those aged 55 and older in the United States?

    A. Macular degeneration

    B. Cataracts

    C. Retinal detachment

    D. *Toxocariasis*

    E. Acute angle closure glaucoma

17. A 30-year-old married woman complains of an increasing, tender lump at the opening of the vagina. The lump appeared within the last 2 days and is very painful when pressure is applied against the vagina. The woman denies any new sexual encounters. Pelvic examination reveals a large, exquisitely tender Bartholin gland. Which of the following is the most appropriate next step?

    A. Antibiotics

    B. Excision

    C. Marsupialization

    D. Sitz baths

    E. Word catheter placement

18. A 19-year-old HIV-positive pregnant woman had been taking a protease inhibitor during the last 2 months of her pregnancy. She delivered a full-term, apparently healthy infant. Which of the following tests should be done to determine if the infant has been infected with HIV?

    A. ELISA at 1 week postdelivery

    B. ELISA at 3 months postdelivery

    C. PCR for HIV provirus

    D. RT-PCR analysis

    E. Western blot for antibody to HIV

19. A 20-year-old woman is having an acute asthma exacerbation. Which of the following is the most appropriate intervention?

    A. Inhaled beta-2 agonist

    B. Inhaled corticosteroid

    C. Systemic corticosteroid

    D. Leukotriene modifier

    E. Cromolyn

20. A 16-year-old woman complains of abdominal pain and greasy stools. She also reports a history of recurrent lung infections. Which of the following is most consistent with the history?

    A. Asthma

    B. Irritable bowel syndrome

    C. Diverticulosis

    D. Cystic fibrosis

    E. Sarcoidosis

21. A 5-year-old mentally retarded boy presents with choreoathetosis. He bites down on his lips and fingers, resulting in multiple lacerations. His parents have wrapped his hands to prevent further injury. Which of the following is also frequently associated with this disease?

    A. Cataracts

    B. Dislocated lenses

    C. Hyperuricemia

    D. Pancreatic insufficiency

    E. Renal proximal tubule defect

22. Which of the following recommendations is appropriate for individuals prone to keloids?

    A. Avoid cold environments

    B. Avoid cosmetic surgical procedures

    C. Avoid wool-containing products

    D. Increase sun exposure

    E. Use hypoallergenic soaps and detergents

23. An obese 40-year-old female smoker had a pulmonary embolism caused by a deep venous thrombosis 2 years ago. You recommend all of the following **EXCEPT**?

    A. Smoking cessation

    B. Weight reduction

    C. Stop taking oral contraceptive pills

    D. Increase activity level

    E. Thrombolytics

24. A 75-year-old man had a 5-year history of progressive mental deterioration that eventually led to his placement in a nursing home. By the time of his death, the man was completely unable to feed or otherwise care for himself. Autopsy demonstrated a shrunken brain. One of the findings on microscopic examination of the brain was the presence of amyloid around small brain vessels. Which of the following is the most likely diagnosis?

    A. Lewy body disease

    B. Alzheimer's disease

    C. Huntington's disease

    D. Creutzfeldt-Jakob disease

    E. Frontotemporal dementia

25. A patient notices that his urine is occasionally red-colored in the morning. Dipstick urinalysis demonstrates microscopic hematuria. Peripheral blood studies demonstrate anemia, leukopenia, and thrombocytopenia. A bone marrow biopsy is unremarkable, and no morphologic abnormalities of blood cells are noted on review of the peripheral smear. A negative Coombs test rules out autoimmune hemolytic anemia. Sucrose lysis test result on erythrocytes is positive. Which of the following has been implicated in the pathogenesis of the patient's condition?

    A. *bcl-2*

    B. Decay accelerating factor (DAF)

    C. Heinz bodies

    D. Methylmalonic acid

    E. Spectrin

26. A female baby is normal at birth but develops a severe hemolytic anemia after age 6 months. Peripheral blood smear shows a microcytic, hypochromic anemia with numerous target cells and increased reticulocytes. Hemoglobin electrophoresis at 9 months of age demonstrates hemoglobin F of 90%, increased hemoglobin A_2, and decreased hemoglobin A. Which of the following is the most likely diagnosis?

    A. Alpha-thalassemia trait

    B. Beta-thalassemia major

    C. Beta-thalassemia minor

    D. Hemoglobin H (Hb H) disease

    E. Hydrops fetalis

27. A 26-year-old woman has been having chronic pelvic pain for over 1 year. The pain is exacerbated during, but not limited to, menstruation. Ultrasound examination is equivocal for adnexal masses. Endoscopy of the pelvis shows multiple red-brown nodules up to 1 cm in diameter over the serosal surfaces of the ovaries, fallopian tubes, and uterus. Which of the following is the most likely diagnosis?

    A. Endometrial cancer

    B. Endometriosis

    C. Germ cell tumor of ovary

    D. Ovarian cystadenoma

    E. Pelvic inflammatory disease

28. A 4-year-old presents with a sore throat, fever, and rash. The rash developed today and appears on physical examination as fine, punctuate erythematous lesions that blanch on pressure. The lesions are located on the face, along skin folds, and on chest, back, and buttocks. The oropharynx is erythematous with enlarged tonsils. Palatal petechiae and strawberry tongue are also noted. Which of the following is the most likely diagnosis?

    A. Kawasaki disease

    B. Scarlet fever

    C. Rubeola

    D. Rubella

    E. Erythema toxicum

29. A patient takes warfarin for a deep vein thrombosis. Which of the following is considered a therapeutic international normalized ratio (INR) for this patient?

    A. 1.0 to 2.0

    B. 1.5 to 2.5

    C. 2.0 to 3.0

    D. 2.5 to 3.5

    E. 3.0 to 4.0

30. A 6-year-old Asian boy is evaluated by a neurologist. The child had initially appeared well, but two years previously had begun to have frequent falls and difficulty climbing stairs. Physical examination reveals an abnormal gait characterized by waddling, walking on the toes, and lordosis. The calf muscles appear enlarged, although weak. A maternal uncle had similar problems that led to him being confined to a wheelchair by age 12 and to his death by age 18. Calf muscle biopsy demonstrates replacement of much of the muscle tissue by fibrofatty tissue. The basis of this boy's disease is thought to be which of the following?

    A. An abnormal protein in the cytoskeleton of the cell membrane

    B. An autoimmune attack on acetylcholine receptors in the postsynaptic neuromuscular junction

    C. Defects in mitochondrial enzymes

    D. A mutation affecting ion channels in the membrane conduction system

    E. Mutations in the calcium-release channels of the sarcoplasmic reticulum

31. A middle-aged woman complains of generalized weakness and bruising easily. The patient also reports that she is unable to concentrate for an extended period of time. Her husband comments that she has become increasingly moody. Physical examination reveals truncal obesity, a rounded, plethoric face; dorsal cervical fat pads, and slender distal extremities. The skin is thin with purple striae, and multiple bruises are present. Her blood pressure is 166/94 mm Hg. What is the most appropriate test to order to screen for the suspected diagnosis?

    A. Dexamethasone suppression test

    B. Schilling test

    C. 24-hour urine collection for vanillylmandelic acid

    D. Adrenocorticotropin hormone stimulation test

    E. Urea breath test

32. What is the first-line treatment for asymptomatic patients with ventricular tachycardia and normal left ventricular function?

    A. Cardioversion

    B. Amiodarone

    C. Defibrillation

    D. Procainamide

    E. Adenosine

33. A 40-year-old textile worker complains of chest tightness. He notices that his symptoms occur usually during Monday afternoon. Which of the following is the most likely diagnosis?

    A. Silicosis

    B. Byssinosis

    C. Asbestosis

    D. Berylliosis

    E. Talcosis

34. A 7-year-old Hispanic boy is taken to a pediatrician because of difficulty walking. Physical examination demonstrates a mass near the knee. Radiologic studies show a lytic bone lesion of the medulla of the femur, with extension into the cortical bone and soft tissues. A periosteal reaction and new bone formation with concentric layers of bony deposition are seen. Biopsy demonstrates a small, round cell tumor with rare groups of tumor cells arranged in circles around a central fibrillary space. This patient's tumor is most similar to which of the following soft tissue tumors?

   A. Chondromyxoid fibroma

   B. Malignant fibrous histiocytoma

   C. Nodular fasciitis

   D. Primitive neuroectodermal tumor

   E. Round cell-type liposarcoma

35. A pregnant woman who is at the end of her second trimester is diagnosed with preeclampsia. Two weeks later she presents to the emergency room convulsing. The convulsions are stopped with magnesium sulfate and the patient is stabilized. Which of the following is the next step in the management of the patient?

   A. Admit to hospital for monitoring

   B. Discharge home and follow up with physician every 2 days

   C. Discharge home with strict instruction of bed rest for the remainder of the pregnancy

   D. Prepare for delivery

   E. Recommend normal salt intake and increased water intake

36. A patient is seen in the emergency department and is diagnosed with a tension pneumothorax. Which of the following is the most appropriate next step?

   A. Tube thoracostomy

   B. Admit to hospital

   C. Insertion of a large-bore needle into the pleural space through the second anterior intercostal space

   D. Pulmonary consultation

   E. Instillation of a sclerosing agent

37. A 65-year-old man presents to the emergency department after a fall. Radiologic studies demonstrate a new fracture of a vertebra that occurred at a site where a 1.5-cm diameter lytic lesion in the bone was present. Biopsy of this area demonstrates a hematologic malignancy. Which of the following hematologic disorders is most likely the cause of this man's lytic bone lesion?

   A. Acute lymphoblastic leukemia

   B. Chronic lymphocytic leukemia

   C. Chronic myelogenous leukemia

   D. Multiple myeloma

   E. Polycythemia vera

38. During an automobile accident, a child's posterior pituitary is severely damaged. Which of the following would most likely be seen?

   A. Addison disease

   B. Decreased skin pigmentation

   C. Decreased thyroid function

   D. Diabetes insipidus

   E. Dwarfism

39. A 32-year-old woman with increased frequency of urination, suprapubic pain, and dysuria for the past 3 days comes to the emergency department. She has no fever, nausea, or vomiting. A Gram stain reveals gram-negative rods. Which of the following is the most likely pathogen?

   A. *Escherichia coli*

   B. *Neisseria gonorrhoeae*

   C. *Shigella dysenteriae*

   D. *Streptococcus pneumoniae*

   E. *Treponema pallidum*

40. A 25-year-old patient is seen for "hay fever" symptoms. On examination, a small nasal polyp is discovered. Which of the following is the most appropriate treatment for the nasal polyp?

    A. Antibiotics

    B. Nasal corticosteroids

    C. Surgical intervention

    D. Ethmoidectomy

    E. Antihistamine

41. Which of the following conditions is considered a reversible obstructive lung disease?

    A. Emphysema

    B. Chronic bronchitis

    C. Asbestosis

    D. Sarcoidosis

    E. Asthma

42. A 30-year-old man has been fasting for religious reasons for several days. His blood glucose level is now about 60% of its normal value, but he does not feel lightheaded because his brain has reduced its need for serum glucose by using which of the following substances as an alternate energy source?

    A. Apoprotein B

    B. Beta-carotene

    C. Beta-hydroxybutyrate

    D. C-reactive protein

    E. Coenzyme A

43. Which of the following organisms causes pneumonia exclusively in immunocompromised individuals?

    A. *Diplococcus*

    B. *Pneumocystis carinii*

    C. *Mycoplasma pneumoniae*

    D. *Legionella pneumophila*

    E. Influenza virus

44. Which of the following statements regarding the pneumococcal vaccine is false?

    A. Revaccination is recommended to all adults

    B. Recommended for asplenic patients

    C. May give with all other vaccines

    D. Recommended for adults 65 years and older

    E. Recommended for adults less than 65 years of age with chronic liver disease

45. A patient with a history of intravenous drug use is diagnosed with endocarditis. Blood cultures are drawn. Which of the following organisms do you suspect caused the infection?

    A. *Streptococcus viridans*

    B. Yeast

    C. *Staphylococcus aureus*

    D. *Enterococcus viridans*

    E. *Eikenella corrodens*

46. Deficiency of which of the following factors usually predisposes to thrombosis rather than bleeding?

    A. V

    B. VIII

    C. IX

    D. X

    E. XII

47. Patients taking ethambutol should be warned about which of the following side effects?

    A. Clinical hepatitis

    B. Retrobulbar neuritis

    C. Orange discoloration of bodily fluids

    D. Photosensitive dermatitis

    E. Hyperuricemia

48. In the nephron, most reabsorption of sodium occurs in which of the following structures?

    A. Ascending loop

    B. Collecting duct

    C. Distal convoluted tubule

    D. Proximal convoluted tubule

    E. Sodium is reabsorbed evenly throughout the nephron

49. Which of the following carbohydrates can be absorbed by the enterocytes of the small intestine?

    A. Amylose

    B. Galactose

    C. Lactose

    D. Maltose

    E. Sucrose

50. Which of the following substances can be converted to glucose to supply the needs of the brain during starvation?

    A. Acetoacetate

    B. Acetone

    C. Amino acids

    D. Beta-hydroxybutyrate

    E. Fatty acids

51. Which of the following is the most appropriate treatment for hypersensitivity pneumonitis?

    A. Levofloxacin

    B. Ipratropium bromide

    C. Albuterol

    D. Oral corticosteroids

    E. Clarithromycin

52. A 43-year-old woman presents with a small, nontender breast mass. Physical examination reveals a firm, mobile mass well demarcated from the surrounding breast tissue mass. Fine needle aspiration shows nonbloody, watery fluid. Which of the following is the most likely diagnosis?

    A. Abscess

    B. Cyst

    C. Fibroadenoma

    D. Malignancy

    E. Mastitis

53. A patient complains of fatigue and shortness of breath. Objective findings note an elevated jugular venous pressure and a Kussmaul sign. There is low voltage on the EKG with nonspecific repolarization changes. An echocardiogram shows impaired diastolic filling with preserved contractile function. You suspect which of the following diagnoses?

    A. Restrictive cardiomyopathy

    B. Dilated cardiomyopathy

    C. Hypertrophic cardiomyopathy

    D. Rheumatic heart disease

    E. Pericardial effusion

54. Which of the following is the most important intervention for the leading cause of cancer deaths in the United States?

    A. Weight loss

    B. Colonoscopy

    C. Annual physical examinations

    D. Controlled hypertension

    E. Smoking cessation

55. A patient was administered trimethaphan during surgery. This drug will most likely cause which of the following responses?

    A. Accommodation

    B. Hypertension

    C. Peristalsis

    D. Pupillary constriction

    E. Tachycardia

56. An obese man complains of excessive daytime sleepiness. He states that he gets 8 hours of sleep a night but never feels well rested. Which of the following is the most appropriate intervention at this time?

    A. Uvulopalatopharyngoplasty

    B. Weight loss

    C. Nasal continuous positive airway pressure

    D. Nasal septoplasty

    E. Tracheostomy

57. A 35-year-old woman complains of fatigue, abdominal discomfort, and nausea. Upon questioning, she states that her menses is a week late; however, she had a tubal ligation several years ago. A urine hCG is positive. Which of the following is the most appropriate next step?

    A. Counsel patient on prenatal care

    B. Discuss all possible courses of action, including continuation of pregnancy, termination, and adoption

    C. Measure serum hCG level

    D. Perform ultrasound

    E. Schedule an appointment with an obstetrician

58. Laboratory results show eosinophilia. Which of the following should be on your differential diagnosis?

    A. Pharyngitis

    B. Pneumococcal pneumonia

    C. Cushing syndrome

    D. Status post-CABG

    E. Allergic rhinitis

59. A patient has a pleural effusion, and the fluid is classified as a transudate. Which of the following diagnosis should be on your differential?

    A. Cirrhosis

    B. Pneumonia

    C. Tuberculosis

    D. Mesothelioma

    E. Systemic lupus erythematosus

60. Which of the following does the enzyme-linked immunosorbent assay detect in the HIV-positive patient?

    A. Antibodies to viral antigens

    B. CD_4^+ count

    C. p24 antigen

    D. Reverse transcriptase activity

    E. Viral RNA

End of Block 4

Block 5

For the following neoplasms, select the most commonly associated predisposing conditions (choices A–E).

A. Actinic keratosis

B. Barrett esophagus

C. Paget disease of bone

D. Plummer-Vinson syndrome

E. Xeroderma pigmentosum

1. Melanoma

2. Esophageal adenocarcinoma

3. A 27-year-old man is fired from his job as a celebrity assistant for stealing 20 pairs of the actress's shoes. He has a prior history of stealing women's high-heeled shoes and has been fired from many jobs, and arrested numerous times for this behavior. He is intensely sexually aroused by women's shoes and has tried to stop this behavior, but his urges are overwhelming. He is heterosexual, married with 2 children, and does not desire to be a woman. Which of the following is the most likely diagnosis?

A. Exhibitionism

B. Fetishism

C. Frotteurism

D. Gender identity disorder

E. Pedophilia

4. A 40-year-old male smoker complains of pain in both of his feet, primarily in the toes. He describes the pain as burning. He also notes the pain at rest. The patient reports he has had the same pain in the past but it resolved by itself. Physical examination of the lower extremities reveals cool distal feet, and small, red, tender cords. The pulsation of the left dorsalis pedis is barely palpable and the right dorsalis pedis is absent. The history and physical examination are most consistent with which of the following?

A. Raynaud disease

B. Diabetic neuropathy

C. Venous insufficiency

D. Thromboangiitis obliterans

E. Morton neuroma

5. Which of the following is used in the management of gestational diabetes?

A. Metformin

B. Glyburide

C. Insulin therapy

D. Pioglitazone

E. Acarbose

6. Which of the following has low levels of factor IX coagulant activity?

A. G6PD

B. Hemophilia A

C. Hemophilia B

D. Sickle cell anemia

E. Thalassemia

7. Which of the following is associated with an exudative pleural effusion?

A. Congestive heart failure

B. Cirrhosis

C. Pneumonia

D. Increased hydrostatic pressure

E. Nephrotic syndrome

8. Before starting a patient on isotretinoin for cystic acne, all of the following tests should be obtained **EXCEPT?**

   A. Cholesterol

   B. Hemoglobin and hematocrit

   C. Liver function test

   D. Serum pregnancy test

   E. Triglycerides

9. A patient known to have gallstones presents with sharp, right upper quadrant pain that started after the evening meal and lasted all night. He has had nausea, but has not vomited. Physical examination reveals low-grade temperature, RUQ pain with a positive Murphy's sign, and equivocal rebound tenderness. The WBC is 14,000/mm³, and there is an elevated total bilirubin level. Liver enzyme tests are normal. Which of the following is the most likely diagnosis?

   A. Acute hepatitis

   B. Acute pancreatitis

   C. Common duct obstruction

   D. Acute cholecystitis

   E. Acute pyelonephritis

10. A 5-year-old girl is brought in by her parents for perianal itching, especially at night. The child reports she feels like "something is crawling" in the anal region. Which of the following laboratory examinations is most useful in establishing a diagnosis?

    A. Anoscopy

    B. Complete blood count

    C. Scotch tape test

    D. Stool culture

    E. Urinalysis

11. Initial investigation for cervical cancer is best accomplished by which of the following?

    A. Bimanual examination

    B. Colposcopy

    C. Conization of the cervix

    D. Endometrium biopsy

    E. Pap smear

12. The estimated date of confinement can be determined by which of the following?

    A. Add 7 days to the first day of the last menstrual period, subtract 3 months, and add 9 months

    B. Add 7 days to the first day of the last menstrual period, subtract 3 months, and add 1 year

    C. Add 7 days to the last day of the last menstrual period, subtract 3 months, and add 1 year

    D. Subtract 3 days from the last day of the last menstrual period, subtract 3 months, and add 1 year

    E. Subtract 7 days from the last day of the last menstrual period, subtract 3 months, and add 1 year

13. A 60-year-old man suddenly becomes completely blind in one eye, and angiography demonstrates occlusion of the central retinal artery. Which of the following is the most likely cause of the occlusion?

    A. Atheroma or embolism

    B. Cranial (temporal) arteritis

    C. Hypertension

    D. Polycythemia vera

    E. Tumor

14. During surgical removal of an invasive glioma from the skull base, cranial nerves IX and X are accidentally cut bilaterally. What would be the immediate change in the patient's hemodynamic condition?

    A. Bradycardia with hypertension

    B. Bradycardia with hypotension

    C. Sinus arrhythmia with hypotension

    D. Tachycardia with hypertension

    E. Tachycardia with hypotension

15. A 29-year-old woman comes in because of a rash on her foot. She insists on removing her pants and not putting on a hospital gown. She sits on the edge of the examination table, making extravagant hand gestures as she speaks, and is inappropriately flirtatious with the physician assistant. Before she leaves the examination room, she puts on her unusually large pink hat and matching suit. Which of the following is the most likely diagnosis?

    A. Borderline personality disorder

    B. Delirium

    C. Dependent personality disorder

    D. Histrionic personality disorder

    E. Narcissistic personality disorder

16. A tall, thin, 21-year-old woman complains of increasing fatigue over the last 6 months. Her last visit to the doctor was over 2 years ago. On physical examination, auscultation reveals a midsystolic click best heard at the apex. What is the most appropriate diagnostic test to order?

    A. Echocardiogram

    B. EKG

    C. Angiography

    D. Chest x-ray

    E. Holter monitor

17. During the history-taking of a patient with chest pain, which of the following findings helps differentiate angina pectoris from myocardial infarction?

    A. Substernal chest pain/discomfort

    B. Radiation to the left shoulder

    C. Pain described as "squeezing"

    D. History of heart disease

    E. Pain immediately relieved by rest

18. Which of the following is the most common cause of Cushing syndrome?

    A. Glucocorticoid therapy

    B. Pituitary adenoma

    C. Small cell lung carcinoma

    D. Adrenal adenoma

    E. Adrenal carcinoma

19. Which of the following is consistent with objective findings of thalassemia?

    A. Decreased vibratory and position sense

    B. Increased total iron binding capacity (TIBC)

    C. Microcytosis

    D. Presence of spherocytes on peripheral smear

    E. Serum folate level <3 ng/mL

20. A patient with COPD complains of fever, cough, and pleuritic pain. A chest radiograph shows patchy alveolar infiltrates, and he is diagnosed with pneumonia. You order a sputum culture. Which of the following organisms is most likely responsible for the pneumonia?

    A. *Pseudomonas aeruginosa*

    B. *Mycoplasma pneumoniae*

    C. *Haemophilus influenzae*

    D. *Staphylococcus aureus*

    E. *Klebsiella pneumoniae*

21. A 45-year-old man has a lesion on his face. The lesion is a shiny, red nodule with telangiectasias, a central ulcer, and rolled borders. Which of the following is the most appropriate step in the diagnosis?

    A. Cryotherapy

    B. Curettage and electrodesiccation

    C. Radiotherapy

    D. Shave or punch biopsy

    E. Watchful waiting

22. A 62-year-old man complains of lower abdominal pain, weight loss, and decreased stool frequency for the past 6 months. His fecal occult blood test result is positive, and there is a family history of Lynch syndrome. Which of the following is the most likely diagnosis?

    A. Colon carcinoma

    B. Diverticulitis

    C. Irritable bowel syndrome

    D. Ulcerative colitis

    E. Diverticulosis

23. Which of the following physical examination findings is consistent with a diagnosis of candidiasis?

    A. Gray discharge with a fishy odor

    B. Green, frothy, malodorous discharge

    C. Nonodorous, white, curd-like discharge

    D. Small, grouped vesicles on an erythematous base

    E. Yellow, creamy discharge

24. A pregnant woman has lower-than-normal levels of maternal serum alpha-fetoprotein. This may indicate which of the following?

    A. Anencephaly

    B. Fetal renal failure

    C. Fetal trisomy

    D. Gastrointestinal tract obstruction

    E. Spina bifida

25. A 42-year-old obese woman experiences episodic abdominal pain. She notes that the pain increases after the ingestion of a fatty meal. The action of which of the following hormones is responsible for the post-prandial intensification of her symptoms?

    A. Cholecystokinin (CCK)

    B. Gastrin

    C. Pepsin

    D. Secretin

    E. Somatostatin

26. If it is dangerous for an infant to ingest a product containing aspartame, he most likely has which of the following genetic disorders?

    A. Hyperornithemia

    B. Hyperuricemia

    C. Hypervalinemia

    D. Phenylketonuria

    E. Wilson disease

27. Following the administration of theophylline, an asthmatic patient begins to see an increase in diaphragmatic contractility. This "signal" to increase stimulation is transmitted to the diaphragm by which of the following nerves?

    A. Axillary

    B. Phrenic

    C. Recurrent laryngeal

    D. Suprascapular

    E. Thoracodorsal

28. In addition to causing beriberi, thiamine deficiency can lead to the development of which of the following?

    A. Carotenemia

    B. Korsakoff syndrome

    C. Pellagra

    D. Pernicious anemia

    E. Scurvy

29. When is cardioversion indicated as first-line treatment?

    A. Unstable ventricular tachycardia

    B. Ventricular fibrillation

    C. Chronic atrial fibrillation

    D. Multifocal atrial tachycardia

    E. Unstable bradycardia

30. Which of the following is associated with a nonpregnant state?

    A. Breast tenderness

    B. Increased urinary frequency

    C. Pink vagina

    D. Quickening

    E. Softening of the cervix

31. A 69-year-old man presents with unilateral hearing loss. A lesion in which of the following structures could be responsible for this loss?

    A. Inferior colliculus

    B. Lateral lemniscus

    C. Medial geniculate body

    D. Medial lemniscus

    E. Organ of Corti

32. Which of the following medications has a positive inotropic effect, has a negative chronotropic effect, and decreases the conduction velocity through the AV node?

    A. Digoxin

    B. Diltiazem

    C. Lisinopril

    D. Metoprolol

    E. Terazosin

33. A 38-year-old man reports chest tightness with strenuous activity. The tightness is located across the anterior chest and is immediately relieved by rest. Which of the following is the most appropriate diagnostic procedure to confirm the diagnosis?

    A. Resting EKG

    B. Echocardiography

    C. Angiography

    D. Stress exercise test

    E. Holter monitor

34. A 60-year-old woman complains of "painful bones," fatigue, and abdominal pain. Her medical history is significant for hypertension and nephrolithiasis. Laboratory findings show elevated serum calcium and low phosphorus. Which of the following is the most likely diagnosis?

    A. Osteomalacia

    B. Hyperthyroidism

    C. Osteoporosis

    D. Paget disease

    E. Hyperparathyroidism

35. A patient has a lobar pneumonia. Which of the following would you expect to find on physical examination?

    A. A decrease in tactile fremitus

    B. Hyperresonance on percussion

    C. Egophony

    D. Cheyne-Stokes breathing

    E. Breath sounds predominately vesicular

36. A 58-year-old man has a 15-year history of recurrent duodenal ulcer. His ulcer heals promptly with H2RAs, but recurs within 3 months of stopping. There is no history of NSAID or steroid use. *Helicobacter pylori* testing is negative. What would management of this patient include at this time?

    A. Long-term treatment with H2RAs

    B. Treating with omeprazole instead

    C. Considering treatment for *H. pylori* infection

    D. Fasting serum gastrin level

    E. Antacid therapy

37. Autoimmune attack on which of the following structures is thought to contribute to the pathophysiology of pemphigus vulgaris?

    A. Actin microfilaments

    B. Desmosomes

    C. Gap junctions

    D. Microtubules

    E. Tight junctions

38. Which of the following infections would be most likely to occur in a male infant with severe combined immunodeficiency (SCID)?

    A. Bacterial infection

    B. Viral infection

    C. Fungal infection

    D. Parasitic infection

    E. All of the above

39. Women who have a normal BMI should gain approximately how much weight during pregnancy?

    A. 20 to 30 lb

    B. 25 to 35 lb

    C. 35 to 45 lb

    D. 40 to 50 lb

    E. 45 to 55 lb

40. Which of the following is a major risk factor associated with thromboembolus formation?

    A. Laminar flow

    B. Hypocoagulability

    C. Injury to endothelial cells

    D. Decreased levels of factor V

    E. Thrombocytopenia

41. All of the following will raise cholesterol levels **EXCEPT**?

    A. Bananas

    B. Tuna fish

    C. Chicken

    D. Whole-wheat bread

    E. Ham

42. A 24-year-old woman with a history of allergic rhinitis is involved in a motor vehicle accident and sustains a splenic laceration. She undergoes surgery and is then transfused with 4 units of Rh- and ABO-compatible blood. As the transfusion progresses, she develops signs and symptoms consistent with anaphylaxis. Which of the following pre-existing conditions best accounts for these symptoms?

    A. AIDS

    B. C1 esterase inhibitor deficiency

    C. DiGeorge syndrome

    D. Selective IgA deficiency

    E. Wiskott-Aldrich syndrome

43. For the treatment of hypercholesterolemia, which of the following medications is not systemically absorbed?

    A. Atorvastatin

    B. Cholestyramine

    C. Gemfibrozil

    D. Niacin

    E. Fenofibrate

44. Which of the following conditions is associated with a lifelong requirement for administration of parenteral vitamin B_{12}?

    A. Megaloblastic anemia

    B. Removal of colon

    C. Removal of gallbladder

    D. Removal of ileum

    E. Removal of jejunum

45. Which of the following is associated with lower HDL cholesterol levels?

    A. Smoking

    B. Losing weight

    C. Estrogen therapy

    D. Physical activity

    E. Insulin therapy

46. A patient is seen in the emergency room with a blood pressure of 234/130 mm Hg. There are signs of hypertensive encephalopathy. Which of the following is the most appropriate therapy?

    A. Oral labetalol

    B. Sublingual nitroglycerin

    C. Clonidine

    D. Sodium nitroprusside

    E. Captopril

47. A woman in her midfifties complains of a dull ache in both her lower extremities. The discomfort is made worse with prolonged standing. Bilateral lower extremity pitting edema is noted. The skin examination of the lower extremities reveals the skin to be shiny, atrophic, and brownish in pigmentation. The pulses of the lower extremities are normal. There is a small ulcer at the medial malleolus. Which of the following are consistent with the history and objective findings?

    A. Chronic arterial insufficiency

    B. Cellulitis

    C. Chronic venous insufficiency

    D. Lymphatic stasis

    E. Orthostatic edema

48. Which of the following disorders will typically cause an elevation in unconjugated bilirubin?

    A. Cholelithiasis

    B. Viral hepatitis

    C. Rotor's syndrome

    D. Hemolytic anemia

    E. Kernicterus

49. A 40-year-old, formerly obese woman presents to her physician. She was very proud of having lost 80 lb during the previous 2 years, but has now noticed that her "hair is falling out." On questioning, she reports having followed a strict, fat-free diet. Her alopecia is probably related to a deficiency of which of the following vitamins?

    A. A

    B. C

    C. D

    D. E

    E. K

50. A patient develops psoriasis. A biopsy shows increased proliferation and incomplete keratinization of keratinocytes. In which of the following locations would the increased level of proliferation responsible for this condition be observed?

    A. Dermal papilla

    B. Stratum basale

    C. Stratum corneum

    D. Stratum granulosum

    E. Stratum lucidum

51. A patient complains of a persistent cough and shortness of breath with exertion. She also states she has been fatigued and reports night sweats. A chest radiograph shows bilateral hilar adenopathy. A biopsy shows noncaseating granulomas. Which of the following is the most likely diagnosis?

    A. Pneumonia

    B. Tuberculosis

    C. Sarcoidosis

    D. Squamous cell lung cancer

    E. Bronchiectasis

52. A patient's arterial blood gas results are as follows:

    pH 7.65

    P_{CO_2} 20 mm Hg

    P_{O_2} 70 mm Hg

    HCO_3^- 26 mEq

    What is your interpretation of the result?

    A. Respiratory alkalosis

    B. Metabolic acidosis

    C. Respiratory acidosis

    D. Metabolic alkalosis

    E. Normal ABG

53. A 38-year-old swimmer complains of right ear pain and discharge. Examination findings note a purulent discharge in the right ear canal and surrounding erythema and edema of the ear canal. The tympanic membrane is mildly erythematous and moves with pneumatic otoscopy. Which of the following is the most likely diagnosis?

    A. Cerumen impaction

    B. Acute otitis media

    C. Otitis externa

    D. Serous otitis media

    E. Mastoiditis

54. Which of the following is the most appropriate treatment intervention for latent tuberculosis in a 25-year-old healthy man?

    A. No treatment necessary

    B. Isoniazid for 9 months

    C. Isoniazid, rifampin, pyrazinamide for 2 months

    D. Isoniazid, rifampin, pyrazinamide for 2 months, then isoniazid and rifampin for 4 months

    E. Rifampin and pyrazinamide for 2 months

55. Which of the following coagulation tests would most likely be abnormal in a patient with vitamin C deficiency?

    A. Bleeding time

    B. Fibrinogen levels

    C. Platelet count

    D. PT (prothrombin time)

    E. PTT (partial thromboplastin time)

56. Which of the following is observed on the physical examination for a patient with entropion?

    A. Drooping of the upper eyelid

    B. The margin of the lower eyelid is turned inward

    C. Puffy eyelids secondary to herniated fat

    D. A protrusion of the eyeball forward

    E. Retracted eyelid

57. A patient is diagnosed with *Mycoplasma* pneumonia. Which of the following is the most appropriate treatment?

    A. Levofloxacin

    B. Augmentin

    C. Clarithromycin

    D. Ciprofloxacin

    E. Penicillin

58. A 54-year-old African American man presents to an urgent care clinic with a very painful and swollen left first metatarsal joint, which woke him up this morning. The patient admits to previous similar episodes and states that he had some meat loaf for his dinner last night accompanied by "about a six-pack" of beer. A joint aspiration would most likely show which of the following?

    A. WBC 500/mm^3 (56% monocytes/40% lymphocytes)

    B. WBC 5500/mm^3 (90% PMNs), negatively birefringent crystals

    C. WBC 7000/mm^3 (90% PMNs), positively birefringent crystals

    D. WBC 20,000/mm^3 (74% PMNs), thin fluid

    E. WBC 67,000/mm^3 (96% PMNs), cloudy fluid

59. A person is in a closed-in garage with the car running, unaware of the danger. This person will develop a condition that is most similar to which of the following?

    A. Anemic hypoxia

    B. Circulatory hypoxia

    C. Histotoxic hypoxia

    D. Hypoxic hypoxia

    E. Obstructive apnea

60. Which of the following is considered an emergency requiring immediate referral to an ophthalmologist?

    A. Macular degeneration

    B. Cataracts

    C. Acute angle closure glaucoma

    D. Diabetic retinopathy

    E. Pinguecula

End of Block 5

Test 1 Answers and Explanations

ANSWER KEY

Block 1

1. A
2. B
3. E
4. D
5. B
6. D
7. C
8. B
9. A
10. A
11. B
12. E
13. A
14. D
15. B
16. D
17. D
18. E
19. D
20. E
21. A
22. B
23. E
24. D
25. C
26. E
27. C
28. E
29. B
30. D
31. B
32. B
33. E
34. E
35. B
36. D
37. B
38. D
39. D
40. C
41. A
42. B
43. E
44. C
45. D
46. B
47. B
48. D
49. A
50. D
51. C
52. C
53. E
54. E
55. A
56. B
57. B
58. A
59. E
60. B

Block 2

1. E
2. D
3. D
4. B
5. A
6. B
7. B
8. D
9. D
10. C
11. D
12. C
13. D
14. E
15. D
16. A
17. E
18. D
19. D
20. D
21. D
22. C
23. B
24. A
25. D
26. B
27. B
28. C
29. D
30. A
31. E
32. A
33. E
34. E
35. A
36. D
37. E
38. C
39. D
40. A
41. D
42. A
43. D
44. A
45. C
46. D
47. A
48. D
49. D
50. C
51. C
52. E
53. C
54. E
55. D
56. A
57. E
58. C
59. C
60. B

Block 3

1. A
2. A
3. B
4. A
5. C
6. D
7. C
8. E
9. A
10. E
11. D
12. A
13. D
14. D
15. E
16. A
17. C
18. D
19. C
20. D
21. C
22. B
23. D
24. B
25. A
26. D
27. E
28. A
29. C
30. E
31. C
32. D
33. C
34. A
35. E
36. A
37. E
38. C
39. B
40. E
41. B
42. C
43. A
44. B
45. B
46. D
47. C
48. C
49. D
50. A
51. B
52. A
53. E
54. D
55. D
56. D
57. B
58. D
59. D
60. A

Block 4

1. B
2. A
3. C
4. E
5. C
6. B
7. D
8. C
9. A
10. B
11. B
12. A
13. D
14. B
15. B
16. A
17. E
18. C
19. A
20. D
21. C
22. B
23. E
24. B
25. B
26. B
27. B
28. B
29. C
30. A
31. A
32. D
33. B
34. D
35. D
36. C
37. D
38. D
39. A
40. B
41. E
42. C
43. B
44. A
45. C

46. E
47. B
48. D
49. B
50. C
51. D
52. B
53. A
54. E
55. E
56. B
57. D
58. E
59. A
60. A

Block 5

1. E
2. B
3. B
4. D
5. C
6. C
7. C
8. B
9. D
10. C
11. E
12. B
13. A
14. D
15. D
16. A
17. E
18. A
19. C
20. C
21. D
22. A
23. C
24. C
25. A
26. D
27. B
28. B
29. A
30. C

31. E
32. A
33. D
34. E
35. C
36. D
37. B
38. E
39. B
40. C
41. A
42. D
43. B
44. D
45. A
46. D
47. C
48. D
49. A
50. B
51. C
52. A
53. C
54. B
55. A
56. B
57. C
58. B
59. A
60. C

Block 1

1. **The correct answer is A.** The first heart sound (S1) is caused by the closing of the mitral and tricuspid valves. The systolic interval separates S1 from the second heart sound (S2). S2 is produced by the closing of the aortic and pulmonic valves (**choice C**). Diastole follows S2. **Choices B, D, and E** are physiologically incorrect.

2. **The correct answer is B.** TSH is the most sensitive test for primary hypothyroidism. Triiodothyronine (**choice A**), thyroxine (**choice C**), triiodothyronine uptake (**choice D**), and thyroxine-binding globulin (**choice E**) may be used in the workup of hypothyroidism, but these tests are not as sensitive as the TSH.

3. **The correct answer is E.** Lead poisoning inhibits porphobilinogen synthetase and heme synthesis. The anemia is usually microcytic, with basophilic stippling, ringed sideroblasts, and increased serum iron. Symptoms include metabolic acidosis and abdominal pain with constipation, and it may eventually lead to shock, coma, and death.

   Anemia of chronic disease (**choice A**) will show either normocytic or microcytic anemia. Folate deficiency (**choice B**) will show a macrocytic anemia with hypersegmented neutrophils. Hereditary spherocytosis (**choice C**) causes a normocytic anemia with spherocytes in the peripheral blood smear, and iron-deficiency anemia (**choice D**) will show a microcytic, hypochromic anemia.

4. **The correct answer is D.** Heart failure, uremia, and respiratory depression can cause Cheyne-Stokes breathing.

   Kussmaul breathing (**choice A**) is characterized by a deep, rapid, labored breathing caused by the stimulation of the respiratory center from acidosis, as seen in diabetic ketoacidosis.

   Obstructive breathing (**choice B**) is seen in obstructive lung disease, such as COPD. The expiration phase is prolonged because there is an increased resistance to air flow caused by the narrow airways.

   Ataxic breathing (**choice C**) is characterized by an unpredictable irregularity consisting of shallow or deep breaths with short apneic periods. Brain damage and respiratory depression can cause ataxic breathing.

   Tachypnea (**choice E**) is characterized by rapid shallow breathing. There are numerous causes of tachypnea.

5. **The correct answer is B.** A small, discolored spot on the skin that lacks depression or elevation (**choice A**) describes a macule; an elevated, fluid-filled, circumscribed lesion smaller than 0.5 cm in diameter (**choice C**) describes a vesicle; a well-demarcated, plateau-like, elevated lesion larger than 0.5 cm in diameter (**choice D**) describes a plaque; and an elevated, fluid-filled, circumscribed lesion larger than 0.5 cm in diameter (**choice E**) describes a bulla.

6. **The correct answer is D.** Although all of the answers are potentially correct, severe postprandial pain, accompanied by bloody diarrhea, in a patient with a history consistent with atherosclerosis is most likely mesenteric ischemia. The postprandial nature and sudden onset of symptoms with eating represent ischemia of the mesenteric vessels.

   Acute cholecystitis (**choice A**) may present with postprandial pain, but typically occurs 2 to 4 hours after the meal. The pain is usually, though not always, in the right upper quadrant. Cholecystitis is not accompanied by hematochezia.

   Diverticulitis (**choice B**) may present similarly. The patient will have abdominal pain, typically in the LLQ, and may also have hematochezia. However, with the history of postprandial exacerbation, mesenteric ischemia is more likely.

   Pancreatitis (**choice C**) may present as diffuse abdominal pain, typically in the epigastrium. However, there is no history of risk factors suggestive of acute pancreatitis. The most common risk factors for pancreatitis include gallstones, alcohol abuse, and infectious etiologies.

   Pyelonephritis (**choice E**) presents with fever and flank pain.

7. **The correct answer is C.** The patient has a classic presentation of Lyme disease. He has a history of a tick bite. A week later he developed erythema migrans—"lesion has a red border with central clearing"—a typical manifestation of stage I Lyme disease. Doxycycline is considered first-line treatment for Lyme disease.

   Acetaminophen (**choice A**) does not have antibacterial properties.

   High-dose IV antibiotics, such as ceftriaxone (**choice B**), are used to treat stage II or III Lyme disease.

   Erythromycin (**choice D**) is used for patients who are allergic to penicillin.

   Rifampin (**choice E**) may be used in conjunction with doxycycline but not as lone therapy.

8. **The correct answer is B.** Screening for group B streptococci (GBS) should occur late in pregnancy to determine if the mother will have GBS at the time of delivery. Pregnant women who have a positive vaginal culture for GBS should be offered antibiotics at the time of labor or membrane rupture.

9. **The correct answer is A.** The clinical history suggests trigeminal neuralgia, which is characterized by extreme pain along the distributions of the maxillary and mandibular subdivisions of the fifth cranial nerve. The trigeminal nerve is derived from the first branchial arch.

    The second branchial arch (**choice B**) gives rise to the muscles of facial expression and is innervated by the facial nerve, cranial nerve VII. The third branchial arch (**choice C**) is innervated by the ninth cranial nerve, the glossopharyngeal, which innervates the stylopharyngeus muscle. The fourth and sixth branchial arch (**choices D and E**) give rise to most pharyngeal constrictor muscles and are innervated by the tenth cranial nerve, the vagus nerve.

10. **The correct answer is A.** The time to the onset, intensity, and duration of acute withdrawal symptoms secondary to opiate abuse are influenced by several factors, including the amount taken on a daily basis, the length of the drug abuse, and the half-life of the opiate. The most common signs and symptoms of withdrawal are often opposite to the acute effects of drug abuse. With this concept in mind, bradypnea would not be expected in a withdrawal situation because bradypnea and respiratory depression are seen with abuse of opiates. In fact opiate withdrawal signs and symptoms include mild to moderate increases in the respiratory rate.

    Common signs and symptoms of withdrawal that an opiate abuser might experience include diarrhea (**choice B**), piloerection (**choice C**), rhinorrhea (**choice D**), and sweating (**choice E**). Other common signs and symptoms include coughing, lacrimation, and muscle twitching, as well as elevations in body temperature and blood pressure.

11. **The correct answer is B.** Acetaminophen is a non-narcotic analgesic and antipyretic used for the temporary relief of mild to moderate pain and as a fever-reducing agent. Acetaminophen is commonly combined with various narcotic preparations for additional pain relief. Aspirin is classified as a salicylate analgesic/NSAID and antipyretic. It is commonly used in the treatment of mild to moderate pain and can be used as a fever-reducing agent in adults; however, its

use in children is not recommended due to the risk of Reye syndrome. Furthermore, aspirin can be used to prevent the recurrence of myocardial infarction, stroke, and transient ischemic attacks (TIAs). One of the disadvantages of using acetaminophen over aspirin in the treatment of pain is that acetaminophen does not have as much anti-inflammatory effect. Therefore, acetaminophen should not be used in the treatment of pain caused by inflammation.

Some advantages of using acetaminophen over aspirin include a decreased effect on uric acid excretion (**choice A**). Aspirin is known to decrease the tubular reabsorption of uric acid.

Use of aspirin, especially on a chronic basis, is associated with gastric irritation (**choice C**); acetaminophen is associated with a much lower incidence of gastric irritation. This gastric irritation can be substantial, especially in patients with peptic ulcer disease.

Aspirin is used clinically to prevent the recurrence of myocardial infarction, stroke, and TIAs. Aspirin is used in these conditions because of its antiplatelet effects, which alters the bleeding times. However, when a patient's bleeding time is altered, there is an increased risk for occult blood loss. Acetaminophen is not associated with occult blood loss (**choice D**) because it does not alter bleeding times (**choice E**).

12. **The correct answer is E.** Tetralogy of Fallot has primarily a right-to-left shunt caused by the right ventricular outflow obstruction. Blood ends up bypassing the pulmonary artery and goes to the aorta.

    Choices A, B, C, and D are the four main components of tetralogy of Fallot.

13. **The correct answer is A.** A fasting plasma glucose greater than or equal to 126 mg/dL establishes a diagnosis of diabetes mellitus. Alternatively, a patient showing symptoms of diabetes mellitus with a random plasma glucose of 200 mg/dL should be classified as having diabetes mellitus.

    The patient is hyperglycemic (**choice B**); however, the most appropriate conclusion that you should make is that the patient is diabetic.

14. **The correct answer is D. Choice A** is consistent with chronic myeloid leukemia. **Choice B** is consistent with chronic lymphocytic leukemia. **Choice C** is consistent with hairy cell leukemia, and **choice E** is consistent with multiple myeloma.

15. **The correct answer is B. Choice A** is consistent with metabolic alkalosis; **choice C** is consistent with respiratory alkalosis; **choice D** is considered normal; and **choice E** is consistent with metabolic acidosis.

16. **The correct answer is D.** Seborrheic keratosis begins as a small papule or plaque. It slowly progresses to a plaque with a greasy, wart-like, stuck-on appearance. The plaque may be brown, gray, black, or skin colored.

    Actinic keratosis **(choice A)** occurs mostly on sun-exposed areas of the skin and is the most common premalignant skin lesion. Isolated single lesions or multiple scattered, discrete, hyperpigmented lesions that are rough and scaly are common. Lesions are usually smaller than 1 cm and are oval or round.

    Basal cell carcinoma **(choice B)** is commonly seen in fair-skinned individuals. It can present as a pearl-like nodule or papule. Central ulceration with raised borders is also common.

    Rosacea **(choice C)** has multiple stages of evolution. It begins as persistent erythema with telangiectases and progresses to persistent erythema with papules, pustules, and nodules.

    Vitiligo **(choice E)** presents as hypopigmented macules ranging from 5 mm to 5 cm or larger. As the disease progresses, the macules gradually enlarge.

17. **The correct answer is D.** Achalasia is a primary disorder of esophageal motility and typically presents with dysphagia for *both* solids and liquids. Diagnosis is made with manometry studies, although barium swallow may be warranted to rule out an esophageal mass or tumor.

    Achalasia is not accompanied by a fever **(choice A)**. If a patient has a fever, an infectious etiology should be investigated.

    Regurgitation of predigested food **(choice B)** typically represents a Zenker diverticulum. Barium swallow would demonstrate this abnormality.

    Epigastric pain **(choice C)** is typically not present with achalasia, although the patient may have a sense of pressure or fullness in the upper chest due to the dysphagia.

    Hematemesis **(choice E)** is seen with Mallory-Weiss tears, esophageal varices, peptic ulcers, erosive gastritis/esophagitis, and vascular malformation.

18. **The correct answer is E.** *Rickettsia rickettsii* are small pleomorphic coccobacilli that can cause Rocky Mountain spotted fever. Ticks are both reservoirs and vectors of the condition.

    Bordetella pertussis **(choice A)** is a gram-negative coccobacillus. It is a respiratory tract pathogen and is responsible for whooping cough.

    Borrelia burgdorferi **(choice B)** is a spirochete. The organism is transmitted by ticks and causes Lyme disease.

    Corynebacterium **(choice C)** is a gram-positive bacterium. *Corynebacterium* species cause diphtheria or skin infections.

    Rickettsia prowazekii **(choice D)** is responsible for typhus.

19. **The correct answer is D.** Absence of menses **(choice A)** describes amenorrhea. Difficult and painful menstruation **(choice B)** describes dysmenorrhea. Excessive menstrual bleeding **(choice C)** describes menorrhagia, and irregular menstrual bleeding between periods **(choice E)** describes metrorrhagia.

20. **The correct answer is E.** In fractures of the floor of the orbit, the adjacent extraocular muscles may become entrapped within the fracture (so-called blowout fracture), thereby immobilizing them. This is especially true for the inferior rectus muscle. In this instance, the ability of the globe to elevate (cornea moved upward) is impeded by the entrapped rectus muscle so that an upward gaze results in incongruent retinal images and hence, the patient reports double vision. The muscles that promote convergence **(choice A**; primarily the medial recti) would not be impeded in their actions under the circumstances described above. The inferior rectus is not involved in divergence **(choice B)**. A leftward gaze **(choice C)** would involve the left lateral rectus and the right medial rectus muscles. The right inferior rectus does not contribute to this movement. Although the inferior rectus is entrapped, so as to limit elevation of the right eye, it would not impede the action of the superior oblique in depressing the globe **(choice D)**.

21. **The correct answer is A.** Transplant rejection can be hyperacute (within minutes to hours), acute (usually within days, although it may appear later), or chronic (appearing 4 to 6 months after transplantation). Most acute rejection reactions are controlled, to some extent, by immunosuppressive therapy, so chronic rejection is more commonly seen. The patient described in this question is experiencing gradual renal failure over months, suggesting chronic rejection of the renal allograft. A renal biopsy from a patient experiencing chronic rejection typically shows intimal fibrosis in the vessels with fibrosis and tubular atrophy in the renal

interstitium. Glomeruli may show ischemic changes or may appear normal.

Linear deposition of immunoglobulin and complement in glomeruli (**choice B**) is a feature of Goodpasture syndrome (not a transplant rejection syndrome). Neutrophils, immunoglobulin, and complement in blood vessel walls (**choice C**) are typical of hyperacute rejection, due to previous sensitization to an antigen found in the transplant. A T-cell infiltrate (CD4-positive and CD8-positive T cells) with interstitial edema (**choice D**) and hemorrhage characterizes acute cellular rejection of an allograft. Acute rejection may occur during the initial months following a transplant; however, rise in serum creatinine would be more sudden, rather than progressive as in chronic rejection. Intimal thickening of vessels (**choice E**) due to proliferation of fibroblasts, myocytes, and foamy macrophages is a feature of subacute vasculitis, a common form of acute rejection generally seen in the first few months after transplantation.

22. **The correct answer is B.** Methyldopa is the drug of choice and is classified in category B. Benazepril (**choice A**), an ACE inhibitor, is a high-risk drug in pregnancy. Amlodipine (**choice C**) is a calcium-channel blocker and is in pregnancy risk group C. Atenolol (**choice D**) is in pregnancy risk category C. Atenolol appears to be safe and effective in late pregnancy but is not first-line therapy. Losartan (**choice E**) cannot be used because it is in category D, which can cause injury or death in a fetus in the second or third trimester.

23. **The correct answer is E.** The Somogyi effect is a phenomenon where hypoglycemia causes a surge of counterregulatory hormones to produce hyperglycemia in the morning. It is usually seen in patients with insulin-dependent diabetes mellitus, especially where an insulin with a long-acting component is being used. It is also referred to as rebound hyperglycemia.

24. **The correct answer is D.** Idiopathic thrombocytopenic purpura is initially treated with prednisone. After the platelet count returns to normal, prednisone can be tapered and discontinued; in some cases, however, a low maintenance dose of prednisone is necessary to keep thrombocytopenia from returning.

Heparin (**choice A**) is an anticoagulant, thus it doesn't have a mechanism of action to treat ITP. Factor VIII (**choice B**) is an antihemorrhagic, and plasmapheresis (**choice C**) is a therapy that aims to remove antibodies or inflammatory mediators from the blood. It is only a supportive therapy, since the underlying cause is not treated.

Splenectomy (**choice E**) is considered definitive treatment but should be reserved for patients who fail to respond to prednisone initially or patients who require a long-term high-maintenance dose of prednisone.

25. **The correct answer is C.** Atopy is the strongest identifiable predisposing factor to the development of asthma. The remaining answer choices are not immune-mediated conditions.

26. **The correct answer is E.** Molluscum contagiosum is caused by an epidermal viral infection. It is transmitted by skin-to-skin contact and therefore commonly seen in children and sexually active adults. The lesions are frequently umbilicated, skin-colored papules.

Condylomata acuminata (**choice A**) is caused by human papillomavirus. It affects mucous membranes and presents with cauliflower-like lesions.

Folliculitis (**choice B**) is an inflammatory condition of the hair follicles. It presents with tender pimples and/or pustules.

Herpes simplex (**choice C**) is a viral infection that causes genital herpes. It is a sexually transmitted disease with primary infections and recurrences. Patients commonly are asymptomatic. Active disease presents with erythematous and grouped vesicles, itching, dysuria, and genital irritation.

Hidradenitis suppurativa (**choice D**) is a chronic disease affecting apocrine glands in the axillae and anogenital region. The lesions are highly tender, erythematous nodules or abscesses. Some of the lesions may drain purulent material. In addition to the nodules and abscesses, comedones (especially paired ones) are common.

27. **The correct answer is C.** Although duodenal ulcers are more common than are gastric ulcers, the history of worsening pain with food (a result of increased HCl secretion) is suggestive of a gastric ulcer. This patient should have endoscopy or UGI double contrast imaging to evaluate the gastric mucosa.

Gastroesophageal reflux disease (**choice A**) is certainly a possibility in this patient, but should not be accompanied by significant weight loss.

Acute pancreatitis (**choice B**) can cause all of these symptoms but is more sudden in its presentation. Other symptoms may include nausea, vomiting, and abdominal pain that radiates to the back.

Esophageal spasms (**choice D**) typically cause dysphagia for solids and liquids.

The pain of a duodenal ulcer (**choice E**) is often relieved with a meal.

28. **The correct answer is E.** There are three stages of syphilis (infective agent is a spirochete, *Treponema pallidum*). The primary stage is characterized by a chancre, which is characteristically infectious and painless, as well as regional adenopathy.

    Patients with chancroid (**choice A**) may present with painful ulcers.

    Genital warts (**choice B**) are soft, moist, or flesh-colored. They appear in the genital area within weeks or months after infection. They may sometimes be pedunculated clusters that resemble cauliflower-like bumps, and can be raised or flat, small or large.

    Patients with gonorrhea (**choice C**) usually present with a burning sensation during urination or a white, yellow, or green discharge from the penis.

    Herpes simplex (**choice D**) is an acute viral disease marked by groups of vesicles on the skin in the form of cold sores or located on the genitalia.

29. **The correct answer is B.** The letter *G* in the answer choices stands for gravida and refers to the number of pregnancies. The letter *P* stands for parity and is the outcome of prior pregnancies. There is only one outcome per pregnancy, even if there are twins. The numbers following *P* represent the number of term pregnancies, the number of premature pregnancies, the number of abortions (including ectopic pregnancies and spontaneous or therapeutic abortions), and the number of living children, respectively.

30. **The correct answer is D.** This patient most likely has cytomegalovirus (CMV) retinitis. The best drug treatment for this infection is ganciclovir. Acyclovir (**choice A**) is not effective in CMV infections. It is used more for HSV type 1 and 2 infections. Amantadine (**choice B**) can be used in the treatment of influenza A virus. Flucytosine (**choice C**) is an antifungal agent. Zidovudine (**choice E**) is used in the treatment of AIDS.

31. **The correct answer is B.** Viral meningitis is relatively common, accounting for 10,000 cases of meningitis per year in the U.S. The majority of cases occur in individuals younger than 30 years. Usually, the symptoms are relatively mild, and death is uncommon. Enteroviruses, arboviruses, and type 2 herpes simplex virus are the most common causes of viral meningitis.

Also, up to 10% of HIV patients develop an acute meningitis, typically at the time of seroconversion.

Adenovirus (**choice A**) infection is associated with upper respiratory tract infections (URTIs), sinusitis, ocular disease, enteric infections, and bladder infections. It does not typically cause aseptic meningitis.

Human papillomaviruses (**choice C**) are associated with warts on the skin and genital areas. Poxviruses (**choice D**) include the causative agents of smallpox, cowpox, and molluscum contagiosum. These agents do not typically cause meningitis. Reoviruses (**choice E**) cause URTIs, hepatitis, gastroenteritis, and encephalitis, but not meningitis.

32. **The correct answer is B.** Cluster headaches are more common in males, present with severe, sharp or stabbing pain located around the orbit of the eye, and may occur multiple times per day.

    Tension headaches (**choice A**) present as mild to moderate dull pain, lasting hours, and are described as a tightness or pressure across the head.

    Migraine headaches (**choice C**) present as moderate to severe pain, lasting hours to days, with throbbing or pulsating pain with associated nausea and vomiting.

    Subdural hematoma (**choice D**) presents after head trauma with a worsening headache and confusion.

    Subarachnoid bleed (**choice E**) presents as a thunderclap headache or worst headache of a patient's life. The pain is pulsatile towards the back of the head.

33. **The correct answer is E.** Triamterene is grouped in the category of potassium-sparing diuretics. Along with spironolactone and amiloride, these diuretic agents may cause excess renal retention of potassium. In this manner, use of these drugs may increase potassium levels and cause hyperkalemia. Acetazolamide (**choice A**) is a carbonic anhydrase inhibitor that initially causes a moderate amount of potassium loss. This would predispose the patient to hypokalemia. Furosemide (**choice B**) is a loop diuretic that causes a moderate to severe loss of potassium. Hydrochlorothiazide and metolazone (**choices C and D**) are thiazide diuretics that cause moderate amounts of potassium loss.

34. **The correct answer is E.** Children and adults with coarctation of the aorta are often asymptomatic. The blood pressure is higher in the upper extremities than in the lower extremities. There are absent or weak femoral pulses. The murmur is usually systolic and can be heard anywhere on the anterior chest but is maximal over the left back.

In contrast to the physical findings of coarctation of the aorta, patent ductus arteriosus (**choice A**) has a continuous, machinery-like murmur over the pulmonary region and a widened pulse pressure.

An atrial septal defect (**choice B**) is often asymptomatic until middle age. There may be a systolic ejection murmur over the pulmonic area and a widely split S2 that does not vary with breathing.

In transposition of the great arteries (**choice C**), cyanosis is typically noted in the first few days of life. The lesion must be treated or the prognosis is very poor.

The clinical features of a ventricular septal defect (**choice D**) depend on the size of the defect. There may be a loud, harsh systolic murmur best heard at the left sternal border.

35. **The correct answer is B.** Hemophilia A is characterized by a reduction in the factor VIII coagulation activity. Partial thromboplastin time is prolonged. Bleeding time, fibrinogen levels, and factor VIII:R antigen levels are normal.

Laboratory evaluation of disseminated intravascular coagulation (**choice A**) shows hypofibrinogenemia, thrombocytopenia, and fibrin degradation products.

Laboratory evaluation of idiopathic thrombocytopenic purpura (**choice C**) shows isolated thrombocytopenia and normal coagulation studies.

Thrombocytopenia and fragmented red blood cells on the peripheral smear are characteristic of thrombotic thrombocytopenic purpura (**choice D**). Partial thromboplastin time, prothrombin time, and fibrinogen levels are normal.

Laboratory evaluation of von Willebrand disease (**choice E**) shows reduction in the von Willebrand factor levels, a prolonged bleeding time either at baseline or post challenge with aspirin, prolonged partial thromboplastin time, and normal levels of platelets.

36. **The correct answer is D.** Chronic bronchitis can cause cor pulmonale. Signs and symptoms associated with cor pulmonale are shortness of breath, swelling of the ankles, cyanosis, and chest discomfort. Chronic hypoxia results in vasoconstriction and pulmonary hypertension. The ensuing right heart failure is referred to as cor pulmonale.

Bronchiolitis is typically seen in children less than 2 years of age. Bronchiolitis obliterans (**choice A**) can occur in adults. Signs and symptoms include shortness of breath, cough, and crackles on chest auscultation.

Pneumonia (**choice B**) can present with fever, cough, shortness of breath, chest discomfort, and rales on chest auscultation.

A lung abscess (**choice C**) is an infectious cause and should not result in cardiac failure. The clinical presentation should be consistent with that of pneumonia.

Bronchiectasis (**choice E**) can present with chronic productive cough, hemoptysis, and recurrent pneumonia.

37. **The correct answer is B.** There are two different strains of herpes simplex viruses. Herpes simplex virus type 1 (HSV-1) is normally associated with infections of the lips, mouth, and face. It is the most common herpes simplex and is transmitted by contact with infected saliva. Herpes simplex virus type 2 (HSV-2) is sexually transmitted and is usually associated with genital ulcers or sores. Once the virus is acquired, it spreads to nerve cells and remains dormant. It may periodically reactivate and cause symptoms. Flares may be caused by overexposure to sunlight, fever, stress, acute illness, and medications, or by conditions that weaken the immune system. Laboratory examinations would yield a giant, multinucleated keratinocyte on a Giemsa-stained smear.

Choice A is consistent with atopic dermatitis; **choice C** is consistent with tinea versicolor; **choice D** is consistent with scabies; and **choice E** is consistent with erythema nodosum.

38. **The correct answer is D.** This is the classic presentation of irritable bowel syndrome. To diagnose a patient with irritable bowel syndrome, organic disease must be excluded. Physical examination and laboratory evaluation often yield normal results.

Inflammatory bowel syndromes, such as ulcerative colitis (**choice A**) and Crohn disease (**choice B**), may present with intermittent cramps and diarrhea, but the diarrheal stools are typically accompanied by mucus or blood. The patient with inflammatory bowel disease is often ill-appearing and may have an elevated sedimentation rate or C-reactive protein during active disease. Anemia and varying degrees of weight loss may be present.

Viral gastroenteritis (**choice C**) is an acute illness typically presenting with diarrhea, occasionally with vomiting, and is self-limiting. The chronic nature of this patient's symptoms rules out a viral gastroenteritis.

Diverticulitis (**choice E**) often presents in older patients. Essentially, it is the result of an infection of the diverticulum. Clinically, it should present with fever and abdominal tenderness accompanied by an elevated white blood cell count. As these are not seen in this patient, diverticulitis can be excluded.

39. **The correct answer is D.** The patient has signs and symptoms of bacterial vaginosis and should be treated with metronidazole.

Ceftriaxone (**choice A**) may be used to treat gonorrhea; clotrimazole (**choice B**) may be used to treat candidiasis; acyclovir (**choice C**) may be used to treat herpes infections; and podophyllum resin (**choice E**) may be used to treat genital warts.

40. **The correct answer is C.** Painless vaginal bleeding is a sign of placenta previa.

Abruptio placentae (**choice A**) is characterized by painful vaginal bleeding with uterine tenderness and increased tone.

Uterine atony (**choice B**) presents postpartum with bleeding.

Preeclampsia (**choice D**) is characterized by hypertension, proteinuria, and edema during pregnancy.

Premature rupture of membranes (**choice E**) is characterized by amniotic fluid leaking from the vagina. The leak can be either a slow trickle or a rush of fluid. The amniotic fluid is from a rupture in the amniotic sac, which occurs before the fetus is full-term.

41. **The correct answer is A.** All the agents listed can infect the eyeball. The agent specifically associated with contact lens use is *Acanthamoeba*, which can infect lens solution. This amoeba is dangerous because it causes an intractable ulcerative keratitis that may progress to uveitis. If the lesion is suspected, the clinical laboratory should be notified and specific directions for collecting samples for culture obtained. The parasites may be difficult to see in histologic sections or corneal scrapings.

Cytomegalovirus (**choice B**) and herpes simplex (**choice C**) infections are most often seen in immunocompromised patients, particularly AIDS patients. Circulating larvae of the helminth *Toxocara* (**choice D**) can lodge in the eye (particularly in the vitreous or retina); *Toxocara* infections are seen more commonly in children. Toxoplasmosis (**choice E**) of the eye is most often congenital, but it can be acquired.

42. **The correct answer is B.** This patient most likely has an injured peroneal nerve. This nerve travels around the neck of the fibula on the lateral aspect of the leg. The peroneal nerve innervates the dorsiflexors of the toes and foot and the muscles that evert the foot. Injury to the lateral leg leads to a foot drop and weakness of foot eversion.

An injury or lesion at the inguinal ligament (**choice A**) would lead to damage of the lateral femoral cutaneous nerve, which does not innervate any muscles. It presents with dysesthesia of the lateral thigh.

An injury or lesion near the medial malleolus (**choice C**) would lead to damage to the distal tibial nerve, which innervates toe flexors and other intrinsic muscles of the foot. Injury to the tibial nerve at the medial malleolus presents with pain and numbness of the sole and weakness of the toe flexors.

An injury or lesion near the sciatic notch (**choice D**) would lead to damage of the sciatic nerve, which innervates the hamstring muscles, hip abductors, and all of the muscles below the knee. Such an injury would present with severe disability, including severe lower leg and hamstring weakness and a "flail foot." The individual would have weakness with foot inversion and eversion, toe dorsiflexion, and plantar flexion.

An injury or lesion proximal to the inguinal ligament (**choice E**) would lead to damage to the femoral nerve, which innervates the iliopsoas and quadriceps muscles of the thigh. A femoral nerve injury would present with knee-buckling, an absent knee-jerk reflex, and weak anterior thigh muscles with atrophy.

43. **The correct answer is E.** Before jumping into treatment recommendations, the provider needs to gain more information. What has the patient tried to do to quit smoking in the past? How long was she able to abstain? What situations or occasions make it harder to avoid smoking? After a more complete understanding of her history, the provider should next detail the range of options available and help her choose the one that is best suited to her temperament, needs, and lifestyle.

Giving medication without conversation (**choice A**) is premature. And although bupropion has been shown to help smokers, especially depressed smokers, to quit, its effectiveness for teenagers is unproven.

Although **choice B** is a great treatment option for teenagers, treatment recommendations are premature.

Bringing the parents into the discussion (**choice C**) may have the virtue of helping them address their own smoking habit, but needlessly complicates the interaction with the patient.

Simple encouragement without assistance (**choice D**) is not likely to foster the intended result.

44. **The correct answer is C.** Mitral regurgitation is consistent with the history and objective findings. Mitral regurgitation can cause left-sided heart failure; the patient's shortness of breath is a symptom of left-sided heart failure.

    The murmur of tricuspid regurgitation (**choice A**) is holosystolic at the right or left sternal border. Jugular venous distention is also noted.

    The murmur of aortic stenosis (**choice B**) is a harsh midsystolic murmur that radiates to the neck and is best heard at the right second intercostal space.

    Aortic regurgitation (**choice D**) and tricuspid stenosis (**choice E**) are diastolic murmurs.

45. **The correct answer is choice D.** The patient's recent fasting plasma glucose results of 142 mg/dL and 150 mg/dL classify his condition as diabetes mellitus type 2. All patients with new-onset type 2 diabetes should have an initial trial of diet and exercise therapy with subsequent follow-up to evaluate glycemic control.

46. **The correct answer is B.** Polycythemia vera is a myeloproliferative disorder that causes an overproduction of primarily red blood cells. Phlebotomy is the treatment of choice.

    Heparin (**choice A**) is an anticoagulant; thus, it doesn't have a mechanism of action to treat polycythemia vera. Plasmapheresis (**choice C**) is a therapy that aims to remove antibodies or inflammatory mediators from the blood. It is only a supportive therapy because the underlying cause is not treated. Prednisone (**choice D**) is inappropriate for treatment. Splenectomy (**choice E**) is considered for patients with symptomatic splenomegaly.

47. **The correct answer is B.** Osteoarthritis presents with pain relieved by rest and morning stiffness that resolves in 30–60 minutes. It is typically due to wear and tear on a joint.

    Gout (**choice A**) is most commonly noted in males and presents with acute onset of pain involving small joints.

    Reiter's syndrome (**choice C**) presents with arthritis, urethritis/cervicitis, and conjunctivitis. It may be due to infection with *Chlamydia* and post dysentery.

    Rheumatoid arthritis (**choice D**) presents with joint pain involving PIP, MCP, wrist, knee, and ankles. Morning stiffness lasts longer than 60 minutes.

    Calcium pyrophosphate deposition disease, or pseudogout (**choice E**), presents with acute onset of painful, red joints. It typically involves the knee, wrist, or shoulder.

48. **The correct answer is D.** Pityriasis versicolor is caused by the yeast *Malassezia furfur* and presents with hypo- or hyperpigmented lesions that have yellow-green fluorescence with Wood's lamp.

    Mupirocin (**choice A**) is an antibacterial agent used primarily for impetigo. It is ineffective against a fungal infection.

    Oral acyclovir (**choice B**) is used for the suppression of recurrent herpes symptoms. Oral corticosteroid (**choice C**) is an inappropriate treatment because prolonged oral corticosteroid use may lead to pityriasis versicolor. Topical retinoid application (**choice E**) is usually used as a treatment for acne vulgaris.

49. **The correct answer is A.** Ultrasound of the gallbladder, although less sensitive than the hepatobiliary iminodiacetic acid (HIDA) scan, is readily available and is the preferred initial study. The ultrasound will help the clinician visualize inflammation, pericholecystic fluid, and gallbladder wall thickening. A radiographic Murphy sign has a 90% positive predictive value. Other benefits to right upper quadrant ultrasound include availability, low cost, and lack of radiation exposure.

    Oral cholecystography (**choice B**) has been replaced by gallbladder ultrasound, CT scan of the abdomen, and the HIDA scan.

    ERCP (**choice C**) is indicated if the patient has symptoms consistent with choledocholithiasis or cholangitis—it is a therapeutic procedure and is not preferred as a diagnostic tool.

    Exploratory surgery (**choice D**) would not be indicated as a diagnostic study, given the aforementioned history. If gallstones are confirmed and a surgical procedure is decided upon, a laparoscopic cholecystectomy would be in order.

    Although the complete blood cell count (**choice E**) will confirm the presence of an infection, it is not useful for the confirmation of acute cholecystis.

50. **The correct answer is D.** Retinoblastomas are rare, aggressive, malignant neoplasms derived from embryonic neuronal cells. These tumors present in early childhood, often within the first 3 months of life. Retinoblastomas are very dangerous because they can metastasize widely via a hematogenous route and because they show a marked propensity to invade the

optic nerve and tract into the brain, where they quickly become inoperable. The pathologist should pay particular attention to the cut end of the optic nerve to make sure that the entire retinoblastoma was removed.

51. **The correct answer is C.** The patient has subclinical hypothyroidism. Subclinical hypothyroidism is characterized by an elevated TSH and normal levels of free T_4, normal T_4, and T_3. If patients have detectable antithyroid antibodies, treatment with levothyroxine should be initiated. Patients with detectable antithyroid antibodies are likely to convert to overt hypothyroidism in the future.

52. **The correct answer is C.** The sound lateralizes to the unaffected ear during the Weber test. During the Rinne test, air conduction is greater than bone conduction on the right side.

    Choices A, B, D, and E are characteristics of conductive hearing loss.

53. **The correct answer is E.** Right ventricle enlargement occurs because there is an increase in the pulmonary pressure. Right ventricular hypertrophy causes right axis deviation.

    Choice A describes an EKG finding of a pulmonary embolus.

    Right ventricular, not left ventricular (**choice B**), hypertrophy is associated with COPD.

    Choice C is incorrect. COPD patients may exhibit multifocal atrial tachycardia.

54. **The correct answer is E.** A prodrome of fever, cough, conjunctivitis, coryza, malaise, and Koplik spots precedes the exanthem. Koplik spots are pathognomonic for rubeola, more commonly known as the measles.

    Erythema infectiosum (**choice A**) is caused by the human parvovirus B19. A prodrome of fever, malaise, and coryza is common in children. The exanthem, consisting of erythematous plaques, starts on the face and gives a "slapped cheeks" appearance. The facial rash then fades, and a reticular rash on the neck, trunk, and arms appears. The condition is self-limiting and resolves in 2 to 3 weeks.

    Mumps (**choice B**) is a viral infection affecting the salivary glands. Clinical manifestations include facial swelling and parotid tenderness.

Roseola (**choice C**) presents with high fever for 3 to 7 days. As the fever subsides, a maculopapular rash appears.

Rubella (**choice D**) has no prodrome in children. It causes a fine, pink, maculopapular exanthem that starts on the face and spreads toward the trunk and extremities. The rash lasts approximately 3 days.

55. **The correct answer is A.** Oxygen is the only proven therapy to correct hypoxemia in COPD. Cromolyn sulfate (**choice B**) and albuterol (**choice D**) may be useful in the treatment of asthma. Ipratropium bromide (**choice C**) and oral corticosteroids (**choice E**) are appropriate for acute exacerbations of COPD.

56. **The correct answer is B.** Hydrochlorothiazide should be used cautiously in diabetic patients.

    Propranolol (**choice A**) can cause hypoglycemia. Benazepril (**choice C**) can cause a nonproductive cough and hyperkalemia. Clonidine (**choice D**) can cause rebound hypertension with abrupt cessation. Terazosin (**choice E**) can cause hypotension and syncope after the first dose.

57. **The correct answer is B.** Normally, stretching of muscle results in a reflex contraction: the harder the stretch, the stronger the contraction. At a certain point, when the tension becomes too great, the contracting muscle suddenly relaxes. The reflex that underlies this sudden muscle relaxation is called the Golgi tendon organ (GTO) reflex, also known as the inverse stretch reflex or autogenic inhibition. The GTO is an extensive arborization of nerve endings (encapsulated by a connective tissue sheath and located near the muscle attachment) that is connected in series with the extrafusal skeletal muscle fibers. As a result, GTOs respond to muscle tension rather than muscle length. Increased tension leads to stimulation of Ib afferents, which inhibit the homonymous muscle via spinal interneurons.

    Free nerve endings (**choice A**) are unmyelinated, unencapsulated nerve endings that penetrate the epidermis. These types of receptors respond to pain and temperature.

    Merkel disks (**choice C**) are composed of specialized tactile epidermal cells and their associated nerve endings. They are located in the basal layer of the epithelium and are slowly adapting receptors that respond to touch and pressure.

Muscle spindles (**choice D**) are spindle-shaped bundles of muscle fibers (intrafusal fibers) that are encapsulated by connective tissue. Muscle spindles are arranged in parallel with extrafusal skeletal muscle fibers, so they sense the length of the muscle. They are innervated by group Ia and II sensory afferent neurons.

Pacinian corpuscles (**choice E**) are unmyelinated nerve endings surrounded by thin, concentric layers of epithelioid fibroblasts. In transverse section, this receptor resembles a sliced onion. They are found primarily in the deep layer of the dermis, loose connective tissue, male and female genitalia, mesentery, and visceral ligaments. They are rapidly adapting receptors that respond to touch and pressure.

58. **The correct answer is A.** An example of a biguanide is metformin. The mechanism of action is inhibition of hepatic gluconeogenesis.

Stimulation of pancreatic insulin release (**choice B**) is consistent with sulfonylureas.

Increased insulin sensitivity (**choice C**) is consistent with thiazolidinediones.

The delay of carbohydrate digestion (**choice D**) is consistent with alpha glucosidase inhibitors.

Promotion of liver gluconeogenesis (**choice E**) is consistent with glucagons.

59. **The correct answer is E.** Pregnancy, PID, and purulent cervicitis are absolute contraindications to IUD use.

Choices A, B, C, and D are relative contraindications to IUD use.

60. **The correct answer is B.** Cystic fibrosis is an autosomal recessive disease in which there is a mutation on chromosome 7 that encodes for the normal transport of chloride channels across the epithelial membranes. In the lungs, failure to transport chloride into the airway lumen also decreases transport of sodium and water, leading to excessively viscous secretions. Mucoid impaction causes obstruction and secondary infection, which results in fibrosis and cyst formation, leading to bronchiectasis with a predilection for the upper lobes. X-ray film will show tubular, air-filled structures that extend to near the edges of the lung fields.

X-ray evidence of severe overinflation and air trapping is characteristic of patients with asthma (**choice A**).

Increased lung markings may be seen on an x-ray when a person has chronic bronchitis (**choice C**).

Changes in the lungs may not be noticed on x-ray findings in the early stages of emphysema (**choice D**).

X-ray examination of the chest may reveal certain abnormal changes associated with pneumonia (**choice E**). Localized shadows obscuring areas of the lung may indicate a bacterial pneumonia, while streaky- or patchy-appearing changes in the x-ray picture may indicate viral or *Mycoplasma* pneumonia.

Block 2

1. **The correct answer is E.** The diagnosis of syphilis can be made by direct visualization of the organism in clinical specimens or by serology. *Treponema pallidum*, the causative agent, can be visualized using direct darkfield microscopy, immunofluorescence, immunoperoxidase, or silver staining. It cannot be visualized using a Gram stain (**choice B**) or a Giemsa stain (**choice C**).

   Serology is the mainstay of the diagnosis of syphilis, because the tests are relatively inexpensive and easy to perform. However, these are indirect tests because they detect the host immune response to infection. There are two types of serologic tests for syphilis: nontreponemal tests and treponemal tests.

   Specific treponemal tests, such as the fluorescent treponemal antibody absorption (FTA-ABS) test (**choice A**) and *T. pallidum* enzyme immunoassay (TP-EIA) (**choice D**) are more complex to perform. They use *T. pallidum* antigens and test for the presence of antibodies against these antigens. These tests are excellent for diagnosing secondary and tertiary syphilis; 100% of those who have secondary syphilis test positive, and approximately 98+% of those with untreated tertiary syphilis test positive. Between 65 and 85% of those with primary syphilis test positive. Although the FTA-ABS test has 98% specificity, false-positive reactions can occur in certain states, such as mixed connective tissue disease, diabetes mellitus, pregnancy, and alcoholic cirrhosis. Specific treponemal tests are not often used to monitor response to treatment, as they may remain reactive for years or even indefinitely following eradication of infection.

2. **The correct answer is D.** The symptoms in the question describe a condition called trigeminal neuralgia. The trigeminal nerve has three divisions. The mandibular division (V3) provides sensory innervation to the lower third of the face up to the ears. It also provides the motor fibers to the muscles of mastication. A lesion to the sensory fibers of the mandibular division of the trigeminal nerve is the cause of the pain described.

   Lesions of the olfactory nerve (CN I) (**choice A**) cause anosmia. Lesions of the optic nerve (CN II) (**choice B**) cause visual field defects and loss of light reflex.

   Lesions of the trochlear nerve (CN IV) (**choice C**) cause weakness looking down with adducted eye, trouble walking down stairs, and the head tilt away from the lesioned side.

   Lesions of the facial nerve (CN VII) (**choice E**) can involve drooping of the corner of the mouth, inability to shut the eye or wrinkle the forehead, loss of blink reflex, hyperacusis, alteration or loss of taste from the tongue, and a dry eye.

3. **The correct answer is D.** Osteogenic cells are mesenchymal-like cells in adult bone that differentiate into bone-forming osteoblasts for remodeling and repair.

   Interstitial lamellae (**choice A**) are wedges of compact bone located between the cylindrical osteons.

   Osteoclasts (**choice B**) are large, motile, multinucleated cells found on bone surfaces at the sites of resorption.

   Osteocytes (**choice C**) are mature bone cells that occupy lacunae in the solid matrix.

   Osteons (**choice E**) are composed of concentric lamellae around a central neurovascular canal.

4. **The correct answer is B.** Beta-blockers, such as atenolol, can mask the signs of hypoglycemia (e.g., tachycardia) and should be used cautiously in diabetic patients.

   Clonidine, nifedipine, benazepril, and terazosin (**choices A, C, D, and E**) can be used in hypertensive diabetic patients.

5. **The correct answer is A.** First-degree heart block is usually asymptomatic and often seen in young individuals, in athletes, and in individuals with increased vagal tone. First-degree heart block is defined as an increase of the PR interval >0.21 sec with all atrial impulses conducted.

   Permanent pacing (**choice C**) is incorrect; indications for permanent pacing are symptomatic bradycardia, Mobitz type II atrioventricular block, or complete heart block.

   Patients with atrial fibrillation, not first-degree heart block, are treated prophylactically with warfarin (**choice D**) to prevent the development of an embolus.

   Mobitz type I heart block (**choice E**) is characterized by a progressive lengthening of the PR interval until a P wave fails to produce a QRS response (a blocked beat).

6. **The correct answer is B.** Acromegaly is caused by excessive growth hormone. It causes enlargement of the hands and feet. A soft, doughy, sweaty handshake is characteristic of acromegaly. Other findings include bony changes of facial features, widening of tooth spacing, and insulin resistance. Hypertrophy of pharyngeal and laryngeal tissue also causes a change in voice.

The physical examination findings of **choice A** are consistent with Graves disease. Similarly, the characteristics found in **choice C** indicate Cushing syndrome, **choice D**, Addison disease, and **choice E**, ovarian hyperthecosis.

7. **The correct answer is B.** Hodgkin disease can present with a painless lymphadenopathy in the cervical or supraclavicular region. Patients may also be symptomatic with fever, weight loss, dry cough, and pruritus.

   Hairy cell leukemia (**choice A**) rarely causes lymphadenopathy. Patients may present with a gradual onset of fatigue, infection, and symptoms related to splenomegaly.

   Patients with multiple myeloma (**choice C**) often present with one or more of the following: bone pain, fatigue, neurologic complications, confusion, recurrent infections, and/or nausea and vomiting.

   Patients with polycythemia vera (**choice D**) present with symptoms relating to the increased viscosity of the blood and abnormal platelet functions. Symptoms may include headaches, bleeding abnormalities, pruritus, and fatigue.

   Patients with von Willebrand disease (**choice E**) often present with mucosal bleeding, and aspirin exacerbates bleeding.

8. **The correct answer is D.** *Staphylococcus aureus* is one of the most common causes of abscesses. *Mycoplasma pneumoniae* (**choice B**) may lead to bullous myringitis. *Haemophilus influenzae* and *Streptococcus pneumoniae* (**choices C and E**) may result in lobar pneumonia. Finally, *Chlamydia pneumonia* (**choice A**) can cause interstitial pneumonia.

9. **The correct answer is D.** Oral isotretinoin suppresses sebaceous follicle epithelium desquamation and the production of sebum, thus reducing the colonization of *Propionibacterium acnes* and decreasing inflammation.

   Oral tetracycline (**choice E**), benzoyl peroxide topical gel (**choice A**), clindamycin (**choice B**), and comedone removal (**choice C**) may be used to treat mild to moderate acne.

10. **The correct answer is C.** Oropharyngeal dysphagia is usually due to neuromuscular conditions that make the complex process of swallowing difficult. There is frequently associated dysphonia or dysarthria.

    Esophageal spasm (**choice A**) causes dysphagia for both solids and liquids. It is episodic and unpredictable. This dysphagia occurs after food is swallowed, in the esophageal phase.

Esophageal cancer (**choice B**) causes dysphagia for solids. The mass effect of the tumor makes it difficult to swallow boluses of food, but liquids can pass through the lumen. There is usually associated weight loss, and this dysphagia occurs after food is swallowed, in the esophageal phase.

Schatzki ring (**choice D**) causes a mechanical obstruction that is intermittent and nonprogressive. This dysphagia occurs after food is swallowed, in the esophageal phase.

Achalasia (**choice E**) often presents with dysphagia to both solids and liquids. A multitude of conditions can result in achalasia, including esophageal tumors, Zenker diverticulum, Chagas disease, nutcracker esophagus, and diffuse esophageal spasm.

11. **The correct answer is D.** Contraindications to varicella vaccine include pregnancy; history of a serious allergic reaction to neomycin or gelatin; anyone who is unable to fight a serious infection, including cancer patients and AIDS patients; and anyone undergoing treatment with oral steroids, including asthmatics.

    The varicella vaccine does not contain egg (**choice B**). Children between 12 and 18 months of age (**choice A**), anyone with a history of mild, intermittent asthma (**choice C**), and a 25-year-old with no prior history of chickenpox (**choice E**) should all receive the vaccine.

12. **The correct answer is choice C.** Fibrocystic disease is seen most commonly in women 30 to 50 years of age. It typically presents as bilateral breast changes described as "lumpy" or "rope-like" by the patient. Tenderness and increase of breast size is common premenstrually. Further investigation is warranted in all masses and breast changes.

    Choice A is consistent with certain endocrine disorders and adverse effects of several antipsychotic medications and other drugs. **Choice B** is consistent with carcinoma of the breast, and **choice D** is consistent with mastitis. **Choice E** is consistent with fibroadenoma of the breast.

13. **The correct answer is D.** The blood fluke *Schistosoma haematobium* is found in the Middle East and Africa. The eggs of the organism are passed in feces and hatch in the water. The free-swimming miracidia must find a hospitable snail, where they can develop into cercariae. Once they leave the snail host, the free-swimming larvae (cercariae) penetrate the skin of the human host. Adults migrate to the renal veins, copulate throughout life, and produce eggs, which are passed in urine. It is the eggs of *Schistosoma haematobium*

that cause the pathology. They induce cell-mediated immunity and the formation of granulomas in the bladder. Symptoms of *Schistosoma haematobium* infection include hematuria, widespread fibrosis, and, eventually, calcification of the bladder, dilation of the ureters due to stenosis of the ureteric orifices, and squamous carcinoma of the bladder.

Ingestion of eggs (**choice A**) in contaminated water is an unlikely way of acquiring a helminth. In the life cycle of organisms that infect a host via eggs, the ingestion of the eggs usually occurs when fecal material is used as fertilizer and contaminates foodstuff.

Ingestion of larvae (**choice B**) in meat is the means by which such parasites as tapeworms and the nematode *Trichinella* are acquired.

Ingestion of oocysts from fecal contamination (**choice C**) is the means of acquiring *Cryptosporidium* or *Toxoplasma gondii*. The oocyst of *Cryptosporidium* is the form of the organism that survives in the environment. It is acquired by ingestion of fecally contaminated food or water. Infection with *Toxoplasma gondii* can be acquired through the ingestion of the oocysts that are shed in cat feces.

Mosquito transmission of microfilariae (**choice E**) is the means by which the agents of lymphatic filariasis are acquired.

14. **The correct answer is E.** The patient has a long tract sign and a cranial nerve sign, both of which are features of a brain stem lesion. The cranial nerve involved is CN V (facial numbness and jaw deviation) and localizes the lesion to the rostral pons on the right, the site of emergence of CN V from the brain stem. The corticospinal tract on the right also is involved, causing left spastic hemiparesis and the Babinski sign on the left.

A lesion of the left cervical spinal cord (**choice A**) might produce one or more long tract signs but no cranial nerve deficits.

Cerebellopontine angle syndrome (**choice B**) usually is caused by an acoustic neuroma (schwannoma) of CN VIII. As the tumor grows, it exerts pressure on the lateral caudal pons where CN VII emerges and may expand to compress the CN V anteriorly. This patient would have signs and symptoms of compression of all of these nerves but no long tract signs because the lesion location is outside of the brainstem.

Right cerebral hemisphere (**choice C**) lesions result in contralateral sensory or motor defects in the body and limbs but no cranial nerve deficits like those seen in this patient.

Right midbrain (**choice D**) lesions affect the fibers of CN III, together with corticobulbar and corticospinal fibers in the medial aspect of the cerebral peduncle. Third nerve lesions result in ptosis, mydriasis, and external strabismus. Although corticospinal tract lesions produce contralateral spastic hemiparesis, the corticobulbar fibers result in a contralateral lower face weakness that involves drooping of the corner of the mouth.

15. **The correct answer is D.** This patient has hypochondriasis, which is characterized by misinterpretation of minor physical symptoms and chronic fears of having a serious medical condition. The fear remains despite a full medical evaluation and reassurance. These individuals are treated with regularly scheduled short appointments.

Body dysmorphic disorder (**choice A**) is the preoccupation with a perceived defect in appearance. This patient has not indicated that she believes that she has a problem with her appearance.

Malingering (**choice B**) is defined as a person producing symptoms with full conscious intent to deceive. The person knows what she is doing and why. The goal is secondary gain, that is, getting money, attention, drugs, etc. The symptom presentation is not florid enough here and the secondary gain is not obvious.

Patients with conversion disorder (**choice C**) experience sensory or motor dysfunction that cannot be explained by a physical or neurologic cause.

Somatization disorder (**choice E**) is characterized by multiple somatic complaints that are not due to a general medical condition. The patient must have pain in at least four different body sites, two gastrointestinal symptoms, one sexual symptom, and one pseudoneurologic symptom. Some of these symptoms must begin before 30 years of age, they must occur over a period of several years, and the patient must experience an impairment in functioning. This patient only has one symptom and therefore does not meet these criteria.

16. **The correct answer is A.** When you ask the patient to roll onto the left side, the left ventricle becomes closer to the chest wall, accentuating the sound of the murmur. Murmurs arising from the mitral valve are best heard at the apex. The bell of the stethoscope is more sensitive to low-pitched sounds, such as mitral stenosis murmurs.

Choice B accentuates aortic murmurs. The diaphragm of the stethoscope picks up higher-pitched sounds, such as aortic murmurs.

Choice **C** is incorrect. The stethoscope should be placed at the apex, not the left sternal border.

Choice **D** is incorrect because it describes the patient position best suited for aortic murmurs, but the use of the bell and the placement of the stethoscope are used for mitral murmurs.

Choice **E** is incorrect because it describes the patient position best suited for aortic murmurs, the use of the diaphragm used with aortic murmurs, and the placement of the stethoscope used in mitral murmurs.

17. **The correct answer is E.** Dexamethasone suppression (**choice A**) is used to diagnose Cushing disease. Antidiuretic hormone (**choice B**) is helpful in the diagnosis of diabetes insipidus, SIADH, or urine concentration disorders. The Schilling test (**choice C**) is used to diagnose pernicious anemia, and the direct Coombs test (**choice D**) is helpful for diagnosing hemolytic diseases.

18. **The correct answer is D.** Patients with sickle cell anemia end up becoming functionally asplenic and therefore would benefit greatly from a pneumococcal vaccination. The spleen plays a role in protecting against life-threatening infections, particularly those with encapsulated organisms like the pneumococcus. The spleen protects children from serious infection by producing immune factors and by filtering bacteria out of the bloodstream.

Choices **A, B, C,** and **E** are deficiencies that do not greatly increase chances of a pneumococcal infection.

19. **The correct answer is D.** *Mycoplasma* is typically seen in younger patients, and bullous myringitis is a common complication. It should be treated with macrolides, doxycycline, or a quinolone.

20. **The correct answer is D.** A keloid is hyperplastic scar tissue that occurs after a cutaneous injury and often expands beyond the site of injury. No treatments have been completely effective in treating keloids. Intralesional injections of triamcinolone acetonide may relieve itching and reduce the volume of the keloid.

Excision (**choice C**) and curettage (**choice B**) of keloids typically cause the lesion to reappear and be larger than the original lesion. Therefore, they are not recommended.

Antibiotics (**choice A**) and topical corticosteroids (**choice E**) are not recommended in the management of keloids. Because a keloid is not of bacterial origin, antibiotics are ineffective. Corticosteroids are effective in reducing keloid size only if they are directly injected

into the base of the keloid. However, topical corticosteroids are not considered effective in management.

21. **The correct answer is D.** Pancreatic cancer frequently presents as painless jaundice. A Courvoisier sign is the presence of a palpable "gallbladder"; or as in this case, a palpable pancreatic head tumor. Other reasons for a Courvoisier sign are a Klatskin tumor, a calcified (or porcelain) gallbladder, or cholangiocarcinoma. The significant weight loss in this patient is ominous for pancreatic cancer. The disease has a poor prognosis with median survival of 9 to 12 months. Diagnostic testing should include an abdominal CT scan and elevated CA-19-9. Treatment options include the Whipple procedure (pancreaticoduodenectomy) and adjuvant chemoradiation.

Chronic cholecystitis (**choice A**) may present as intermittent or chronic RUQ pain with radiation to the back. Jaundice may be present, but significant weight loss would not be likely.

Gastric ulcer (**choice B**) may present with epigastric pain. Weight loss may accompany an ulcer, but more likely a gastric cancer. Jaundice is not a presenting sign of ulcerative disease of the stomach.

An hepatic abscess (**choice C**) may present with pain, typically in the RUQ. Jaundice could occur if the abscess occluded the cystic duct, but it is unlikely that an hepatic abscess would be palpable or accompanied by significant weight loss.

Acute cholecystitis (**choice E**) would not present over the course of 4 months. Further, a positive Murphy sign would be expected on the physical examination.

22. **The correct answer is C.** The patient has classic signs and symptoms of *Trichomonas vaginalis*. *Trichomonas vaginalis* is a protozoal flagellate that is sexually transmitted. It causes vaginal itching and irritation. The characteristic discharge is malodorous, green, and frothy. Microscopic examination of the wet mount shows flagellated motile organisms, which confirms the diagnosis. Treatment of choice is metronidazole. Any partner should be treated simultaneously.

Ceftriaxone (**choice A**) may be used to treat gonorrhea. Doxycycline (**choice B**) may be used to treat chlamydia. Miconazole (**choice D**) may be used to treat candidiasis. Penicillin (**choice E**) may be used to treat syphilis.

23. **The correct answer is B.** Rheumatic heart disease most frequently affects the mitral valve, causing stenosis and/or regurgitation. Most cases of acquired mitral stenosis result from rheumatic heart disease. Mitral

stenosis is produced by inflammation of the valve leaflets, leading to deposition of fibrin on the cusps, fusion of the leaflet commissures, and formation of the classic "fishmouth deformity" of the valve.

Tricuspid involvement (**choice A**) occurs only in association with mitral or aortic valve involvement and accounts for approximately 10% of cases.

The aortic valve (**choices C and D**) is affected less frequently than the mitral valve. It is usually a combined lesion with mitral valve involvement.

The pulmonic valve (**choice E**) is rarely affected.

24. **The correct answer is A.** Standing causes a decrease of venous return to the heart, which causes a decrease in left ventricular volume and a decrease in vascular tone. The decrease in left ventricular volume causes earlier mitral prolapse in systole. Squatting causes increased filling of the left ventricle. This stretches the ventricle and allows the floppy leaflets of the mitral valve to approximate (fit together) more accurately. Thus, there is less regurgitant flow and a less intense murmur with squatting.

Standing decreases the murmur intensity of aortic stenosis (**choice B**).

Choices D and E are incorrect because squatting decreases the prolapse of the mitral valve and increases the murmur intensity of aortic stenosis.

25. **The correct answer is D.** The uterine fundus is palpable at the pubic symphysis by 12 to 15 weeks. It reaches the umbilicus by 20 to 22 weeks and stops ascending at the xiphisternum by 36 to 38 weeks.

26. **The correct answer is B.** The patient is experiencing paroxysmal supraventricular tachycardia (PSVT). This is the most common paroxysmal tachycardia. It often occurs in patients without heart disease. Patients are usually aware of their rapid heart action. Some may experience shortness of breath or mild chest pain. The diagnosis is suspected from the history of abrupt onset and abrupt termination of palpations, and the EKG further confirms the diagnosis. Adenosine has a rapid onset of action and is the first-line drug therapy.

Lidocaine (**choice A**) is an antiarrhythmic and is often used in ventricular arrhythmias.

Verapamil (**choice C**) is a calcium channel blocker. It is used to treat PSVT but is not considered the first-line treatment.

Intravenous propranolol (**choice D**) may be used if the patient fails to respond to adenosine.

Amiodarone (**choice E**) is not used to treat PSVT.

27. **The correct answer is B. Choices A, C, D, and E** are characteristics of chronic bronchitis; however, the diagnosis can be made only when there is sputum production for longer than 3 months of the year for longer than 2 successive years.

28. **The correct answer is C.** Spirometry is helpful in assessing the extent and severity of airway obstruction. As air flow obstruction increases, the patient will not be able to expire as forcefully or as quickly, resulting in a decreased FEV_1 and thus a decreased FEV_1:FVC ratio. It also assesses the results of therapy.

Choices A, B, D, and E are incorrect. Chest radiographs, sputum cultures, EKGs, and blood gases may be obtained during exacerbations of the disease but are not typically performed on a routine basis.

29. **The correct answer is D.** Neural tube defects result from failure of the primitive neural tube to close, which may affect either end of the neuraxis and lead to anomalies involving both the neural tissue and overlying skin and bone. Anencephaly and encephalocele may develop at the cranial end, whereas various forms of spina bifida, myelomeningocele, and meningocele occur at the caudal end. Folate deficiency has been linked to neural tube defects. Elevated alpha-fetoprotein in the maternal blood allows antenatal diagnosis.

Arnold-Chiari malformations (**choice A**), which affect the craniospinal junction, have two forms. Type 1 is frequent but usually asymptomatic and consists of downward displacement of the cerebellar tonsils. Type 2 is much more complex and manifests with early signs and symptoms of hydrocephalus.

Germinal matrix hemorrhage (**choice B**) is one cause of perinatal brain injury and consists of hemorrhage within the germinal matrix, the periventricular layer of neuronal and glial precursors. This injury affects premature infants and may lead to significant neurologic impairment or death.

Holoprosencephaly (**choice C**) is a severe malformation in which lack of separation between hemispheres leads to a single central ventricle. It is usually associated with trisomy 13.

Syringomyelia (**choice E**) refers to the formation of an ependymal-lined cavity within the spinal cord, parallel to and connected with the central canal. It is associated with Arnold-Chiari type 1, traumas, or spinal tumors, and leads to progressive neurologic deficits.

30. **The correct answer is A.** The patient has psoriasis. This chronic disease, which affects 1 to 2% of people in the U.S., typically involves the elbows, knees, scalp, intergluteal cleft, penis, and lumbosacral area. Well-established lesions show extensive parakeratotic scales overlying a thinned or absent stratum granulosum. The mitotic rate in the underlying epidermis is increased, and mitotic figures can be seen well above the basal cell layer. Collections of neutrophils (Munro abscesses) can be seen within the parakeratotic stratum corneum. The pathogenesis of psoriasis is not well understood, but evidence has been accumulating that autoimmunity may play a role. The theory is that exogenous or endogenous damage to the stratum corneum of the skin exposes antigens against which complement-fixing autoantibodies are directed. Activation of the complement cascade draws neutrophils to the site, further damaging the stratum corneum and perpetuating the process. The damage also triggers release of proliferative factors for epidermal cells, leading to increased epithelial turnover, hyperplasia, and scale formation (an alternative theory is that the underlying process begins with an enhanced ability of the endothelial cells of the superficial dermal microvessels to recruit neutrophils).

Bacterial (**choice B**) or fungal (**choice C**) diseases may trigger psoriasis but are not the primary etiologies. Psoriasis is not associated with granuloma formation (**choice D**), but rather with the formation of microabscesses (Munro abscesses—see above) in the stratum corneum. Large vessel vasculitis (**choice E**) does not seem to play a role in the pathogenesis of psoriasis.

31. **The correct answer is E.** Category X drugs are contraindicated in pregnancy, and drug risk clearly outweighs potential benefits.

Category A (**choice A**) drugs are safe for use in pregnancy and demonstrate no risk to the fetus.

Category B (**choice B**) drugs demonstrate no risk to the fetus in animal studies, and either there are no human studies or human studies failed to demonstrate risk.

Category C (**choice C**) drugs have shown adverse effects in animal studies, but there are no studies in humans.

Category N (**choice D**) drugs have not been classified into a specific category.

32. **The correct answer is A.** The histopathologic change described here is squamous metaplasia, which may be induced by vitamin A deficiency in different types of epithelial membranes, including conjunctiva, respiratory airways, and the urinary tract. This change is probably related to the fact that vitamin A and retinoids play an important role in regulating epithelial differentiation.

Vitamin B_{12} deficiency (**choice B**) results in megaloblastic anemia and degeneration of the posterolateral tracts of the spinal cord. Vitamin C deficiency (**choice C**) causes scurvy, a syndrome characterized by vascular fragility and bleeding diathesis, with resultant recurrent hemorrhage in the gums, skin, and joints. Vitamin D deficiency (**choice D**) results in two different clinical pictures depending on the patient's age, i.e., rickets in children and osteomalacia in adults.

Vitamin E (**choice E**) is a major free radical scavenger. For obscure reasons, deficiency of vitamin E results in degeneration of the ascending axons in the posterior spinal column and spinocerebellar tract.

33. **The correct answer is E.** The Health Belief Model reminds us that adherence is the consequence of the patient thinking the disease is serious and that he or she personally is threatened by it. The likelihood of action is determined by *1)* cues to action, *2)* perceived benefits of action, and *3)* reducing barriers to action. The postcard is a simple cue to action, reminding the patient of the treatment to which they agreed. It is simple, but also empirically, the most effective method for gaining adherence of all the options presented here. To get the action, cue the action.

A joint consultation (**choice A**) is not a bad idea, but it will take some time to set up. Schedules can be full and convenient time may be hard to come by. In addition, bringing in the spouse takes the locus of responsibility off the patient. Getting personal commitment, and reminding the patient of it, is the best way to gain adherence.

As a part of informed consent procedures, **choice B** should already have been done before the treatment was selected. In addition, highlighting the potential difficulties of the treatment is likely to decrease, not enhance, adherence.

The question tells us that the patient already knows that the disease is serious. Information is useful to get a patient's attention and educate him as to the important facts about his disease. However, in this specific case, sufficient information has already been given. In addition, key information should be transmitted directly by the physician, not indirectly by means of a pamphlet (**choice C**).

The question tells us that the patient already knows that he is susceptible. Reinforcing that perception (**choice D**) is unlikely to produce the desired adherence. There is also a risk that the fear induced will be too great, causing the patient to slip into denial.

34. **The correct answer is E.** Terfenadine, which belongs to the piperidine drug class, is the only drug listed that does not cross the blood-brain barrier and therefore does not cause sedation. Other drugs from the same class include astemizole and loratadine. All the other choices have some degree of sedation as a side effect and therefore would not be recommended for someone who is flying an airplane or operating any kind of machinery.

35. **The correct answer is A.** Long-term corticosteroid use can cause osteopenia with vertebral compression fractures. This can be minimized with oral calcium supplementation.

    Vitamin D supplementation is also recommended, as well as weight-bearing exercise in moderation. Bisphosphonates are also widely used and recommended for prevention and treatment of glucocorticoid-induced bone loss. Estrogen therapy in postmenopausal women is no longer recommended as first-line therapy because of the increased risk of breast cancer, stroke, and venous thromboembolism. Use of calcitonin and thiazide diuretics is controversial, so these are not considered first-line therapies.

    Carotene (**choice B**) is an antioxidant and has no role in the amelioration of bone loss due to long-term corticosteroid treatment. Some patients with lupus develop hemolytic anemia, and extranutritional support with folate (**choice C**) or iron (**choice D**) may be helpful. However, the anemia is a feature of the disease itself, rather than of the steroid therapy. Supplementation with vitamin B$_{12}$ (cobalamin; **choice E**) is not indicated with glucocorticoid therapy.

36. **The correct answer is D.** The inferior leads are II, III, and aVF. The ST elevation indicates the acuteness of the infarct.

    A posterior infarction (**choice A**) would show a large R wave in V1 and V2. There may be a Q wave in V6.

    A lateral infarction (**choice B**) would show Q waves in I and aVL.

    An anterior infarction (**choice C**) would show Q waves in V1, V2, V3, or V4.

A subendocardial infarction (**choice E**) involves only a small area of myocardium just beneath the endocardial lining. It is a type of non–Q wave infarction; hence, there will be no Q waves on the EKG. It causes flat depression of the ST segment.

37. **The correct answer is E.** The combination of ipratropium and albuterol is considered first-line therapy. Although oxygen, corticosteroids, and antibiotics are often used in the treatment of acute COPD exacerbations, the combination of β$_2$-adrenergics and anticholinergics are the first-line therapy.

    Albuterol (**choice B**) is considered second-line treatment.

    Theophylline (**choice C**) is considered fourth-line treatment.

    Methylprednisolone sodium succinate (**choice D**) is considered third-line treatment.

38. **The correct answer is C.** Pityriasis rosea is thought to be caused by human herpesvirus 7. A single herald patch appears 1 to 2 weeks prior to the exanthem, which typically consists of fine-scaling papules and plaques in a Christmas tree distribution. The exanthem is usually on the trunk and proximal arms. The face is usually spared.

    Lichen simplex chronicus (**choice A**) results from chronic rubbing of an area. A solid plaque develops from the confluence of small papules. There is hyperpigmentation of the area.

    Nummular eczema (**choice B**) causes round erythematous plaques from the coalesced small vesicles and papules. The plaques are approximately 4 to 5 cm in diameter.

    Pityriasis versicolor (**choice D**) is caused by yeast. It results in well-demarcated, round or oval macules that vary in size. Fine scaling can be noted when lesions are gently abraded. The macules are hypopigmented on tanned white skin and are brown on darker-skinned individuals.

    Shingles (**choice E**) is caused by a reactivation of the varicella-zoster virus. It results in painful vesicles and bullae with erythematous bases in a dermatomal distribution.

39. **The correct answer is D.** A Mallory-Weiss tear presents as hematemesis, most frequently after a protracted bout of emesis. It is not related to cirrhotic liver disease. Most frequently, this is a previously healthy patient. It is almost always self-limited.

Cancer of the stomach (**choice A**) may present as vague abdominal pain. Because this cancer presents so late, there is frequently anemia and weight loss.

A duodenal ulcer (**choice B**) is more common than a gastric ulcer and frequently presents with pain *relieved by eating.* The duodenum secretes bicarbonate to neutralize the hydrochloric acid produced when the patient eats. In this case, the bicarbonate secretion improves the patient's pain.

A gastric ulcer (**choice C**) may present very similarly. It is less common than a duodenal ulcer. Frequently, the pain is made *worse* with food and milk because of the production of hydrochloric acid in response to a food bolus, which will irritate the stomach ulcer.

Acute pancreatitis (**choice E**) can present with epigastric pain. The presentation is often sudden. Other symptoms include nausea, vomiting, and abdominal pain that radiates to the back.

40. **The correct answer is A.** Caplan syndrome is a pneumoconiosis plus rheumatoid arthritis. Pneumoconiosis is an occupation-associated disease related to coal mining. The disease varies from simple anthracosis—in which the carbon pigment accumulates in macrophages along the pleural lymphatics, causing no reaction—to progressive massive pulmonary fibrosis, increased respiratory distress, pulmonary hypertension, and cor pulmonale.

Goodpasture syndrome (**choice B**) is a glomerular disease characterized by the production of antibodies directed against the basement membrane, which results in damage of the lungs and the kidneys.

Plumbism (**choice C**) is a toxic condition produced by the absorption of excessive lead into the system.

Von Gierke disease (**choice D**) is a hereditary deficiency of glucose-6-phosphatase and is characterized by severe hypoglycemia, lactic acidosis, hepatomegaly, hyperlipidemia, hyperuricemia, and short stature.

WAGR syndrome (**choice E**) is a genetic syndrome that includes *W*ilms tumor (kidney cancer), *a*niridia, *g*enitourinary anomalies, and mental *r*etardation.

41. **The correct answer is D.** People who are infected with HIV have a poor immune response to herpesvirus 8 (HHV8), which is likely the reason why HIV-infected patients are at high risk of contracting Kaposi sarcoma. In the last 20 years the vast majority of Kaposi sarcoma cases have developed in association with human immunodeficiency virus (HIV) infection and acquired immunodeficiency syndrome (AIDS), especially among homosexual men. Kaposi sarcoma is a cancer that develops in the connective tissues such as cartilage, bone, fat, muscle, blood vessels, or fibrous tissues. These lesions appear as raised blotches or nodules that may be purple, brown, or red in color. Sometimes the disease causes painful swelling, especially in the legs, groin area, or skin around the eyes.

Epstein-Barr virus (**choice A**) in an HIV-infected person multiplies and causes infection throughout the body. Symptoms include headache, change in mental status, cough, abdominal cramps, diarrhea, and vision changes such as spots, floaters, or tunnel vision.

Herpes simplex type I (**choice B**) typically causes cold sores or blisters on the mouth and face, and herpes simplex type II (**choice C**) causes similar sores that typically appear on the genitals and anal area.

Human papilloma virus (**choice E**) is associated with squamous cell carcinoma of the anus.

42. **The correct answer is A.** Propylthiouracil is the treatment of choice for hyperthyroidism in pregnant and lactating women.

Methimazole (**choice B**) is not completely contraindicated during pregnancy, although propylthiouracil is the treatment of choice. Methimazole has been noted to be expressed in breast milk at a higher degree than is propylthiouracil.

Radioactive iodine (**choice C**) leaves a remnant of radioactivity posttreatment, increasing the risk of radiation exposure to the fetus.

Surgery (**choice D**) is reserved for pregnant women who cannot take antithyroid medication, i.e., allergy or the need for high doses of antithyroid medication to control the disease. The preferred time to operate is during the second trimester because the risks of miscarriage (during the first trimester) or premature labor and delivery (third trimester) are minimized.

Propranolol (**choice E**) is a category C drug, so the fetal risk is not established.

43. **The correct answer is D.** Heparin is delivered intravenously and has a quicker onset of action. This allows immediate anticoagulation and treatment of the clot. Warfarin takes several days to reach its effectiveness.

The two drugs should be started at the same time. Once warfarin reaches a therapeutic level for 24 hours, heparin can be discontinued.

The patient would not be anticoagulated for several days if only warfarin therapy (**choice A**) was initiated.

Insertion of a vena cava filter (**choice B**) is recommended in patients with contraindication to anticoagulation therapy.

Heparin therapy (**choice C**) is delivered by continuous intravenous infusion and requires hospitalization. It is not used on an outpatient basis. However, there are low-molecular-weight heparin preparations that can be delivered via injection and can be used in some cases.

Streptokinase (**choice E**) is a fibrinolytic agent used in the treatment of myocardial infarction and pulmonary embolism.

44. **The correct answer is A.** Smoking and the resultant pulmonary damage can lead to chronic bronchitis and eventually COPD.

Deficiency of alpha 1-antitrypsin (**choice D**) can lead to emphysema. Pneumonia (**choice C**), air pollution (**choice B**), and allergies (**choice E**) can cause pulmonary dysfunction but do not result in chronic bronchitis.

45. **The correct answer is C.** Premature ejaculation is the most common orgasm disorder in men.

Anorgasmia (**choice A**) is the inability to achieve orgasm in women. The presented patient is a man.

Dyspareunia (**choice B**) is a sexual pain disorder that can occur in men or women, although it is much more common in women. Because it is not an orgasm disorder, it is the wrong answer.

Retarded ejaculation (**choice D**), the inability to achieve orgasm, is an orgasm disorder, but it is not as common as premature ejaculation. Retarded ejaculation has been reported as a side effect of SSRI medication in approximately 15% of male patients.

Secondary impotence (**choice E**) is fairly common, with an incidence that can approach 70% in elderly men. It is a sexual arousal disorder, however, and therefore not the correct answer.

46. **The correct answer is D.** Each of the four cardiac valves can be auscultated at various positions on the chest. The right second intercostal space is the anatomic position for the auscultation of the aortic valve.

The inferior border of the heart (**choice A**) extends from the sixth right costal cartilage to the fifth left

intercostal space at the midclavicular line; none of the cardiac valves are auscultated at this anatomic position. The left second intercostal space (**choice B**) is the anatomic position for the auscultation of the pulmonary valve. The left fifth intercostal space (**choice C**) is the anatomic position for the auscultation of the mitral valve. The xiphisternal junction (**choice E**) is the anatomic position for the auscultation of the tricuspid valve.

47. **The correct answer is A.** Holter monitoring is used to document suspected rhythm disturbances. A Holter monitor continuously records an EKG for a prolonged period, typically 24 hours.

Because a rhythm disturbance has not been diagnosed, a stress test (**choice B**) is inappropriate in this situation. Stress tests are valuable in diagnosing ischemic heart disease, and are also helpful in further investigating physiologic mechanisms, such as arrhythmias and dysfunctioning heart valves in previously diagnosed patients.

Echocardiogram (**choice C**) is incorrect because it is used primarily to examine the morphology and function of the heart. It is not likely that an echocardiogram will catch an occasional rhythm disturbance during the study.

Prescribing beta-blockers (**choice D**) is incorrect. Beta-blockers can be used to control the rate of a rhythm; however, the rhythm disturbance in this case is not known.

Radioablation (**choice E**) is used to treat known rhythm disturbances, such as atrial fibrillation.

48. **The correct answer is D.** The symptoms presented—excitement, paranoia, random behavior, moist skin, and dry mouth—are all classic signs of amphetamine use. "Track marks" suggest that the patient has been injecting the drugs intravenously.

Barbiturate intoxication (**choice A**) results in slowed movement, slurred speech, stumbling gait, and, if severe enough, stupor and coma. This is the opposite of the pattern presented here.

Diazepam (**choice B**), because it increases GABA, should result in calmer behavior, not the more agitated behavior described here.

Heroin (**choice C**) results in slow, lethargic behavior, the opposite of what is described here. Heroin is often injected, resulting in "track marks," but the rest of the description rules out heroin intoxication.

Phencyclidine (PCP) (**choice E**) results in very aggressive, violent behavior. Users are often paranoid, excessively strong, and impervious to pain. The patient described here is not elevated to this level.

49. **The correct answer is D.** This patient has failed empiric treatment and should be endoscoped to biopsy and evaluate the gastric ulcer. If *Helicobacter pylori* testing (or empiric treatment) was not done at initial diagnosis, *H. pylori* culture should be done at endoscopy.

In regard to **choices A and B**, this patient has failed outpatient treatment and must be further evaluated.

Repeat upper gastrointestinal imaging (**choice C**) is not the intervention of choice. If the gastric ulcer is not healed (which this patient's history suggests), it should be biopsied at this time.

Surgical intervention such as vagotomy (**choice E**) is recommended in some cases when patients do not respond to medication and endoscopic therapy. It would be premature in this case.

50. **The correct answer is C.** The home ovulation urine test is screening for the LH surge that occurs prior to ovulation to increase the chances of fertilization.

Follicle-stimulating hormone (FSH; **choice A**) stimulates follicular (ovum/egg) growth of the ovary, prepares ovarian follicles for action by luteinizing hormone (LH), and enhances the LH-induced ovarian release of estrogen.

Human chorionic gonadotropin (HCG) (**choice B**) is a peptide hormone produced in pregnancy, which is made by the embryo soon after conception and later by the trophoblast (part of the placenta). Its role is to prevent the disintegration of the corpus luteum of the ovary and thereby maintain progesterone production critical for pregnancy in humans.

Progesterone (**choice D**) is responsible for preparing and maintaining the lining of the uterus in preparation for the fertilized egg. Progesterone secreted from the ovary is necessary for the survival of the ovum and the resulting embryo until the placenta takes over this production.

Prolactin (**choice E**) affects breast milk protein synthesis and excretion in ducts and lobules, whereas high levels also have a contraceptive effect.

51. **The correct answer is C.** This patient has Graves disease, which is the most common form of hyperthyroidism. Levothyroxine is used for treatment of hypothyroid conditions.

Antithyroid drugs such as propylthiouracil (PTU; **choice A**) or methimazole are common agents used in the treatment of Graves disease.

Patients with Graves disease often have characteristic exophthalmos, causing excessive dryness to the eyes. Therefore, methylcellulose eyedrops (**choice B**) would be a necessary treatment for a patient with that finding.

Radioactive iodine (**choice D**) is the treatment of choice for patients who are older than age 21 and would be a good initial choice for this particular patient.

Propranolol (**choice E**) is an adjunctive therapy used in Graves disease to alleviate the beta-adrenergic symptoms of hyperthyroidism (tachycardia, tremor).

52. **The correct answer is E.** Amaurosis fugax causes transient unilateral blindness secondary to retinal emboli. The patient typically describes the event as a vertical curtain passing across the visual field with unilateral blindness lasting a few minutes. Then a similar vertical curtain passes over the visual field and vision is restored.

Central retinal vein occlusion (**choice A**) presents with abrupt onset of painless, unilateral, severe visual loss. Ophthalmoscopic examination shows venous dilation, disc swelling, and retinal hemorrhages.

Central retinal artery occlusion (**choice B**) presents as sudden unilateral, painless visual loss. Typically, patients can barely count fingers in front of their face from the affected eye. Ophthalmology examination shows pallid swelling of the retina with a cherry-red spot at the fovea.

Retinal detachment (**choice C**) is characterized by abrupt, painless, unilateral blurred vision getting progressively worse. The patient may experience flashes of light, floaters, and describe the visual loss as "a curtain came over my eye." Ophthalmoscopic evaluation reveals the retina hanging in the vitreous.

Patients with open angle glaucoma (**choice D**) are asymptomatic at the early stages. Open angle glaucoma insidiously progresses. Patients have gradual peripheral vision loss.

53. **The correct answer is C.** Muffled heart sounds, shortness of breath, and tachycardia are suggestive of cardiac tamponade. A >10 mm Hg decline in systolic blood pressure during inspiration is pulsus paradoxus. It is a classic finding in cardiac tamponade. Pulsus paradoxus also occurs in restrictive lung disease.

54. **The correct answer is E.** The diagnosis of classic Wernicke triad (ophthalmoplegia, ataxia, and global confusion) and Korsakoff psychosis is considered to be a medical emergency that necessitates the immediate administration of thiamine, or vitamin B_1. Biotin (**choice A**) acts as a carrier of "activated carboxyl" groups for three key enzymes that catalyze carboxylation reactions. Symptoms of biotin deficiency are alopecia, skin and bowel inflammation, and muscle pain. Niacin (**choice B**), or vitamin B_3, is converted to nicotinamide, which is then incorporated into the coenzymes NAD^+ and $NADP^+$. Pellagra is a condition associated with a deficiency of niacin, which can result in the development of diarrhea, dermatitis, and dementia. Pyridoxine (**choice C**), or vitamin B_6, is associated with the coenzyme pyridoxal phosphate. A deficiency in pyridoxine can lead to the development of peripheral neuropathy and dermatitis. Riboflavin (**choice D**), or vitamin B_2, is responsible for maintaining proper levels of both flavin mononucleotide (FMN) and flavin adenine dinucleotide (FAD). Individuals deficient in riboflavin are likely to present with lesions of the lips, mouth, skin, and genitalia.

55. **The correct answer is D.** The most common etiology of pharyngitis is viral.

All other choices are causes of pharyngitis. Group A beta-hemolytic *Streptococcus* (**choice A**) is the most common bacterial cause, accounting for 15 to 30% of cases in children and 5 to 10% of cases in adults.

56. **The correct answer is A.** Women who undergo fertility treatment with ovarian stimulation are at an increased risk for ectopic pregnancy. Sharp pelvic pain, irregular bleeding, and an adnexal mass are classic signs of an ectopic pregnancy.

Endometrial cancer (**choice B**) most frequently affects women between 50 to 70 years of age. It often presents with abnormal bleeding.

Endometriosis (**choice C**) is caused by the growth of the endometrium outside of the uterus. It may cause infertility. Symptoms vary, depending on the location of the endometrial implants. Symptoms may include aching pain prior to menstruation, abnormal bleeding, fatigue, pain with intercourse, and painful bowel movements.

History of pelvic inflammatory disease (**choice D**) is a risk factor for ectopic pregnancy.

Uterine prolapse (**choice E**) commonly results from the injury of the pelvic floor muscles during vaginal deliveries. Uterine prolapse may also be caused by

aging and menopause, which may weaken the pelvic floor muscles. Symptoms may include vaginal pain or heaviness, difficulty urinating, pain with intercourse, and low back pain.

57. **The correct answer is E.** Squamous cell carcinoma is associated with ultraviolet radiation and human papillomavirus infection.

Actinic keratosis (**choice A**) is primarily seen in fair-skinned individuals with a history of prolonged or repeated sun exposure.

Emotional stress and exposure to hot, humid weather may be a precipitating factor for patients with dyshidrosis (**choice B**).

Seborrheic dermatitis (**choice C**) may be associated with a pre-psoriasis state. In addition, Parkinson disease, facial paralysis, and HIV-infected individuals have an increased incidence of seborrheic dermatitis.

Seborrheic keratosis (**choice D**) is hereditary and usually does not occur before 30 years of age.

58. **The correct answer is C.** If a pregnant woman is exposed to a possible rubella-infected person, hemagglutination-inhibiting rubella antibody level must be drawn. If the tests are positive, there is no need for concern. If the tests are negative, a follow-up test must be done.

Live attenuated rubella virus vaccine (**choice A**) should be administered to all infants. Therapeutic abortion (**choice B**) is an option for a pregnant woman with a rubella infection.

Counseling (**choice D**) on possible manifestations of an infant acquiring rubella infection in utero and on whether to proceed or terminate the pregnancy is important in confirmed rubella cases in pregnant women.

Acetaminophen (**choice E**) is recommended for symptomatic relief for nonpregnant rubella-infected women.

59. **The correct answer is C.** Chronic venous insufficiency (**choice A**) is incorrect. Venous insufficiency can be caused by phlebitis or leg trauma. Typically, there is ankle edema and the skin is shiny and thin. Later in the course there are pigmentation changes.

Thrombophlebitis of the deep veins (**choice B**) occurs unilaterally. There is pain in the calf or thigh associated with edema.

Livedo reticularis (**choice D**) is a vasospastic disorder. There is a mottled discoloration of large areas of extremities, which is more pronounced in cold weather.

This case presents with a venous disorder. Arterial occlusion (**choice E**) of an extremity results in pain, pallor, pulselessness, poikilothermia, paresthesias, and paralysis.

60. **The correct answer is B.** Infection with hepatitis B virus (HBV) at birth or a very young age is associated with chronic HBV infection and the development of hepatocellular carcinoma later in life. In fact, infants born to hepatitis B surface antigen (HB$_s$Ag)–positive mothers are commonly infected, and approximately 90% become chronic carriers of the virus. In chronic carriers, hepatocellular carcinoma develops at an incidence more than 200 times higher than in noncarriers. The current recommendation for infants born of HB$_s$Ag-positive mothers is administration of hepatitis B immunoglobulin (HBIg) in the delivery room, with the first dose of the hepatitis B vaccine given at the same time or within 1 week. The second and third doses of the vaccine are then given at 1 and 6 months. With this protocol, 94% protection is achieved.

Epstein-Barr virus (EBV; **choice A**) is the agent of heterophile-positive infectious mononucleosis. In children, primary EBV infection is often asymptomatic.

The measles virus (**choice C**) often causes a more severe disease in adults. The incidence of complications, including pneumonia, bacterial superinfection of the respiratory tract, bronchospasm, and hepatitis, is much higher in adults older than 20 years than in children.

Poliovirus (**choice D**) causes asymptomatic or inapparent infections 95% of the time. Frank paralysis occurs in approximately 0.1% of all poliovirus infections. However, the probability of paralysis increases with increasing age.

Varicella-zoster virus (**choice E**) is the agent of chickenpox and shingles. In immunocompetent children, it is a benign illness with a mortality of less than 2 per 100,000 cases. This risk is increased more than 15-fold in adults. Much of the increase is due to varicella pneumonitis, a complication that occurs more frequently in adults than in children.

Block 3

1. **The correct answer is A.** Warfarin acts via the liver to delay coagulation by interfering with the action of vitamin K-related factors (II, VII, IX, and X), which promotes clotting. Platelet disorders do not affect the action of vitamin K-related factors.

   The ingestion of excessive green, leafy vegetables (**choice B**) increases the body's absorption of vitamin K, which promotes blood clotting.

   Chronic diarrhea (**choice C**), alcoholism (**choice D**), and biliary obstruction (**choice E**) will increase the PT.

2. **The correct answer is A.** The most common cause of urge incontinence is inappropriate and involuntary detrusor muscle contractions.

3. **The correct answer is B.** The "statins" are a class of medications that inhibit the activity of the enzyme HMG-CoA reductase. Medications such as pravastatin and simvastatin produce a reversible inhibition of this enzyme, which subsequently leads to a reduction in LDL, total cholesterol, and triglycerides in patients with familial hypercholesterolemia.

   Chronic inflammation (**choice A**) can be effectively treated with cyclooxygenase inhibitors, including non-steroidal anti-inflammatory drugs, such as naproxen and ibuprofen, and cyclooxygenase-2 inhibitors, such as celecoxib. Essential hypertension (**choice C**) can be treated with angiotensin-converting enzyme (ACE) inhibitors, such as captopril. These agents decrease angiotensin II production and reduce systolic and diastolic blood pressure. Hyperuricemia (**choice D**) can be treated with allopurinol, which inhibits the activity of xanthine oxidase, leading to decreased production of uric acid. One of the treatment measures for type 2 diabetes (**choice E**) is to inhibit the activity of the enzyme alpha-glucosidase. Acarbose, an alpha-glucosidase inhibitor, helps prevent postprandial surges in blood glucose levels.

4. **The correct answer is A.** The patient is presenting with signs and symptoms highly suggestive of type 1 diabetes. The primary source of ketones in the urine is free fatty acid breakdown. Ketone body formation occurs as follows: insulin deficiency → activated lipolysis → increased plasma free fatty acids → increased hepatic fatty acids → accelerated ketogenesis.

   Gluconeogenesis (**choice B**) and glycogenolysis (**choice C**) occur when glucose is needed for the production of ATP in various cells in the body. Protein breakdown (**choice D**) results in the formation of amino acids. Triglyceride breakdown (**choice E**) results in the release of free fatty acids.

5. **The correct answer is C.** Complete transposition of the great arteries is the most common cyanotic lesion seen in an infant during the newborn period.

   Choices A, B, D, and E are acyanotic congenital heart lesions, though severe coarctation of the aorta may present with differential cyanosis, or cyanosis of the lower half of the body.

6. **The correct answer is D.** This patient has classic signs and symptoms of giant cell arteritis. The most serious complication is loss of vision; once it develops, it is typically permanent. Therefore, when giant cell arteritis is clinically suspected, prednisone therapy must be started immediately. Treatment should not be delayed while waiting for results of laboratory or diagnostic tests.

   A temporal artery biopsy (**choice A**) should be obtained promptly to confirm the diagnosis.

   The ESR (**choice B**) is elevated in giant cell arteritis. However, a normal ESR does not exclude a diagnosis of giant cell arteritis.

   The CBC (**choice C**) typically shows a normochromic, normocytic anemia with an elevated platelet count.

   A chest radiograph (**choice E**) is not part of the initial management. Annual chest radiographs in a patient with a history of giant cell arteritis is prudent because there is a markedly increased risk of developing an aortic aneurysm.

7. **The correct answer is C.** Central diabetes insipidus results from an insufficient amount of vasopressin. A vasopressin challenge test would confirm a diagnosis of central diabetes insipidus.

   A urine culture (**choice A**) is used to check for a urinary tract infection. An oral glucose tolerance test (**choice B**) is used to assess diabetes mellitus. Dexamethasone suppression test (**choice D**) is performed when overproduction of cortisol is suspected, and plasma growth hormone levels (**choice E**) are used to measure growth hormone levels.

8. **The correct answer is E.** The child has a classic presentation of erythema infectiosum, which is caused by the human parvovirus B19. The intensely erythematous cheeks, sometimes described as "slapped cheeks," will resolve spontaneously, and a reticular rash on the neck, trunk, and arms will appear. The condition is self-limiting and resolves in 2 to 3 weeks. Treatment consists of symptomatic management of fever, pain, or itching.

Antibiotics (**choice A**) have no activity against parvovirus, the causative organism of erythema infectiosum.

Antiviral therapy (**choice B**) is only effective in certain conditions, such as herpes simplex virus, varicella-zoster virus, cytomegalovirus, and respiratory syncytial virus. There is no effective antiviral with activity against parvovirus B19.

Immunoglobulin (**choice C**) is used in patients in an immunocompromised state. It is not needed in an otherwise healthy patient.

Racemic epinephrine (**choice D**) is used in the management of croup.

9. **The correct answer is A.** This is the classic presentation of squamous cell carcinoma of the esophagus. Smoking and alcohol are risk factors for cancer of the esophagus.

Gastric cancer (**choice B**) may present with weight loss, but instead of dysphagia (difficulty swallowing) the patient will have dyspepsia or epigastric discomfort.

Achalasia (**choice C**) is a primary motility disorder of the esophageal innervation and peristalsis. It most frequently presents with dysphagia for *both* solids and liquids.

An esophageal stricture (**choice D**) may present in a similar manner; however, the dysphagia is intermittent and not progressive. The most common stricture is a Schatzki ring.

Barrett esophagus (**choice E**) is a complication of long-standing reflux disease. Essentially, it is a metaplastic change of the epithelium of the lower esophagus. High-grade dysplasia may progress to adenocarcinoma.

10. **The correct answer is E.** The difficulty with developing a vaccine against influenza A arises because the influenza virus genome is composed of eight strands of single-stranded RNA. Minor shifts (antigenic drift) in surface antigens occur as point mutations in the genes accumulate. However, influenza A can also undergo larger, abrupt changes in antigen expression (antigenic shift) as a consequence of reassortment of some of the RNA fragments between human and nonhuman hosts. Thus, last year's vaccine does not necessarily work against this year's virus. Polysaccharide coats (**choice A**) are a virulence factor of some bacteria, not of viruses. Influenza A can compromise the lungs sufficiently to predispose to secondary infections, producing a functional immunosuppression (**choice B**), but this attribute does not make it difficult to produce vaccines

against the virus. Unlike AIDS, influenza virus does not selectively target lymphocytes (**choice C**). Influenza A, bound to antibody and complement, can be effectively phagocytized (compare with **choice D**).

11. **The correct answer is D.** Serum FSH levels begin to rise prior to menopause and may remain elevated throughout the menopausal transition. FSH levels may also be normal at times in menopausal women, so measurement of serum FSH is not recommended for the diagnosis of menopause. However, of all the answer choices, this is the most correct, as increased FSH is, indeed, suggestive of menopause. LH (**choice B**) is also elevated in menopause.

12. **The correct answer is A.** Wearing waist-high elastic hosiery prevents venous pooling, which can prevent orthostatic hypotension.

Daily use of an alpha blocker (**choice B**) would lower blood pressure and worsen orthostatic hypotension.

Potassium supplementation (**choice C**) would have no effects on blood pressure.

Moving quickly from a sitting to standing (**choice D**) position could worsen hypotension.

Prolonged recumbency (**choice E**) should be avoided as it can cause an inadequate vasoconstrictor reflex response.

13. **The correct answer is D.** This patient likely has cholelithiasis, with possible acute cholecystitis. The typical patient is "fat, female, fertile, and older than 40." The RUQ tenderness on inspiration is called the Murphy sign and is characteristic of biliary inflammation. In this patient, inflammation of the gallbladder might produce irritation of the central diaphragmatic pleura, which is innervated by the phrenic nerve. The dermatome of the nerve root of the phrenic nerve (C3 to C5) includes the right shoulder.

The expiratory motor neurons (**choice A**) are located in the lower medulla. They operate only during forced expiration to initiate contraction in expiratory muscles via alpha motor fibers. The inspiratory motor neurons (**choice B**) are located in the upper part of the medulla and send impulses via alpha motor fibers to the muscles of inspiration. They play no role in the Murphy sign. The intercostal nerves (**choice C**) innervate the costal and peripheral portions of the diaphragmatic pleura. The vagus nerve (**choice E**) mediates the Hering-Breuer (stretch-inflation) reflex of breathing.

14. **The correct answer is D.** Punishment within the operant conditioning paradigm means that an applied stimulus stops a behavior. In this case, the man feels uncomfortable (stimulus) and this results in stopping exercise (response).

Classical conditioning is an old response (salivation) to a new stimulus (bell). Extinction of a classically conditioned response (**choice A**) does not mean that the response goes away, merely that it is no longer evoked by the new stimulus. The dog keeps salivating to the meat, but no longer salivates to the bell.

Extinction in an operant conditioning paradigm (**choice B**) means that a removed stimulus stops a behavior. In the present case, it is the addition of a stimulus (the man feels uncomfortable), not the removal, that stops the behavior.

Negative reinforcement (**choice C**) in an operant conditioning paradigm means that a removed stimulus increases a behavioral response. The present case is the exact opposite—the stimulus is added and the behavior stops.

A secondary reinforcer (**choice E**) is something that has no value in and of itself, but modifies behavior because of what it represents. A dollar is only a piece of paper, but symbolizes so much more. In this case, it is the addition of the discomfort, not the removal of any reinforcer, that stops the behavior.

15. **The correct answer is E.** The pouch of Douglas, also known as the rectouterine pouch, is situated between the rectum, uterus, and posterior fornix of the vagina.

The vesicouterine pouch is found between the bladder (**choice A**) and uterus. There are no pouches between the uterus and the cervix (**choice B**), fallopian tubes (**choice C**), or ovaries (**choice D**).

16. **The correct answer is A.** Hepatocellular carcinoma is associated with aflatoxin exposure. Aflatoxin is produced by *Aspergillus flavus* and *Aspergillus parasiticus*. Arsenic exposure (**choice B**) is associated with squamous cell carcinoma of the skin. Vinyl chloride (**choice E**) is responsible for angiosarcoma of the liver.

17. **The correct answer is C.** Mesothelioma is a result of asbestos exposure. Nitrosamines (**choice D**) can result in esophageal and gastric carcinomas.

18. **The correct answer is choice D.** Hypoparathyroidism most commonly occurs after a thyroidectomy. It is characterized by lethargy, irritability, muscle aches, and tingling around the mouth, hands, and feet.

Hypocalcemia causes patients to have Chvostek's sign and Trousseau phenomenon.

19. **The correct answer is C.** IV drug users are at an increased risk of developing infective endocarditis. Suggestive findings include a Janeway lesion, small hemorrhages on the palms or soles, subungual splinter hemorrhages, fever, and a new onset of a murmur.

Infectious mononucleosis (**choice B**) is incorrect. It presents with malaise, fever, sore throat, and lymphadenopathy. Occasionally, there is a maculopapular rash.

Polymyalgia rheumatica (**choice A**) is characterized by pain and stiffness of the shoulders and pelvic girdle musculature. Constitutional symptoms such as fever and malaise are common.

Scarlet fever (**choice D**) is an exotoxin-mediated disease arising from group A beta-hemolytic streptococcal infection. There are prodromal symptoms of fever, malaise, and sore throat. The rash of scarlet fever is generalized, erythematous, and punctuate and has the texture of sandpaper.

Dermatomyositis (**choice E**) presents with bilateral proximal muscle weakness. The patient will have difficulty rising from a chair. Serum levels of muscle enzymes are elevated. A diffuse, flat, erythematous rash is noted on the neck and upper chest.

20. **The correct answer is D.** Kawasaki disease is treated with high-dose aspirin. Aspirin will lower the fever, help with joint pain, and prevent clot formation. A common complication of the disease is arteritis of the coronary vessels, which, on occasion, can cause myocardial infarction.

Ordinarily, aspirin is not given to children because of its association with Reye syndrome. Acetaminophen (**choice A**) is often used as an antipyretic in children but it does not have antiplatelet activity, as aspirin does.

Ibuprofen (**choice E**) is not an effective treatment (it would only treat the fever).

The etiology of Kawasaki disease is unknown. Antibiotics, such as amoxicillin (**choice B**), are not appropriate.

Diarrhea is a complication of the disease. Oral hydration (**choice C**) would be appropriate to prevent dehydration but it is not the most appropriate treatment.

21. **The correct answer is C.** Triple therapy with a PPI, clarithromycin, and amoxicillin for 10 to 14 days is the accepted therapy. If the patient is allergic to penicillin, metronidazole may be substituted for the amoxicillin.

22. **The correct answer is B.** Bronchogenic adenocarcinoma is only weakly associated with smoking. This disorder is the most common lung cancer seen in non-smokers and in women. Bronchioloalveolar carcinoma (**choice A**) is a relatively uncommon form of carcinoma of the lung. It arises in the lung periphery and does not appear to be clearly related to smoking. Large cell (anaplastic) carcinomas (**choice C**) are unusual and probably represent undifferentiated variants of squamous cell and bronchogenic adenocarcinomas. Small cell (oat cell) carcinoma (**choice D**) is very strongly associated with smoking. Squamous cell carcinoma (**choice E**) is very strongly associated with smoking.

23. **The correct answer is D.** The most important risk to this patient is liver damage by free radical species derived from carbon tetrachloride (CCl_4), notably CCl_3. These species are produced when the hepatic P-450 microsomal system attempts to degrade the CCl_4. They can cause severe, sometimes fatal, fatty liver damage by reacting with the polyenoic (multiple double bonds) acids present in the membrane phospholipids. The reaction is particularly harmful because peroxides are often formed as a by-product. Peroxides can be autocatalytic, in that the peroxide radicals themselves form new free radicals capable of more damage to membranes and other cellular structures. Clinically, patients may have an extremely rapid (30 minutes to 2 hours) decline in hepatic function after the carbon tetrachloride exposure. Other organs are not affected to the same degree because of the relatively lower concentration of the toxic metabolites there.

24. **The correct answer is B.** Wegener granulomatosis is a necrotizing vasculitis that affects small arteries and veins. This disease develops over a period of months and classically involves the nose, sinuses, lungs, and kidneys. Patients usually present with upper or lower respiratory symptoms such as chronic sinusitis, otitis, hemoptysis, nasopharyngeal ulcerations, and bilateral pneumonitis with nodular and cavitary pulmonary infiltrates. Renal manifestations are due to the same process. IgG and complement are found in renal biopsies, but the most specific laboratory finding is the presence of circulating c-ANCA. This form of glomerulonephritis is classified among the pauci-immune glomerulonephritis. The cytoplasmic pattern of ANCA (c-ANCA) is due to antibodies directed against the neutrophil proteinase-3. Treatment is with immunosuppressive drugs such as cyclophosphamide.

None of the other choices are consistent with the clinical history. None of them are related to a necrotizing vasculitis with granulomas affecting small arteries and veins.

25. **The correct answer is A.** Postmenopausal women are susceptible to atrophic vaginitis secondary to decreases in estrogen levels. Symptoms include vaginal soreness or itching, burning on urination, and painful intercourse. Exam reveals thin, pale vaginal walls.

Bacterial vaginosis (**choice B**) is caused by an overgrowth of *Gardnerella* and other anaerobes. It is characterized by a malodorous, grayish discharge. A whiff test is positive.

Patients with cervicitis (**choice C**) often present with discharge, spotting, and cervical erythema. Cervicitis is most frequently caused by sexually transmitted diseases.

Endometrial cancer (**choice D**) most frequently affects women between 50 to 70 years of age. It often presents with abnormal bleeding.

Uterine prolapse (**choice E**) may also be caused by aging and menopause, which may weaken the pelvic floor muscles. Symptoms may include vaginal pain or heaviness, difficulty urinating, pain with intercourse, and low back pain.

26. **The correct answer is D.** Lead poisoning is the most common type of chronic metal poisoning in the United States, primarily affecting children in poor urban areas. Central nervous toxicity includes lethargy, somnolence, cognitive impairment, and behavioral problems and can lead to cerebral edema and encephalopathy. Abdominal pain is one of the most common symptoms. Laboratory findings are characteristic for a microcytic anemia with basophilic stippling. An x-ray of long bones will show lead lines at the epiphyseal plates, and deposits of lead can be seen at the gingivodental line (lead lines). Chelating drugs are the treatment of choice.

As with most large-dose pill ingestions, acetaminophen poisoning (**choice A**) will produce nausea and vomiting. Signs of liver failure are present after the first 72 hours postingestion.

Patients with chronic arsenic poisoning (**choice B**) present with malaise, abdominal pain, peripheral neuropathy, muscular weakness, and skin changes (hyperpigmentation and dermatitis). Arsenic deposits on the fingernails create transverse lines called Mess lines.

Patients with carbon monoxide poisoning (**choice C**) present with a bright, "cherry red" color of the skin, mucosal membranes, and the blood. Symptoms include headache and shortness of breath. Treatment is 100% oxygen.

Abdominal pain, vomiting, and diarrhea are characteristic of mushroom poisoning (**choice E**). Fulminant hepatitis with extensive liver necrosis is a late complication.

27. **The correct answer is E.** *Strongyloides stercoralis* (threadworm) is a nematode that can potentially be lethal because of its unique ability to cause autoinfection. It is widely distributed in the tropics, although in the United States a prevalence of 0.4 to 4% has been estimated in the South. *S. stercoralis* has a complex life cycle. The filariform larvae, the infective stage, penetrate the skin and migrate through the bloodstream. Ultimately, they reside in the small intestine, where eggs are laid in the mucosa. The eggs usually hatch in tissue, and rhabditiform larvae are passed in stool. In the soil, the rhabditiform larvae may undergo the direct development cycle and become the infective form, or they may undergo the indirect development cycle and become free-living adults. Autoinfection of the host is also possible because a relatively short period of time is necessary for rhabditiform larvae to develop into the infective filariform larvae, and this change can occur in the intestine or on the perianal skin. Unlike most other worm infections, in strongyloidiasis the worm burden of the host depends not only on the initial size of the larval inoculum but also on the amount of autoinfection. The symptoms of strongyloidiasis correspond to the three stages of infection. During the dermal stage, there is an immediate hypersensitivity reaction to the migrating worms. Patients may experience symptoms from itching to urticaria. In the migration stage, passage through the lungs can cause Loeffler's syndrome. In the intestinal phase, the parasites may cause superficial damage to the mucosa, leading to intermittent watery diarrhea and burning or colicky abdominal pain. If the host becomes immunosuppressed, such as during cancer chemotherapy or steroid treatment, disseminated infection can occur. This massive larval invasion causes severe generalized abdominal pain, distension, fever, cough, shock, and meningitis or sepsis. Infection with *S. stercoralis* can be eradicated with thiabendazole.

Ingestion of eggs in contaminated water (**choice A**) is an unlikely way of acquiring an intestinal helminth. In the life cycle of most organisms that infect a host through the ingestion of eggs, infection occurs when fecal material is used as fertilizer and contaminates foodstuff.

Ingestion of infected feces (**choice B**) is not the typical means of acquiring a helminth infection. Usually, the fecal material contaminating a food source is unwittingly consumed.

Ingestion of larvae in infected meat (**choice C**) is the means by which parasites, such as tapeworms and the nematode *Trichinella*, are acquired.

Mosquito inoculation of the larvae (**choice D**) is the means by which the agents of lymphatic filariasis are acquired.

28. **The correct answer is A.** An annular pancreas may exert pressure on the duodenum, causing the patient to vomit bile-stained material. This condition is the result of the ventral pancreatic bud's failure to migrate normally.

Esophageal atresia (**choice B**) is diagnosed shortly after birth. Milk cannot reach the stomach and is therefore quickly regurgitated in an undigested state.

The lodging of one or more gallstones (**choice C**) in the extrahepatic biliary apparatus may cause indigestion, severe pain, and jaundice.

Meckel (ileal) diverticulum (**choice D**) is persistence of a portion of the embryonic vitelline duct (yolk stalk). It is usually asymptomatic but may cause bleeding or ulceration because of the presence of ectopic gastric tissue. Pyloric stenosis (**choice E**) is a congenital thickening of the smooth muscle in the wall of the pyloric portion of the stomach. It is usually diagnosed in infants following episodes of projectile vomiting.

29. **The correct answer is C.** Atrial septal defects are often asymptomatic. Larger defects may cause exertional dyspnea. Objective findings include a fixed split S_2 and a grade I-III/VI systolic ejection murmur at the pulmonic area.

Aortic stenosis (**choice A**) is a systolic ejection murmur that is best heard at the right second intercostal space. It often radiates to the neck and down the left sternal border.

The clinical features of a ventricular septal defect (**choice B**) depend on the size of the defect. There may be a loud, harsh, systolic murmur best heard at the left sternal border.

Choices D and E are incorrect. Mitral regurgitation and tricuspid regurgitation are systolic murmurs. A mitral regurgitation murmur is best heard at the apex and radiates to the left axilla. Tricuspid regurgitation is best heard at the lower left sternal border. It radiates to the right of the sternum and xiphoid area.

30. **The correct answer is E.** Patients with sickle cell anemia are at high risk of developing aplastic anemia, especially with parvovirus B19 infection, due to the

fact that by the age of 6 years most of these patients will have no spleen. Autosplenectomy is caused by chronic capillary thrombi as a result of sickle cells blocking small vessels.

CMV (**choice A**) is the most common in utero infection. This disease ranges from infected but no obvious defects to severe cytomegalic inclusion disease (jaundice, hepatosplenomegaly, thrombocytic purpura).

EBV (**choice B**) causes infectious mononucleosis. Epstein-Barr virus has been associated with Burkitt lymphoma, nasopharyngeal carcinoma, and thymus carcinoma.

Gingivostomatitis, keratoconjunctivitis, and meningoencephalitis are the clinical presentations of herpes simplex I (**choice C**).

HPV (**choice D**) serotype 1 and 4 are related to plantar warts; serotype 6 and 11 have been related to anogenital and laryngeal papillomas; and 16 and 18 are related to cervical intraepithelial neoplasias.

31. **The correct answer is C.** The patient has eclampsia; first-line therapy is magnesium sulfate.

Calcium gluconate (**choice A**) is used when there is magnesium toxicity.

Diazepam (**choice B**) may be used in treatment of eclampsia, but it is not considered first-line therapy.

An obstetric consult (**choice D**) is important, but it is not the most appropriate intervention. The seizure must be stopped immediately.

Phenytoin (**choice E**) is an FDA fetal risk D. Phenytoin may be used to treat seizures in nonpregnant individuals.

32. **The correct answer is D.** Platelets (**choice B**) are incorrect. However, heparin can induce transient thrombocytopenia. Patients receiving heparin should have platelet counts measured.

N-acetylcysteine (**choice A**) is the antidote for acetaminophen toxicity.

Vitamin K (**choice C**) is the antidote for an overdose of warfarin.

Flumazenil (**choice E**) is used in the reversal of the sedative effects of benzodiazepines.

33. **The correct answer is C.** A hydatidiform mole can present with severe nausea, vomiting, and vaginal bleeding. The ultrasound will show a "snowstorm appearance," an enlarged uterus, and a lack of a fetus.

An ectopic pregnancy (**choice A**) may present with spotting and cramping shortly after the first missed period. Objective findings show lower abdominal peritoneal irritation, an enlarged uterus, and a tender mass in one adnexum. Ultrasound will show an enlarged uterus with no fetus.

Hemorrhage (**choice B**) is a complication of a hydatidiform mole.

An intrauterine infection (**choice D**) is a complication of a hydatidiform mole.

34. **The correct answer is A.** During complete heart block, no atrial impulses are conducted to the ventricles; the atria and the ventricles are depolarized by their respective pacemakers, independent of each other. A pacemaker is needed to initiate the impulse. Complete heart block is life-threatening.

Acute inferior wall myocardial infarction can cause heart block; however, empiric thrombolytic therapy (**choice B**) is not appropriate.

Cardioversion (**choice C**) and adenosine (**choice D**) are not appropriate treatments for complete heart block.

Beta-blockers (such as propranolol, **choice E**) can cause varying degrees of heart block.

35. **The correct answer is E.** Following antineoplastic therapy for treatment of acute lymphocytic leukemia, patients often have a high level of urate secondary to the breakdown of nucleic acids. Therefore, patients are often given allopurinol to decrease plasma urate levels. Allopurinol prevents uric acid formation by inhibiting the enzyme xanthine oxidase. Decreasing uric acid levels will help prevent the formation of kidney stones, as well as block the appearance of other deleterious effects of hyperuricemia. Acarbose is an agent used in the treatment of type 2 diabetes. It inhibits the activity of alpha-glucosidase (**choice A**) in the intestinal tract, thereby helping to prevent postprandial hyperglycemia. Inhibition of angiotensin-converting enzyme (**choice B**) will lower blood pressure and help prevent the "ventricular remodeling" that occurs secondary to congestive heart failure. Beta-lactamase (**choice C**) inhibitors are combined with penicillin antibiotics to help improve their activity against bacteria that produce the enzyme beta-lactamase. Nonsteroidal anti-inflammatory drugs (NSAIDs) inhibit the activity of the enzyme cyclooxygenase (**choice D**), thereby decreasing the production of prostaglandins.

36. **The correct answer is A.** *Bacillus cereus* contaminates grains, such as rice, and produces spores resistant to

quick frying and steaming. If you see the words "fried rice," the odds are that the correct answer is *B. cereus*. *Campylobacter jejuni* (**choice B**) causes enterocolitis with bloody diarrhea, crampy abdominal pain, malaise, and fever. *Clostridium botulinum* (**choice C**) produces a constellation of signs and symptoms, including bulbar palsy, descending weakness or paralysis, progressive respiratory weakness, absence of fever, dry mucous membranes, and autonomic dysfunction. *Clostridium difficile* (**choice D**) causes pseudomembranous colitis, classically resulting from clindamycin use. *Escherichia coli* (**choice E**) comes in a variety of forms. The enterotoxigenic type is the most common cause of traveler's diarrhea.

37. **The correct answer is E.** The patient is presenting with the signs and symptoms of Wernicke's encephalopathy, which consists of the classic triad of ophthalmoplegia, ataxia, and global confusion. This syndrome is considered a medical emergency and necessitates immediate administration of thiamine, or vitamin B_1. Biotin (**choice A**) acts as a carrier of "activated carboxyl" groups for three key enzymes that catalyze carboxylation reactions. Symptoms of biotin deficiency include alopecia, skin and bowel inflammation, and muscle pain. Niacin (**choice B**), or vitamin B_3, is converted to nicotinamide, which is then incorporated into the coenzymes NAD^+ and $NADP^+$. Pellagra, a condition associated with niacin deficiency, leads to diarrhea, dermatitis, and dementia. Pyridoxine (**choice C**), or vitamin B_6, is utilized as the coenzyme pyridoxal phosphate. A deficiency in pyridoxine can lead to peripheral neuropathy and dermatitis. Riboflavin (**choice D**), or vitamin B_2, is responsible for maintaining proper levels of both FMN and FAD. Individuals with riboflavin deficiency are likely to present with lesions of the lips, mouth, skin, and genitalia.

38. **The correct answer is C.** Renin levels increase when there is decreased renal perfusion pressure, as in coarctation of the aorta.

A CBC (**choice A**) is a basic screening panel. It provides hematologic information.

Partial thromboplastin time (**choice B**) and prothrombin time (**choice D**) screen for coagulation disorders.

Total metanephrine (**choice E**) is used to help diagnose pheochromocytoma.

39. **The correct answer is B.** Phlebitis is an inflammation of the vein. It is often caused by local irritation, such as an intravenous line. Warm soaks and NSAIDs are the treatment of choice.

Anticoagulation (**choices A and C**) is the treatment for thrombophlebitis.

Antibiotics (such as cephalexin, **choice D**) are not an appropriate treatment for phlebitis. Antibiotics should be use in septic thrombophlebitis.

Excision of the involved vein (**choice E**) is used in the treatment of septic thrombophlebitis.

40. **The correct answer is E.** The patient has mild preeclampsia and should be managed with strict bed rest. A normal salt intake and an increased water intake should be advised. The patient should be instructed to lie on her left side to lessen intravascular dehydration and to increase urine output.

41. **The correct answer is B.** A toxin-secreting bacterium, *Clostridium botulinum,* causes botulism. The toxin blocks the release of acetylcholine at autonomic synapses and neuromuscular junctions, causing sudden muscle weakness. Spores of *Clostridium botulinum* have been found in honey and canned goods.

Adenovirus infection (**choice A**) would present with respiratory and gastrointestinal symptoms. Congenital hypothyroidism (**choice C**) usually presents at birth. The infant may have coarse facial features as well as an enlarged tongue. Congenital myasthenia gravis (**choice D**) usually presents at or close to birth. Reye's syndrome (**choice E**) usually is suspected after a viral illness or prolonged exposure to NSAIDs.

42. **The correct answer is C.** Most folliculitis is caused by the common organism *Staphylococcus aureus.* However, "hot-tub" folliculitis is caused by *Pseudomonas aeruginosa. Pseudomonas* survives in hot tubs, especially those made of wood, unless the pH and chlorine content are strictly controlled.

Choices A, B, D, and E are incorrect. They can all be causes of folliculitis, although *P. aeruginosa* is the most common organism, causing perifollicular lesions with some pustules that are associated with hot tub use.

43. **The correct answer is A.** Immunity to hepatitis B infection is conferred by antibody against the hepatitis B surface antigen (HB_sAg). The hepatitis B vaccine is a noninfectious subunit vaccine that is composed of hepatitis B surface antigen (HB_sAg) produced in yeast cells using recombinant DNA techniques. Because it is a subunit vaccine, a response is only raised to HB_sAg, which accounts for the absence of antibodies to other viral components that occur during natural infection.

Choice B cannot be a true statement because at the resolution of a natural hepatitis B infection, antibodies against hepatitis B e antigen (HB_eAg) and hepatitis B c antigen (HB_cAg) are also seen.

Choice C cannot be a true statement because chronic carriers are incapable of making antibodies against HB_sAg.

Choice D cannot be correct because the donor lacks any other hepatitis B virus antigens or antibodies against them. Of special note, he lacks anti-HB_cAg. Presence of this antibody in the sera is evidence that the patient has been infected with hepatitis B virus. Even during the "window period," when other antibodies against the virus and viral antigens may not be detectable, antibody against HB_cAg will be detectable.

Choice E cannot be correct because there is no serologic evidence that he is infected with hepatitis B virus.

44. **The correct answer is B.** In a patient with MVP who complains of chest pain or palpitations, beta-blockers may be effective therapy.

   Patients with MVP and mitral valve regurgitation are at risk for stroke. It has been recommended that patients with redundant and thickened mitral valves use low-dose aspirin (**choice C**) daily.

   Most asymptomatic patients with MVP require no therapy (**choice D**).

   Patients with MVP may also have mitral valve regurgitation. Mitral valve regurgitation may be treated with mitral valve repair (**choice A**). In chronic mitral valve regurgitation, digitalis therapy may be of some benefit.

   In MVP, digitalis therapy (**choice E**) is of little use because contractile function is essentially normal.

45. **The correct answer is B.** An L/S (lecithin to sphingomyelin) ratio of 2:1 usually indicates pulmonary maturity.

   Choices A, C, D, and E are all risk factors for hyaline membrane disease.

46. **The correct answer is D.** If the patient does not have any contraindications to surgery, the treatment of choice for patients with non–small cell carcinoma is surgical resection. Neoadjuvant therapy may be used in addition to surgical resection.

47. **The correct answer is C.** Patients with an aortic dissection complain of sudden, severe chest pain that radiates to the back. The chest radiograph shows widening of the mediastinum.

Clinical presentation of an aortic dissection can be confused with myocardial infarction (**choice A**). Aortic dissections will have negative cardiac enzymes.

PE (**choice B**) should be on the differential diagnosis when a patient presents with sudden chest pain. Patients with a PE can also have shortness of breath, hemoptysis, or syncope. The chest radiograph frequently shows pleural effusions, atelectasis, and parenchymal infiltrates that are nonspecific.

Cor pulmonale (**choice D**) is characterized by right ventricular hypertrophy and subsequent right ventricle failure. Signs and symptoms include dyspnea on exertion, chronic cough, wheezing, and easy fatigability.

Constrictive pericarditis (**choice E**) often presents with progressive fatigue, dyspnea, and weakness. A chest radiograph may show cardiomegaly.

48. **The correct answer is C.** Calcium channel blockers, such as amlodipine, are used during vasospasm episodes and are effective prophylactically as well.

   Beta-blockers (such as propranolol, **choice A**) can exacerbate coronary vasospasm.

   Aspirin (**choice B**) is prescribed for patients with angina to avoid coronary thrombosis.

   Streptokinase therapy (**choice D**) and heparin (**choice E**) are inappropriate here. Prinzmetal angina is caused by coronary vasospasm, not a thrombolic event. Thrombolytics or anticoagulation may be used in the treatment of unstable angina.

49. **The correct answer is D.** Choices A, B, C, and E are all relative contraindications to fibrolytic therapy.

50. **The correct answer is A.** Secondary hypertension has a specific cause, such as coarctation of the aorta, pheochromocytoma, renal vascular hypertension, estrogen use, etc. If a patient's blood pressure is nonresponsive to antihypertensives, you must suspect secondary hypertension.

51. **The correct answer is B.** ACE inhibitors, such as benazepril, are nephroprotective and should be prescribed to hypertensive diabetic patients.

   Hydrochlorothiazide (**choice A**) and furosemide (**choice E**) may cause hyperglycemia and should be used cautiously in diabetic patients.

   Atorvastatin (**choice D**) is a lipid-lowering drug. There is no information provided that indicates its use.

52. **The correct answer is A.** Incision and drainage of the abscess is required. An empiric course of penicillin (**choice C**) should be initiated until cultures and sensitivity studies return. If the peritonsillar abscess recurs, tonsillectomy (**choice B**) may be indicated. It is usually performed after the acute infection has subsided. Viscous lidocaine (**choice D**) would only anesthetize the area and treat it symptomatically, and aspirin (**choice E**) would also only treat the patient's symptoms and would increase the chance of bleeding complications during the incision and drainage.

53. **The correct answer is E.** Arterial insufficiency presents with intermittent claudication that progresses to pain at rest. Objective findings show decreased or absent pulses; absent or mild edema; shiny, atrophic skin; and loss of hair over the foot and toes.

Venous insufficiency (**choice A**) is incorrect. Venous insufficiency is caused by chronic obstruction or valvular incompetence of the deep lower veins. Patients complain of a generalized ache in the lower extremities, made worse with prolonged standing and alleviated with elevation of the lower extremities. Typical physical findings include pitting edema and shiny, atrophic, brownish skin. Ulcerations may develop at the side of the ankle, especially medially.

Patients with varicose veins (**choice B**) present with an achiness of the lower extremities. The veins are tortuous and dilated. Because the varicosities are part of the venous system, the patient's pulses are unaffected.

Thrombophlebitis (**choice C**) occurs unilaterally. There is pain in the calf or thigh associated with edema.

Thromboangiitis obliterans (**choice D**), also known as Buerger disease, occurs almost always in young men who smoke. It is an episodic, segmental, inflammatory vaso-occlusive disease of primarily the distal extremities.

54. **The correct answer is D.** This infant is exhibiting passive immunity acquired from his mother in utero. IgG is the only class of immunoglobulins that can cross the placenta. As such, IgG molecules diffuse into the fetal circulation, providing immunity. This circulating maternal IgG protects the newborn during the first 4 to 6 months of life. Note that IgG is also capable of opsonization and complement activation (a feature shared with IgM).

IgA (**choice A**) functions in the secretory immune response. The secretory form of this immunoglobulin (sIgA) is found in tears, colostrum, saliva, breast milk, and other secretions. It is produced by the plasma cells in the lamina propria of the gastrointestinal and respiratory tracts.

IgD (**choice B**) functions as a cell surface antigen receptor on undifferentiated B cells. IgE (**choice C**) is involved in the allergic response and immediate hypersensitivity reactions. The Fc region of IgE binds to the surface of basophils and mast cells. Antigen binding to two IgE molecules leads to mast cell degranulation and the release of leukotrienes, histamine, eosinophil chemotactic factors, and heparin.

IgM (**choice E**) is the first antibody detected in serum after exposure to antigen. IgM circulates as a pentamer and thus has five Fc regions. This structure makes it especially effective in fixing complement.

55. **The correct answer is D.** This patient has not been controlling his blood glucose for several months, as evidenced by his glycosylated hemoglobin (HbA_{1c}), where the goal is <7.0%. His current sugar level is an immediate concern and should be quickly lowered by using a rapid-acting insulin such as insulin lispro or insulin aspart. These rapid-acting insulins will begin to lower blood sugar within 15 minutes of injection.

Glucagon (**choice A**) is used to correct hypoglycemia by raising the blood glucose level quickly and would be contraindicated in this situation.

Metformin (**choice B**) is an oral agent that controls blood glucose by decreasing peripheral insulin resistance. It is a first-line agent of choice in most type 2 diabetics but may not be of immediate use for an extremely elevated blood glucose level that needs to be quickly reduced.

Insulin glargine (**choice C**) is a peakless, long-acting insulin lasting 24 hours. Its onset, however, takes 2 to 4 hours and would not be the best choice in this situation.

Exercise and weight loss (**choice E**) are important nonpharmacologic therapies for all diabetics; such measures increase the cellular glucose uptake by the muscles. However, this mainstay is a lifestyle change that will produce long-term improvement, but will do nothing to immediately lower his blood sugar.

56. **The correct answer is D.** Rosacea is exacerbated by both alcoholic and hot beverages. Both can increase the reactivity of capillaries and lead to telangiectasias.

57. **The correct answer is B.** This patient has chronic digitalis toxicity. A review of medications is crucial.

    Choices A, C, D, and E are correct components of history-taking, but they are not the most useful in this case.

58. **The correct answer is D.** The patient presents with typical symptoms of a rectocele. Patients often complain of a vaginal bulge, pain with intercourse, constipation, and difficulty with evacuation. Women may also report that pressing against the lower back wall of the vagina helps with evacuation.

    Women with a cystocele (**choice A**) may report incomplete bladder emptying or unwanted urine leakage when coughing or laughing. Women may also report pelvic pain and the feeling of a bulge in the vagina.

    An enterocele (**choice B**) frequently is asymptomatic. Some women may have a sense of fullness, pressure, or pain in the pelvis.

    An incompetent cervix (**choice C**) occurs during pregnancy when the cervix opens too early, which may lead to a miscarriage or premature delivery. An incompetent cervix is usually asymptomatic until the miscarriage.

    Uterine prolapse (**choice E**) is often asymptomatic. Symptomatic uterine prolapse may present with low back pain, vaginal fullness, coital difficulty, and voiding and evacuation difficulties.

59. **The correct answer is D.** Nasal oxymetazoline is an over-the-counter medication that when used longer than a few days causes rebound nasal congestion.

60. **The correct answer is A.** Heparin is indicated in the prevention of embolism. Streptokinase (**choice C**) is a thrombolytic and is only used in the acute treatment of a pulmonary embolism in high-risk patients. Warfarin (**choice B**) is not indicated due to its prolonged onset of action. Intermittent pneumatic compression (**choice D**) and postoperative early ambulation (**choice E**) are not indicated unless the patient has active bleeding or at high risk for active bleeding.

Block 4

1. **The correct answer is B.** A pterygium is a benign growth of the conjunctiva. It typically grows from the nasal side of the eye onto the cornea. Risk factors include exposure to sunny, windy, and dusty areas.

   Hordeolum (**choice A**) is a common staphylococcal infection of the lid glands. The symptoms include swelling, redness, and pain. There are two specific types: internal hordeolum is relatively the larger of the two and affects the meibomian glands. It may point toward the skin or toward the conjunctiva. The external hordeolum ("sty") is relatively smaller and more superficial. This is an infection of the glands of Moll or Zeiss, is usually painful, and always points toward the skin side of the lid margin.

   A chalazion (**choice C**) is a small lump in the eyelid caused by obstruction of the meibomian gland. Conjunctivitis (**choice D**) is redness and inflammation of the conjunctiva, which coats the whites of the eye and lines the inside of the eyelids. A cataract (**choice E**) is a clouding of the lens of the eye that affects vision.

2. **The correct answer is A.** Unilateral blindness with normal sympathetic and parasympathetic innervations to both irises does not cause anisocoria.

3. **The correct answer is C.** The presence of sickle cell disease in a question stem is usually a significant clue. This question tests whether you know that patients with sickle cell anemia are more susceptible to osteomyelitis caused by *Salmonella*. (The patient's fever, bone pain, and x-ray results indicate osteomyelitis). Note, however, that *Staphylococcus aureus* (gram-positive coccus) is the most common cause of osteomyelitis in patients with or without sickle cell disease. If it had not been ruled out on bone culture, you should have looked for it in the answer choices.

   Vibrio cholerae (**choice A**), a gram-negative rod, causes severe endotoxin-induced diarrhea with "rice-water" stools and dehydration. *Legionella* (**choice B**), a gram-negative rod, contaminates air-conditioning cooling towers and causes Legionnaire disease. *Pseudomonas* (**choice D**) is a gram-negative rod that colonizes the lungs of patients with cystic fibrosis. *Shigella* (**choice E**) causes bacillary dysentery with abdominal cramps, fever, and mucoid, bloody diarrhea.

4. **The correct answer is E.** Sodium intake should be reduced to 2.3 g of sodium or 6 g of sodium chloride per day.

   Choices A, B, C, and D are lifestyle modifications for hypertension prevention and management set forth by the Joint National Committee on Detection, Education, and Treatment of High Blood Pressure.

5. **The correct answer is C.** Myocardial infarction is the leading cause of death in diabetics. The advanced glycosylated products associated with long-standing diabetes mellitus accelerate the atherosclerotic process. Other risk factors for coronary artery disease (CAD) include hypertension, smoking, hypercholesterolemia, family history of CAD at a young age, male sex, or being a postmenopausal female.

   DKA (**choice A**) carries a high mortality rate for type 1 diabetics. However, this patient had type 2 diabetes, which is associated with hyperosmolar coma, not with DKA. Although the remaining options (**choices B, D, and E**) are all common causes of morbidity and mortality in diabetics, myocardial infarction is the most frequent cause.

6. **The correct answer is B.** Folate can lower the risk of neural tube defects.

   Choices A, C, D, and E are incorrect. Prenatal vitamins may contain an increased dose of iron and folate compared with other multivitamins.

7. **The correct answer is D.** The child has a classic presentation of impetigo. The most appropriate treatment is mupirocin ointment.

8. **The correct answer is C.** Foreign body aspiration is most consistent with this patient's history and physical examination. The abrupt onset of wheezing, the unilateral absence of breath sounds, and a previously well child should make one suspect foreign body aspiration.

   Croup (**choice A**) typically presents with symptoms of an upper respiratory infection for a few days. Then a brassy cough and inspiratory stridor develops. Croup is seen mostly in children 6 months to 3 years of age.

   Pertussis (**choice B**) has three stages: catarrhal, paroxysmal, and convalescent stage. It is most common in children younger than 5 years. During the catarrhal stage, low-grade fever, rhinorrhea, mild cough, wheezing, and conjunctival injection are common. The paroxysmal stage is named for the episodes of cough. During the convalescent stage, the frequency and intensity of the cough decreases.

   Acute epiglottitis (**choice D**) typically occurs in children 2 to 7 years of age. It is characterized by sudden onset of fever and respiratory distress. Patients often have a muffled voice and are in a tripod sitting position leaning forward.

Bronchiolitis (**choice E**) is common in children under 2 years of age. It presents with sneezing, coughing, rhinorrhea, and low-grade fever for several days. Symptoms progress to tachypnea and wheezing. Signs of respiratory distress are common.

9. **The correct answer is A.** Atrial fibrillation is an irregularly irregular rhythm.

A regular irregular rhythm (**choice B**) has a pattern to the irregularity, such as ventricular bigeminy.

An S_3 (**choice C**) is a ventricular gallop. Causes of an S_3 include volume overloading of a ventricle, myocardial failure, or decreased myocardial contractility.

A fourth heart sound, S_4 (**choice D**), occurs in late diastole and is caused by the atrial kick, where the final 20% of the atrial output is delivered to stiff, noncompliant ventricles. Atrial fibrillation does not have an atrial kick and therefore cannot have an S_4.

There is no murmur (**choice E**) associated with atrial fibrillation.

10. **The correct answer is B.** Tissue grafts in which the same individual acts as both donor and recipient are termed autografts. Allografts (**choice A**) refer to tissue transplants from one person to another. Homograft (**choice C**) is a synonym for allograft. Isografts (**choice D**) refer to tissue transplants between genetically identical individuals (e.g., an identical twin donates her kidney to her twin sister). Xenografts (**choice E**) refer to tissue transplants from another species (e.g., baboon heart transplanted into a human).

11. **The correct answer is B.** Retinitis in the setting of HIV is most likely caused by cytomegalovirus (CMV), which is a herpesvirus. Other herpesviruses include herpes simplex, varicella-zoster (chickenpox, shingles), and Epstein-Barr virus (mononucleosis). The adenoviruses (**choice A**) can cause respiratory infections, pharyngitis, gastroenteritis, and conjunctivitis. They do not cause retinitis. The orthomyxoviruses (**choice C**) include the influenza viruses. The paramyxoviruses (**choice D**) include the viruses responsible for croup (parainfluenza), measles (rubeola), mumps, and respiratory syncytial virus. The retroviruses (**choice E**) include HIV; however, retinitis in AIDS patients is usually due to an opportunistic infection with CMV.

12. **The correct answer is A.** Myasthenia gravis is a disease in which autoantibodies to the acetylcholine receptor inactivate receptors at the neuromuscular junction, resulting in muscle weakness. Symptoms generally worsen with repeated use of the muscle.

Treatment measures include inhibiting the enzyme acetylcholinesterase, which is the enzyme in the neuromuscular junction responsible for breaking down acetylcholine. When acetylcholine levels increase, the patient will experience a lessening of the signs and symptoms of this condition.

Inhibition of angiotensin-converting enzymes (**choice B**) will result in a lowering of blood pressure and aid in the prevention of the "ventricular remodeling" that occurs secondary to congestive heart failure. Nonsteroidal antiinflammatory drugs (NSAIDs) inhibit the activity of the enzyme cyclooxygenase (**choice C**), thereby decreasing the production of prostaglandins. DOPA decarboxylase (**choice D**) inhibitors are used in the treatment of Parkinson disease to prevent the peripheral conversion of levodopa to dopamine in the periphery. Phenylalanine hydroxylase (**choice E**) is responsible for the production of tyrosine. Inhibition of this enzyme is detrimental to the patient.

13. **The correct answer is D.** Hereditary fructose intolerance (HFI) results from a deficiency of aldolase B, the enzyme that cleaves fructose-1-phosphate to glyceraldehyde and dihydroxyacetone phosphate. This results in the accumulation of fructose-1-phosphate in the liver, which causes an inhibition of glycogen phosphorylase and aldolase. Glycogen lysis and gluconeogenesis are thereby impaired, resulting in severe hypoglycemia and vomiting. Symptoms can be reversed after removing fructose and sucrose from the diet. Although many pathologic conditions can result in the development of any of the answer choices, some sample "biochemistry-related" disorders are listed below. Galactosemia is an autosomal-recessive disorder resulting from a deficiency of either galactokinase or galactose-1-phosphate uridyl transferase. In both deficiencies, galactose accumulates and is converted to galactitol in the lens of the eye (cataracts [**choice A**]) and nervous system (mental retardation [**choice E**]). Glucose-6-phosphate dehydrogenase deficiency is an X-linked recessive disorder that causes a decrease in NADPH, leading to the development of hemolytic anemia (**choice B**). In uridyl transferase deficiency, galactose-1-phosphate accumulates in the liver, resulting in hepatomegaly (**choice C**).

14. **The correct answer is B.** The patient described here most likely has a diagnosis of obsessive-compulsive anxiety disorder (OCD). Examination of the activity of the brain for OCD patients should reveal increased frontal lobe activity (obsessions) and increased activity in the caudate nucleus (compulsions). Recall that stimulation of the caudate nucleus in dogs produces cleaning and

grooming behavior and that many compulsive behaviors focus on cleaning and straightening up.

Excess activity in the amygdala (**choice A**) is associated with unipolar depression.

Damage to the cerebellum (**choice C**) can result in clumsy, less coordinated behavior. Certain types of learning disabilities also are associated with dysfunctions of the cerebellum. The lack of coordination associated with the use of inhalants is the consequence of action on the cerebellum also.

The hippocampus (**choice D**) holds a map of the inside of the brain, telling us where to locate stored memories, and a map of the world around us, helping us locate ourselves geographically. Atrophy of the hippocampus has been associated with schizophrenia, severe unipolar depression, and Alzheimer dementia.

The pons (**choice E**) is responsible for the initiation of rapid eye movement (REM) sleep by activation to the cortex and enervation to the spinal cord.

15. **The correct answer is B.** A classic clinical and radiographic picture of pneumonia due to *Klebsiella pneumoniae* involves patients who are typically male, older than 48 years, and have a history of chronic alcoholism. The majority of these pneumonias are community-acquired. *Klebsiella pneumoniae* is a large, gram-negative rod that produces a mucoid capsule when grown on agar.

Candida albicans (**choice A**) is an oval yeast that stains strongly gram-positive.

Legionella pneumophila (**choice C**), the cause of Legionnaire disease, is a facultative, intracellular, gram-negative bacterium that is difficult to stain. It will not grow on conventional agar. It must be grown on charcoal yeast extract agar supplemented with iron and cysteine.

Mycoplasma pneumoniae (**choice D**) are prokaryotic cells that lack peptidoglycan and are bounded by a single trilaminar membrane. On Gram stain, they appear gram-negative. They exhibit a "fried egg" colonial morphology on special artificial media. They are an important cause of atypical pneumonia.

Streptococcus pneumoniae (**choice E**) is a very common cause of pneumonia, and alcoholism increases the risk of disease. However, on Gram stain, it is a lancet-shaped, gram-positive diplococci.

16. **The correct answer is A.** Macular degeneration is the leading cause of blindness for those aged 55 and older in the United States. There are no definitive treatments for macular degeneration.

Cataracts (**choice B**), retinal detachment (**choice C**), *Toxocariasis* (**choice D**), and acute angle closure glaucoma (**choice E**) can cause profound visual loss but are not the leading cause of blindness for those aged 55 and older in the United States.

17. **The correct answer is E.** The woman has a symptomatic Bartholin gland abscess. Word catheter placement is used to treat Bartholin gland abscesses and cysts.

Antibiotics (**choice A**) should never be the sole treatment. Antibiotics may be used when there is evidence of cellulitis.

Excision (**choice B**) is reserved for patients who have recurrent Bartholin gland abscesses and have failed conservative treatments. Excision should not be performed when there is an active infection.

Marsupialization (**choice C**) is used to treat Bartholin's duct cysts and should not be used when an abscess is present.

Sitz baths (**choice D**) can be used to treat small, asymptomatic Bartholin duct cysts.

18. **The correct answer is C.** PCR amplification of the HIV proviral DNA provides the ability to detect HIV at early stages of infection, because the viral nucleic acid is present immediately upon exposure. It is used to detect HIV infection in newborns whose mothers are HIV positive.

ELISA testing (**choices A and B**) and Western blot (**choice E**) detect antibodies to HIV in the blood samples. Because antibodies (IgG) are transferred from mother to fetus through the placenta, testing for antibodies in the newborn's blood will provide false positive results and is not a test specific for newborn infection.

RT-PCR analysis (**choice D**) is used to measure the quantity of HIV circulating in the blood (viral load) when monitoring the response to drugs or the status of infection in patients with HIV infection.

19. **The correct answer is A.** A short-acting inhaled beta-2 agonist is used for immediate bronchodilation. It is the initial treatment for acute symptoms.

Inhaled corticosteroids (**choice B**), systemic steroids (**choice C**), leukotriene modifiers (**choice D**), and cromolyn (**choice E**) are used in the long-term control of asthma.

20. **The correct answer is D.** Cystic fibrosis should be suspected in young adults with recurrent lung infections. Complaints of abdominal pain and steatorrhea are also common in patients with cystic fibrosis.

Asthma (**choice A**) presents with episodic shortness of breath, cough, chest tightness, and wheezing.

Characteristics of irritable bowel syndrome (**choice B**) include abdominal pain and alteration in bowel habits.

Patients with diverticulosis (**choice C**) are often asymptomatic. Patients may complain of abdominal pain, diarrhea, and constipation.

Sarcoidosis (**choice E**) varies in clinical manifestations depending on the stage of the disease and the affected organs. Pulmonary complaints include dry cough, chest discomfort, and shortness of breath. Constitutional symptoms are often present.

21. **The correct answer is C.** This child has Lesch-Nyhan disease, resulting from a deficiency of hypoxanthine guanine phosphoribosyl transferase (HGPRT), a purine-salvage enzyme. Lacking the ability to recycle purine bases into purine nucleotides, most purines are converted to uric acid, causing hyperuricemia. A normal individual recycles approximately 90% of all released purines in the body.

    Signs of Lesch-Nyhan disease include mental retardation, spastic cerebral palsy with compulsive biting of hands and lips, and hyperuricemia.

    Cataracts (**choice A**), dislocated lenses (**choice B**), pancreatic insufficiency (**choice D**), and renal proximal tubule defect (**choice E**) are not associated with Lesch-Nyhan disease.

22. **The correct answer is B.** Keloids are hyperplastic scar tissue that occur following a cutaneous injury and often expand beyond the site of injury. Individuals prone to keloids should avoid cosmetic procedures, such as ear piercing.

23. **The correct answer is E.** Thrombolytics are used in the acute management of a pulmonary embolus.

    All the other answer choices should be recommended to the patient.

24. **The correct answer is B.** The patient's presentation is classic of Alzheimer disease, which has an insidious onset beginning usually in the seventh or eighth decade. Progressive memory impairment, especially related to recent events, alterations in mood and behavior, progressive deterioration, aphasia (loss of language skills), and apraxia (loss of learned motor skills) are within the presentation of Alzheimer disease. The pathogenesis of Alzheimer disease is unknown, but there is enough evidence that shows decreased levels of cholinergic nuclei in the neocortical and hippocampal areas of the frontal cortex. This produces an abnormal accumulation of amyloid in the cerebral cortex and basal ganglia, also known as senile plaques.

    Lewy body disease (**choice A**) presents with changes in cognition, recurrent visual hallucinations, and the motor features of Parkinson's disease. Lewy bodies are noted in the brain.

    Huntington's disease (**choice C**) typically presents between the ages of 35 and 45, with changes in personality, cognition, and physical skills. The most common physical symptoms include chorea (jerky, random, uncontrollable movements), abnormal posturing, and difficulties chewing or swallowing.

    Creutzfeld-Jacob disease (**choice D**) is caused by an agent called a prion and presents with progressive dementia, memory loss, personality changes, and hallucinations. Physical symptoms include speech impairment, myoclonus, and coordination dysfunction.

    Frontotemporal dementia (**choice E**) is caused by loss of spindle neurons in the frontal or temporal lobes. It most commonly presents between the ages of 55 and 65, with changes in social and personal behavior, apathy, emotion blunting, and deficits in expressive and receptive language.

25. **The correct answer is B.** Paroxysmal nocturnal hemoglobinuria (PNH) arises as a result of a somatic mutation of the X-linked PIG-A gene that affects the synthesis of the glycosylphosphatidylinositol (GPI) membrane anchor required for several membrane proteins, such as decay accelerating factor (DAF). This mutation produces an abnormal clone of all hematopoietic stem cells and affects the GPI anchored molecules of red blood cells, causing an increased sensitivity for the red blood cells to lysis by complement due to absence of DAF. Clinically, PNH has a variable course of intravascular hemolysis, pancytopenia, and recurrent (usually venous) thromboses. Hemoglobinuria, often on awakening, is a characteristic symptom of PNH.

    Bcl-2 (**choice A**) is a proto-oncogen located on chromosome 18 that is associated with B-cell leukemia and lymphomas.

    Oxidation of hemoglobin forms Heinz bodies (**choice C**), which are seen in glucose-6-phosphate dehydrogenase deficiency.

    Increased levels of methylmalonic acid (**choice D**) are seen in vitamin B_{12} deficiency.

Hereditary spherocytosis is an autosomal dominant disorder that is due to a defect involving spectrin (**choice E**) in red blood cell membranes, which causes a decrease in the RBC surface membrane. Spherocytes are removed in the spleen by macrophages.

26. **The correct answer is B.** Beta-thalassemia major results from the presence of two beta-globin chain genes that are expressed postnatally only, thereby presenting as postnatal, and not prenatal, disease. Microcytic, hypochromic anemia with numerous target cells and increased reticulocytes is characteristic of beta-thalassemia major, also known as Cooley anemia. Also characteristic of this disease are the increased hemoglobin F at 90%, increased hemoglobin A_2, and decreased hemoglobin A. Patients are typically normal at birth, with symptoms developing at about 6 months. Symptoms include severe hemolytic anemia resulting from decreased RBC life span, ineffective erythropoiesis due to intramedullary destruction, and jaundice secondary to hemolysis. Erythroid hyperplasia in the bone marrow causes "crewcut" skull x-ray and increased size of maxilla ("chipmunk face"). Congestive heart failure is the most common cause of death in patients with Cooley anemia.

Alpha-thalassemia trait (**choice A**) results from two deletions in the alpha-globin chain genes, of which there are normally four, and causes prenatal disease since alpha chains are expressed prenatally.

Beta-thalassemia minor (**choice C**) presents with increased hemoglobin A_2 and increased hemoglobin F, but is asymptomatic.

Hemoglobin H disease (**choice D**) results from three deletions in the alpha chain genes, and presents with increased Hb H and Heinz bodies inside red blood cells.

Hydrops fetalis (**choice E**) results from four deletions and therefore the absence of all the alpha chain genes. This condition is lethal in utero.

27. **The correct answer is B.** Endometriosis is characterized by red-brown serosal nodules, known as "powder burns," on sites outside the uterus such as the ovaries, ovarian and uterine ligaments, pouch of Douglas, the serosa of the bowel and bladder, and the peritoneal cavity. Clinical presentation of endometriosis includes chronic pelvic pain with dysmenorrhea (painful menstruation) and dyspareunia (pain during sexual intercourse), rectal pain and constipation, and infertility.

Endometrial carcinoma (**choice A**) shows up as a tan polypoid endometrial mass and commonly presents with postmenopausal vaginal bleeding.

A germ cell tumor of the ovary (**choice C**) contains elements from all three germ cell layers, and therefore appears as an ovarian cyst containing hair, teeth, and greasy material. The vast majority of ovarian germ cell tumors are benign, but complications include torsion, rupture, and malignant transformation.

An ovarian cystadenoma (**choice D**), arising from the ovarian surface epithelium, is the most common benign ovarian tumor and appears as a unilocular, smooth-lined cyst. Therefore, the presence of multiple nodules rules out a cystadenoma.

Pelvic inflammatory disease (**choice E**) is a broad term referring to ascending infection that can progress from the cervix to the endometrium, fallopian tubes, and pelvic cavity. It can present as cervicitis, endometritis, salpingitis, peritonitis, or perihepatitis. The red-brown nodules are not consistent with pelvic inflammatory disease.

28. **The correct answer is B.** Scarlet fever is a toxin-mediated disease that presents with sore throat, high fever, and mucous membrane erythema ("strawberry tongue"). A fine, punctuate pink rash is noted on the upper trunk and extremities.

Kawasaki disease (**choice A**) presents with high fever, bilateral conjunctivitis, strawberry tongue, and cervical lymphadenopathy.

Rubeola, or measles (**choice C**), presents with high fever, dry cough, conjunctivitis, and maculopapular rash on the face, neck, arms, and chest. Koplik spots in the mouth are pathognomonic.

Rubella (**choice D**) presents with mild fever, mild lymphadenopathy, and a rash that begins on the face and moves to the trunk.

Erythema toxicum (**choice E**) is a pustular rash noted on the trunk, face, and extremities in the newborn.

29. **The correct answer is C.** Target INR range of 2.0 to 3.0 is recommended for patients with deep vein thrombosis and prevention of an embolus in patients with atrial fibrillation.

Choices A, B, D, and E are incorrect. A lower therapeutic INR, 1.5 to 2.5, is recommended for patients undergoing a non-hip, noncardiac surgery. Patients with mechanical valves should be anticoagulated to an INR range of 3.0 to 4.5.

30. **The correct answer is A.** The clinical description is typical for the X-linked disease, Duchenne's muscular dystrophy. This condition is due to an abnormal dystrophin, which is a very large (2 million base-pair

gene located in the Xp21 region) structural protein in the cytoskeleton of the cell membrane. The normal gene product is thought to stabilize both the cell membrane and the sarcolemma.

An autoimmune attack on acetylcholine receptors in the postsynaptic neuromuscular junction (**choice B**) is the mechanism of disease production of myasthenia gravis.

Defects in mitochondrial enzymes (**choice C**) underlie the mitochondrial myopathies.

A mutation affecting ion channels in the membrane conduction system (**choice D**) causes many cases of myotonic dystrophy.

Mutations in the calcium-release channels of the sarcoplasmic reticulum (**choice E**) underlie some forms of congenital myopathies.

31. **The correct answer is A.** This patient presents with Cushing syndrome, which is caused by excessive cortisol exposure. The subjective complaints of weakness and lack of concentration are typical. Physical examination reveals hypertension, moon facies (a rounded, plethoric face), and a buffalo hump (dorsal cervical fat pads), all of which are consistent with Cushing syndrome. The dexamethasone suppression test helps to determine the different causes of elevated cortisol and is used to screen for Cushing syndrome.

The Schilling test (**choice B**) is used to diagnose pernicious anemia.

The 24-hour urine collection for vanillylmandelic acid (**choice C**) is used to diagnose pheochromocytoma.

The adrenocorticotropin hormone stimulation test (**choice D**) is used to screen for Addison disease.

The urea breath test (**choice E**) is used to confirm the eradication of *Helicobacter pylori* in cases of peptic ulcer disease.

32. **The correct answer is D.** If the patient is stable, pharmacologic treatment with procainamide or sotalol is the first-line therapy.

Cardioversion (**choice A**) is indicated in an unstable patient with ventricular tachycardia. Amiodarone (**choice B**) may also be used in stable ventricular tachycardia but is not considered first-line therapy. Defibrillation (**choice C**) should never be used to treat ventricular tachycardia. Adenosine (**choice E**) is considered first-line pharmacologic therapy in supraventricular tachycardia.

33. **The correct answer is B.** Byssinosis is caused by the inhalation of cotton dust. People working in factories involved with the treatment of cotton are subject to the disease. It is characterized by chest tightness. Symptoms typically occur after returning to work from the weekend.

Silicosis (**choice A**) is caused by the inhalation of free silica. Persons with occupations such as rock mining, stone cutting, and pottery are at risk.

Asbestosis (**choice C**) is caused by the inhalation of asbestos. Mining, installing insulation, construction, and shipbuilding are occupations associated with asbestos exposure.

Berylliosis (**choice D**) is caused by the inhalation of beryllium from the manufacturing of alloys, ceramics, and electronics.

Talcosis (**choice E**) is caused by the inhalation of magnesium silicate. Talc is used in asbestos, paper, textiles, cosmetics, rubber, and ceramics.

34. **The correct answer is D.** This boy has a Ewing sarcoma, which is a primary, malignant, small, round cell tumor of bone. Like its soft tissue counterpart, primitive neuroectodermal tumor (which often has an indistinguishable appearance on microscopy), Ewing sarcoma shows neural differentiation, as indicated by the Homer-Wright rosettes (cells arranged around a fibrillar core) described in the question stem. Both Ewing sarcoma and primitive neuroectodermal tumor often show the same characteristic translocation t(11;22)(q24;q12). Ewing sarcoma is the most lethal and second-most common malignant tumor of bone in younger patients.

Chondromyxoid fibroma (**choice A**) is a benign, cartilage-producing tumor.

Malignant fibrous histiocytoma (**choice B**) and its benign counterpart, nodular fasciitis (**choice C**), are soft tissue lesions that typically contain abundant spindle-shaped cells.

Liposarcomas (**choice E**) are malignant neoplasms of fat cells and come in many varieties, including round cell; these tumors are not closely related to Ewing's sarcoma.

35. **The correct answer is D.** Once eclampsia has occurred and the patient is stabilized, delivery is mandated. Women with mild preeclampsia are managed with bed rest at home. Women with moderate to severe preeclampsia are hospitalized.

36. **The correct answer is C.** A tension pneumothorax is a life-threatening condition and must be attended to immediately. A large-bore needle is inserted into the pleural space through the second anterior intercostal space to relieve the pressure.

37. **The correct answer is D.** The only hematologic malignancy to commonly cause lytic bone lesions that may develop pathologic fractures is multiple myeloma. The lytic lesions are often multiple and have a characteristic "punched-out" appearance.

    The other hematologic malignancies listed in the choices tend to fill the marrow with abnormal cells but do not destroy bone.

38. **The correct answer is D.** This is a 3-step question. You need to know which hormones are produced in the posterior pituitary, then know the function of each hormone, and finally know which pathologic condition will follow when this "particular" hormone is absent. The posterior pituitary produces antidiuretic hormone (ADH, or vasopressin) and oxytocin. ADH is responsible for maintaining plasma osmolarity and preventing excessive water loss. When ADH is absent, diabetes insipidus can result. This condition is caused by a decrease in the renal reabsorption of water, an increase in serum osmolarity, and the generation of a dilute (hypotonic) urine. All the other conditions can result from a decrease in the secretions of the anterior pituitary.

    Addison's disease (**choice A**) is caused by decreased production of corticosteroids, such as cortisol. The production is decreased secondary to a decrease in the secretion of ACTH.

    Decreased skin pigmentation (**choice B**) can occur when melanocyte-stimulating hormone is not secreted.

    When thyroid-stimulating hormone (TSH) is not secreted, you can expect to see a decreased thyroid function (**choice C**).

    Dwarfism (**choice E**) is a condition that can occur in young children when growth hormone production is decreased.

39. **The correct answer is A.** This patient has the symptoms of a urinary tract infection (UTI). *Escherichia coli* is the leading cause of community-acquired UTIs. The proximity of the urinary tract to the anus facilitates colonization of the tract by fecal flora. Other gram-negative rods causing UTIs include *Enterobacter cloacae*, *Klebsiella pneumoniae*, *Serratia marcescens*,

Proteus mirabilis, and *Pseudomonas aeruginosa*. None of the other choices listed cause UTIs.

40. **The correct answer is B.** Small nasal polyps are initially treated with nasal corticosteroids for 1 to 3 months. When medical management fails, surgical intervention (**choice C**) is warranted. When recurrence is likely, ethmoidectomy (**choice D**) may be considered.

41. **The correct answer is E.** Asthma is considered a reversible obstructive lung disease.

    Emphysema (**choice A**) and chronic bronchitis (**choice B**) are types of obstructive lung diseases. Both conditions may be partially reversible.

    Asbestosis (**choice C**) and sarcoidosis (**choice D**) are classified as restrictive lung diseases.

42. **The correct answer is C.** Ketone bodies, which include acetoacetate, beta-hydroxybutyrate, and acetone, are produced by the liver in the fasting state by beta-oxidation of fatty acids. They are then released into the bloodstream, where they can be used as alternative energy sources for other organs, such as muscle, kidney, and brain. The brain specifically still requires a small amount of circulating glucose to function, but the amount required is reduced when ketone bodies are available.

    Apoprotein B (**choice A**) is one of the proteins that hold lipoproteins together. Beta-carotene (**choice B**) is a vitamin with antioxidant properties. C-reactive protein (**choice D**) is a serum protein produced by the liver that rises during infections and in inflammatory states. Coenzyme A (**choice E**) is found in mitochondria and carries acetyl groups into the citric acid, or tricarboxylic acid, cycle.

43. **The correct answer is B.** *Pneumocystis carinii* pneumonia (PCP) is found exclusively in immunocompromised patients. It is common in AIDS patients, but other immunocompromised individuals may have the disease, as well. It is one of many forms of pneumonia, including bacterial, chemical, and viral. All of the other organisms listed in the question can cause pneumonia; however, only PCP is exclusively found in individuals with damaged immune systems. Note that Legionnaires' disease, caused by *L. pneumophila*, is more common in the elderly and immunocompromised, but it is not exclusive to them. Note also that PCP is currently classified as a fungus and had been formerly classified as a protozoan. PCP pneumonia is usually treated with trimethoprim-sulfamethoxazole.

44. **The correct answer is A.** The vaccine is not recommended to all adults; only those at high risk for infection should receive the vaccination. The pneumococcal vaccine is recommended for all adults 65 years of age and older. It is also recommended for people between the ages of 2 and 64 who have chronic conditions or are immunocompromised. The vaccine may be given with all other vaccines. It is routinely given as a one-time dose; a one-time revaccination is recommended 5 years later for adults at high risk.

45. **The correct answer is C.** Patients who are diagnosed with endocarditis and have a history of IV drug use are susceptible to *Staphylococcus aureus* infections.

    Streptococcus viridans (**choice A**) is the most common organism responsible for endocarditis in patients without a history of IV drug use.

    Yeast (**choice B**), *Enterococcus viridans* (**choice D**), and *Eikenella corrodens* (**choice E**) are less common.

46. **The correct answer is E.** Factor XII is unusual among coagulation factors in that its deficiency is associated with thrombosis rather than hemorrhage. The mechanism appears to be a deficient activation of fibrinolysis, and both thrombophlebitis and myocardial infarction have occurred in severely affected patients. The condition is inherited in an autosomal recessive manner. Many patients with mild-to-moderate factor XII deficiency are never detected; others are identified when a routine preoperative clotting screen demonstrates a greatly prolonged partial thromboplastin time. Deficiency of each of the other factors (**choices A, B, C, and D**) is associated with hemorrhage.

47. **The correct answer is B.** Ethambutol is used in the treatment of tuberculosis. It can cause retrobulbar neuritis, cutaneous reactions, and, rarely, peripheral neuritis.

    The other choices are side effects of other tuberculosis medications. Isoniazid can cause clinical hepatitis (**choice A**). Rifampin causes orange discoloration of bodily fluids (**choice C**). Pyrazinamide can cause a photosensitive dermatitis (**choice D**), and an asymptomatic hyperuricemia (**choice E**) is an expected effect of this drug.

48. **The correct answer is D.** The average American daily sodium intake is about 150 mmol, most of which is excreted by the kidney, with a variable amount lost in sweat. Of the 25 mmol of sodium filtered each day, between 97 and 100% is reabsorbed by various parts of the nephron. Sodium excretion is also regulated by blood pressure independently of plasma sodium concentration. Several mechanisms, including the glomerular filtration rate (GFR) and the renin-angiotensin-aldosterone system, regulate sodium elimination. Greater than 70% of sodium is reabsorbed in the proximal convoluted tubule. In other words, most sodium reabsorbed in the nephron occurs in the proximal convoluted tubule. The ascending loop (**choice A**) reabsorbs 20%, the collecting duct (**choice B**) reabsorbs 3 to 5%, and the distal convoluted tubule (**choice C**) reabsorbs around 5% of the sodium filtered by the nephron.

49. **The correct answer is B.** Only monosaccharides, such as galactose, glucose, and fructose, can be absorbed by the enterocytes of the small intestine. Amylose (**choice A**) is a complex carbohydrate, whereas lactose (**choice C**), maltose (**choice D**), and sucrose (**choice E**) are disaccharides. These compounds must be hydrolyzed into their monosaccharide components before they can be absorbed.

50. **The correct answer is C.** During starvation, the diet is inadequate to provide sufficient glucose to maintain the brain, yet the brain requires glucose as an energy source. Glucose used in the brain during starvation is synthesized from amino acids, primarily derived from muscle protein. This use of amino acids in starvation leads to profound muscle wasting.

    The ketone bodies (acetoacetate [**choice A**], acetone [**choice B**], and beta-hydroxybutyrate [**choice D**]) produced during starvation and diabetic ketoacidosis are derived from adipose triacylglycerols. Although these compounds can be used in biochemical pathways in the brain, they cannot completely replace glucose in that organ. Furthermore, glucose cannot be synthesized from these precursors. Fatty acid (**choice E**) degradation cannot be used to produce glucose. It can be used, however, to produce ketone bodies that can be used by the brain as a source of intermediates for some synthetic pathways.

51. **The correct answer is D.** Hypersensitivity pneumonitis is an immunologically induced inflammation of the lung parenchyma. It is an occupational disease caused by repeated inhalation of a variety of organic agents. Treatment consists of identifying the offending agent, avoidance of further exposure, and oral corticosteroids. If the condition is not treated, it will progress to a chronic pulmonary disease.

52. **The correct answer is B.** Breast cysts are typically nontender, unless they have developed rapidly and are firm, mobile, and well demarcated. Aspiration reveals clear fluid.

Breast abscess (**choice A**) presents with a very tender, warm, erythematous, edematous mass. The mass is fluctuant, and discharge from the mass may be present.

A fibroadenoma (**choice C**) is rubbery, mobile, and has smooth edges. Fibroadenomas are solid breast masses.

A palpable breast malignancy (**choice D**) is often firm with ill-defined margins, nontender, and fixed. Bloody aspirate of a breast mass necessitates further investigation to rule out malignancy.

Signs and symptoms of mastitis (**choice E**) include breast redness, tenderness, increased warmth, and induration, usually in a lactating woman.

53. **The correct answer is A.** The patient's signs and symptoms are consistent with restrictive cardiomyopathy.

Dilated cardiomyopathy (**choice B**) may present with left or biventricular congestive heart failure. The physical exam may show an elevated jugular venous pressure, an S_3, and rales. An echocardiogram will reveal left ventricular dilation and dysfunction.

Hypertrophic cardiomyopathy (**choice C**) may present with dyspnea, chest pain, and syncope. Objective findings show an S_4, a variable systolic murmur, and a sustained apical impulse. An echocardiogram will show left ventricular hypertrophy.

Rheumatic heart disease (**choice D**) typically affects the mitral valve. Symptoms may include that of mitral stenosis. An echocardiogram will show valve thickening with a decreased opening.

Patients with pericardial effusion (**choice E**) may be asymptomatic or may complain of cough and shortness of breath. An echocardiogram will demonstrate the pericardial effusion.

54. **The correct answer is E.** Lung cancer is the leading cause of cancer deaths in the United States. Cigarette smoking is the most important cause of lung cancer. Lung cancer is often asymptomatic and goes undetected for many years.

55. **The correct answer is E.** Trimethaphan is a ganglionic blocker that is sometimes administered during surgery to maintain controlled hypotension and to minimize blood loss. The trick to determining the effect of a ganglionic blocker is to first know the predominant tone of the end organ in question. The blocker will produce the opposite effect of the predominant tone. The vessels, arterioles, and veins are predominantly under sympathetic tone. Most everything else is under parasympathetic tone. The heart is under predominantly parasympathetic control. Parasympathetic stimulation of the heart causes bradycardia. Removal of this tone with trimethaphan would result in tachycardia. The eye is predominantly under parasympathetic control. Parasympathetic stimulation causes the eye to accommodate (focus for near vision; **choice A**). Removal of this tone with trimethaphan would produce focusing for far vision. Arterioles are predominantly under sympathetic control. Sympathetic stimulation produces vasoconstriction and possibly hypertension (**choice B**). Removal of this tone with trimethaphan would produce vasodilatation and hypotension. The gut is predominantly under parasympathetic control, which increases gut motility (**choice C**). Removal of parasympathetic tone with trimethaphan would diminish gut motility. The eye is predominantly under parasympathetic control. Parasympathetic stimulation causes the pupil to constrict (**choice D**). Removal of this tone with trimethaphan would produce mydriasis.

56. **The correct answer is B.** Weight loss, avoidance of alcohol, and hypnotic medications are the initial interventions.

Choices A, C, D, and E are all appropriate interventions that should be pursued if the initial lifestyle modifications are unsuccessful.

57. **The correct answer is D.** Because the woman has had a tubal ligation, she is at risk for an ectopic pregnancy. An ultrasound should be performed immediately to rule out an ectopic pregnancy.

Choices A, B, C, and E are not the best answers. Ectopic pregnancies typically show lower levels of serum hCG than levels expected in a normal pregnancy. Serum hCG should be correlated with ultrasound findings.

Once an intrauterine pregnancy is determined and if the woman has not decided on a course of action, all possible courses of action, including continuation of pregnancy, termination, and adoption, may be presented to her. Prenatal care should begin as early as possible.

58. **The correct answer is E.** Eosinophilia is present in allergic rhinitis. Other causes of eosinophilia include parasitic infection, myeloproliferative disorders, chronic skin disorders, ulcerative colitis, Crohn disease, and many drug reactions. Eosinophilia is typically caused by an increased adrenal steroid production.

This is often seen when the body is put under stress, such as surgery or an acute bacterial infection.

All the other choices listed cause eosinopenia.

59. **The correct answer is A.** Cirrhosis, nephrotic syndrome, and congestive heart failure can cause a transudate pleural effusion.

Pneumonia (**choice B**), tuberculosis (**choice C**), mesothelioma (**choice D**), systemic lupus erythematosus (**choice E**), viral infection, and pulmonary embolus can cause exudate pleural effusions.

60. **The correct answer is A.** The ELISA (enzyme-linked immunosorbent assay) test for HIV antibody is an initial screening test that is used for the diagnosis of infection in patients or for screening donated blood. It is an indirect test for the virus because it does not detect the virus itself. Instead, it looks for the antibody response raised to the viral infection. The advantage to the ELISA is that it is a rapid and relatively inexpensive test. If a person tests positive on an ELISA, however, a Western blot test must be performed to confirm that the positive response is caused by antibodies against HIV proteins. During primary infection, the ELISA may be briefly (2 to 6 weeks) negative. At this time, however, the diagnosis can be established by checking the viral load. During acute infection, there are high levels of viremia ($>10^6$ copies/mL).

CD4$^+$ count (**choice B**) is used as a marker of the immunologic damage caused by HIV. In the early stages of HIV infection, there is a rapid decline in CD4 cells, which stabilizes then continues to decline at an average of approximately 50/mm^3 per year. Destruction of CD4$^+$ lymphocytes is the major cause of the immunodeficiency observed in AIDS, and decreasing CD4$^+$ lymphocyte levels seems to be the best indicator for developing opportunistic infections. For this reason, the CD4 count is the most important predictor of late-stage infection.

p24 antigen (**choice C**) is a core structural protein of HIV. It is detectable 2 to 3 weeks after HIV infection during the initial burst of viral replication. During this time, the blood is highly infectious, and tests for p24 antigen are usually positive. Its presence can be used to screen for acute HIV infection before antibodies appear. When antibodies to HIV become detectable, p24 antigen is no longer detectable because of antigen-antibody complexing and viral clearance.

Reverse transcriptase activity (**choice D**) is not used as an assay in the diagnosis of HIV or in establishing a prognosis for the infection.

The viral load (**choice E**) is the level of HIV RNA in plasma or other body fluids. It is determined by the viral replication rate and is measured by a PCR assay. It can be used to make the diagnosis of primary infection before antibodies appear. Viral load is the most important predictor of progressive disease in the early stage. The lower the viral load, the longer the time to AIDS diagnosis, and the longer the survival time.

Block 5

1. **The correct answer is E.** Xeroderma pigmentosum is an autosomal recessive disorder characterized by cellular insensitivity to ultraviolet light and deficient repair of DNA. The condition results in the development of melanoma, basal cell carcinoma, and squamous cell carcinoma. This should be differentiated from actinic keratosis (**choice A**), which is a predisposing condition only for squamous cell carcinoma of the skin.

2. **The correct answer is B.** Barrett esophagus is a result of chronic gastroesophageal reflux. Distal esophageal squamous cells are replaced with metaplastic columnar epithelium and goblet cells. This condition eventually progresses to esophageal adenocarcinoma in 30% of patients. It should be noted that Plummer-Vinson syndrome (**choice D**) results in squamous cell carcinoma of the esophagus.

3. **The correct answer is B.** This patient has a shoe fetish. A fetish is characterized by sexual arousal derived from fantasy or behavior involving nonliving objects (i.e., shoes). This paraphilia causes significant distress and can produce an impairment of occupational functioning.

   Exhibitionism (**choice A**) is a paraphilia characterized by sexual arousal derived by exposing one's genitals to strangers.

   Frotteurism (**choice C**) is a paraphilia characterized by sexual arousal derived by sexually touching a stranger.

   Gender identity disorder (**choice D**) is characterized by a constant feeling of discomfort with one's assigned gender and persistent desire to be the opposite gender. This patient does not fall into this category because he does not want to be a woman.

   A pedophile (**choice E**) is an individual who is sexually aroused by engaging in, fantasizing about, or viewing sexual acts involving prepubescent children.

4. **The correct answer is D.** Thromboangiitis obliterans, also known as Buerger disease, occurs most often in men who smoke, beginning at age 40–45. It is an episodic, segmental, inflammatory vaso-occlusive disease of primarily the distal extremities.

   Raynaud disease (**choice A**) is seen primarily in young women. It is characterized by intermittent attacks of cyanosis of the hands when exposed to the cold or provoked by an emotional period. The cyanosis remits spontaneously or when the hands are warmed. During this period the hands may swell, throb, and have pares-

thesia. In contrast to thromboangiitis obliterans, there is no impairment of arterial pulsations.

   Diabetic neuropathy (**choice B**) is incorrect. Diabetic neuropathy is a common chronic complication of diabetes. There is often a bilateral, stocking-glove distribution of sensory deficits in the lower extremities. There is a dull perception of pain, vibration, and temperature.

   An early sign of venous insufficiency (**choice C**) is progressive edema of the lower extremities. As venous insufficiency progresses, skin changes occur.

   Morton neuroma (**choice E**) is a benign growth, usually between the third and fourth toes, caused by irritation, pressure, or injury.

5. **The correct answer is C.** Approximately 15% of women with gestational diabetes require insulin therapy during pregnancy. All women with gestational diabetes need to participate in diet-management treatment.

   Metformin (**choice A**) is used to treat non-insulin-dependent diabetes mellitus (NIDDM, or type 2 diabetes). It works in three ways: First, it reduces the amount of glucose produced by the liver; second, it reduces the amount of glucose absorbed from the diet; and third, it increases the efficacy of insulin that the body produces. Metformin has not been shown to cause birth defects or other problems in humans. However, metformin should not be used during pregnancy.

   Glyburide (**choice B**) is an oral drug of the sulfonylurea class that lowers blood glucose. It stimulates the release of insulin from the pancreas, assuming the patient has functional beta cells in the pancreatic islets. Glyburide also plays a role in increasing insulin sensitivity and decreasing hepatic glucose production.

   Pioglitazone (**choice D**) is a thiazolidinedione-type antidiabetic drug that can be used in conjunction with a sulfonylurea. It also increases the insulin activity in the body.

   Acarbose (**choice E**) is an alpha-glucosidase inhibitor. It slows down the digestion of carbohydrates, thereby facilitating better blood glucose control.

6. **The correct answer is C.** Hemophilia B is an X-linked deficiency of factor IX. It often presents with spontaneous bleeding from joints and deep tissues. G6PD (**choice A**) is an episodic hemolytic anemia caused by a hereditary enzyme defect. Oxidative stresses, such as ingestion of sulfa medications, cause the hemolytic anemia. Hemophilia A (**choice B**) has low levels of factor VIII coagulant activity. Sickle cell anemia (**choice D**)

is a hereditary hemolytic anemia in which abnormal hemoglobin causes sickling of red blood cells. Thalassemia (**choice E**) causes a hereditary microcytic anemia. There is abnormal red blood cell morphology.

7. **The correct answer is C.** Congestive heart failure (**choice A**), cirrhosis (**choice B**), increased hydrostatic pressure (**choice D**), and nephrotic syndrome (**choice E**) cause pleural fluid transudates.

8. **The correct answer is B.** Isotretinoin is a teratogenic medication. A serum pregnancy test (**choice D**) should be ordered before starting a female patient on isotretinoin at 1-month intervals. Isotretinoin may cause elevations of liver function tests, cholesterol, and triglycerides (**choices A, C, and E**). These laboratory tests should be drawn before treatment is initiated and 1 month after the initiation of treatment.

9. **The correct answer is D.** Acute cholecystitis is the most likely choice. This may represent a cystic duct obstruction.

   Acute hepatitis (**choice A**) is not likely with normal liver enzyme tests.

   Acute pancreatitis (**choice B**) may occur with a common duct obstruction. In this case, liver enzyme tests would be elevated. With normal liver functions, it is unlikely that there would be accompanying pancreatitis to this patient's cholecystitis.

   With choledocholithiasis (**choice C**; common duct obstruction), the exam should reveal jaundice and biliary colic. However, the absence of jaundice and the presence of normal liver function tests in this case suggest cholecystitis.

   Acute pyelonephritis (**choice E**) presents with fever and flank pain. Costovertebral angle tenderness is often noted on the physical examination. This diagnosis is not appropriate in this case, given the positive Murphy sign and temporal association with meals.

10. **The correct answer is C.** The patient has a pinworm infection, which is caused by *Enterobius vermicularis*. Applying Scotch tape to the perianal region and observing the tape on a slide under a microscope will reveal eggs of the *Enterobius*.

    Choices A, B, D, and E would not be the best initial choices of examination in establishing a diagnosis.

11. **The correct answer is E.** A Pap smear is an initial screening test for cervical cancer. If the test is abnormal, a colposcopy (**choice B**) with cervical biopsy and endocervical curettage may be performed.

A bimanual examination (**choice A**) is performed to evaluate the internal pelvic organs, primarily the uterus and ovaries. Conization of the cervix (**choice C**) is used to treat severe dysplasia and cancer in situ. Endometrium biopsy (**choice D**) is used to detect endometrial cancer.

12. **The correct answer is B,** which describes the Naegele rule for determining the delivery date.

13. **The correct answer is A.** The point of this question is that sometimes the obvious explanation is the correct one. Occlusion of the central retinal artery rapidly causes irreversible blindness with loss of the inner retinal layers. (The photoreceptor rod and cone cells are maintained by the pigment epithelium.) The site of occlusion is typically just posterior to the cribriform plate. A garden-variety atheroma or embolism is overwhelmingly the most common cause of central retinal artery occlusion.

    Despite all of the teaching about the risk of blindness in temporal arteritis (**choice B**), this disorder causes only 10% of central retinal artery occlusions. Hypertension (**choice C**) is more likely to cause bleeding than is thrombosis. Polycythemia vera (**choice D**) could (but rarely) cause occlusion because of increased blood viscosity and a tendency for thrombosis. Tumor (**choice E**) might also cause retinal artery thrombosis, but this would be far rarer than atheroma.

14. **The correct answer is D.** The glossopharyngeal nerve (CN IX) and the vagus nerve (CN X) carry afferent information to the medulla from the carotid sinus and aortic arch baroreceptors, respectively. The firing rate of these neurons increases with increasing blood pressure. Therefore, severing these nerves sends the medulla a false signal that the patient has suddenly lost all blood pressure. This elicits a baroreceptor reflex, resulting in an increase in sympathetic outflow and leading to tachycardia and hypertension.

15. **The correct answer is D.** This patient most likely has histrionic personality disorder. Individuals with this disorder engage in attention-seeking behavior, including inappropriately flirtatious behavior, flamboyant dress, and exaggerated emotional responses. They tend to believe that their relationships are more intimate than they actually are, and they are easily influenced by others. They always want to be the center of attention.

    An individual with borderline personality disorder (**choice A**) suffers from instability in mood, identity, and relationships. He or she may change from loving to hating a person within a single day. Patients with borderline disorder are often self-destructive, and may attempt suicide.

Delirium (**choice B**) is a transient global disorder of cognition producing an acute confusional state. This patient is not confused.

Dependent personality disorder (**choice C**) is characterized by the constant need for emotional support and advice from others. Patients with this disorder fear abandonment.

An individual with narcissistic personality disorder (**choice E**) appears self-centered, and seems to have an unusual sense of entitlement. These patients are grandiose, and have little concern for others. Narcissistic personality would be in the differential for this patient, but the observed behavior is more consistent with histrionic personality disorder.

16. **The correct answer is A.** The patient presents with mitral valve prolapse (MVP). MVP occurs frequently in individuals who are thin and tall. MVP is often asymptomatic, but patients may complain of fatigue, palpitations, dyspnea, or nonspecific chest pain. Echocardiography is the most appropriate diagnostic modality to diagnose MVP. Echocardiography shows one or both leaflets of the mitral valve superior to the annular plane in systole.

Electrocardiogram (**choice B**) is often normal in patients with MVP. An EKG may show nonspecific ST- and T-wave abnormalities.

Angiography (**choice C**) is invasive and would not be used to diagnose MVP. Chest x-ray (**choice D**) is normal in MVP. Holter monitors (**choice E**) are used to diagnose rhythm disturbances.

17. **The correct answer is E.** Angina pectoris occurs during physical exertion or emotional stress and is relieved immediately by rest or nitroglycerin use.

Substernal chest pain/discomfort (**choice A**), radiation to the left shoulder (**choice B**), pain described as "squeezing" (**choice C**), and history of heart disease (**choice D**) can be true of both myocardial infarction and angina pectoris.

18. **The correct answer is A.** Glucocorticoid therapy is the most common cause of Cushing syndrome. Some benign and malignant tumors, including small cell lung carcinomas (**choice C**), adrenal adenomas (**choice D**), and adrenal carcinomas (**choice E**), can cause Cushing syndrome.

Pituitary adenomas (**choice B**) that secrete an excess of ACTH cause Cushing *disease*.

19. **The correct answer is C.** Microcytosis is characteristic of thalassemia. Decreased vibratory and position sense (**choice A**) is suggestive of vitamin B_{12} deficiency. The TIBC (**choice B**) is increased in iron deficiency anemia. Spherocytes on the peripheral smear (**choice D**) is seen in hereditary spherocytosis, and a serum folate level <3 ng/mL (**choice E**) is typically seen in folic acid deficiency.

20. **The correct answer is C.** Patients with COPD are at risk for *Haemophilus influenzae* pneumonia. The other two most common bacterial causes of pneumonia in COPD patients are *Moraxella catarrhalis* and *Streptococcus pneumoniae*.

Pseudomonas aeruginosa (**choice A**) is common in nosocomial infections, cystic fibrosis, and bronchiectasis. *Mycoplasma pneumoniae* (**choice B**) is frequently seen in young adults. *Staphylococcal pneumoniae* (**choice D**) is common in IV drug users, nosocomial infections, nursing homes, cystic fibrosis, and bronchiectasis. *Klebsiella pneumoniae* (**choice E**) is frequently seen in patients who abuse alcohol, in diabetics, and in patients with nosocomial infections.

21. **The correct answer is D.** The description of the lesion given in the vignette is classic for basal cell carcinoma (BCC). The most appropriate next step is a biopsy to confirm the diagnosis and identify the histologic subtype of BCC.

Choices A, B, and C are treatment options for BCC.

Watchful waiting (**choice E**) is inappropriate in this patient because BCC can cause significant morbidity if diagnosis is delayed and treatment is not initiated.

22. **The correct answer is A.** Although the presentation of colon cancer is highly variable, abdominal pain and bowel changes are common presentations. There is an association between colon cancer and various genetic syndromes such as Lynch syndrome, hereditary nonpolyposis, and familial adenomatous polyposis.

Diverticulitis (**choice B**) presents acutely with LLQ pain and fever. It is an acute infection of the bowel secondary to diverticulosis.

Irritable bowel syndrome (**choice C**) is a functional bowel problem. Symptoms must be present for at least 3 months before considering the diagnosis. The pain is usually intermittent, crampy, and associated with a change in stool frequency or form. The pain is relieved with defecation. There is frequently mucus, but no blood. It does not interfere with sleep, and there will not be weight loss or fever.

Ulcerative colitis (**choice D**) will most often present with bloody, mucus-laden stools.

Diverticulosis (**choice E**) does not present with weight loss. It is not associated with Li-Fraumeni syndrome.

23. **The correct answer is C.** Candidiasis causes vaginal itching, dyspareunia, and a nonodorous, white, curd-like discharge. Risk factors include pregnancy, antibiotic treatment, corticosteroid use, oral contraceptives, uncontrolled diabetes, and AIDS.

   Gray discharge with a fishy odor (**choice A**) is consistent with bacterial vaginosis.

   A green, frothy, malodorous discharge (**choice B**) is consistent with a *Trichomonas vaginalis* infection.

   Small, grouped vesicles on an erythematous base (**choice D**) is consistent with a herpetic infection.

   A yellow, creamy discharge (**choice E**) is consistent with a *Chlamydia* infection.

24. **The correct answer is C.** All the other choices listed will have higher-than-normal levels of maternal serum alpha-fetoprotein.

25. **The correct answer is A.** This woman has a risk profile (female, fat, forties) and symptomatology consistent with gallstones (cholelithiasis). As would be expected, contraction of the gallbladder following a fatty meal often exacerbates the pain caused by gallstones. Cholecystokinin (CCK) is the hormone responsible for stimulation of gallbladder contraction; the release of CCK is stimulated by dietary fat. It is produced in the I cells of the duodenum and jejunum. In addition to gallbladder contraction, CCK also stimulates pancreatic enzyme secretion and decreases the rate of gastric emptying.

   Gastrin (**choice B**) is produced by the G cells of the antrum and duodenum. Gastrin stimulates the secretion of HCl from the parietal cells and pepsinogen from the chief cells of the stomach.

   Pepsin (**choice C**) is a protease produced by the chief cells of the stomach (as pepsinogen). It is involved in the digestion of proteins.

   Secretin (**choice D**) is produced by the S cells of the duodenum. It is secreted primarily in response to acidification of the duodenal mucosa.

   Somatostatin (**choice E**) is produced by the D cells of the pancreatic islets and in the gastric and intestinal mucosa.

26. **The correct answer is D.** The administration of any product that contains phenylalanine, such as aspartame, to an individual with any of the hyperphenylalaninemias could be detrimental to his or her general health. The hyperphenylalaninemias result from an impaired conversion of phenylalanine to tyrosine. The most common and clinically important is phenylketonuria, which is characterized by an increased concentration of phenylalanine in blood, increased concentration of phenylalanine and its by-products (such as phenylpyruvate and phenylacetate) in urine, and mental retardation. Phenylketonuria is a condition caused by a deficiency of phenylalanine hydrolase.

   Hyperornithemia (**choice A**) is an inherited disorder of amino acid metabolism that results from a defect of the enzyme ornithine decarboxylase. This condition is associated with mental retardation, neuropsychiatric dysfunction, and protein intolerance.

   Hyperuricemia (**choice B**) is a condition associated with higher than normal blood levels of uric acid. This condition is commonly known as gout. Hypervalinemia (**choice C**) is an inherited disorder of amino acid metabolism that results from a defect of the enzyme valine aminotransferase. This condition is associated with mental retardation, neuropsychiatric dysfunction, and protein intolerance. Wilson's disease (**choice E**) is an autosomal-recessive disorder associated with an abnormality of the hepatic excretion of copper resulting in toxic accumulations of the metal in the brain, liver, and other organs.

27. **The correct answer is B.** The phrenic nerve is a branch of the cervical plexus, which arises from C3, C4, and C5. It is the sole motor nerve to the diaphragm. It crosses the anterior scalene muscle from lateral to medial to enter the thoracic inlet. In other words, after the administration of theophylline, an asthmatic patient begins to see an increase in diaphragmatic contractility secondary to the signal transmitted to the diaphragm by the phrenic nerve.

   The axillary nerve (**choice A**) is primarily involved with the muscles of the shoulder, such as the anterior and posterior segments of the deltoid and teres minor.

   The recurrent laryngeal nerve (**choice C**) is a branch of the vagus nerve. This is a mixed nerve that conveys sensory information from the laryngeal mucosa below the level of the vocal folds and provides motor innervation to all intrinsic muscles of the larynx except the cricothyroid muscle.

The suprascapular nerve (**choice D**) innervates muscles of the shoulder, such as the supraspinatus and the infraspinatus. The thoracodorsal nerve (**choice E**) also innervates muscles of the shoulder, such as the latissimus dorsi.

28. **The correct answer is B.** Beriberi is a condition caused by a deficiency of thiamine. It typically occurs in alcoholics because of impaired absorption. Cardiovascular complications secondary to beriberi include a high output state, biventricular myocardial failure, and retention of sodium. Another complication of thiamine deficiency is Korsakoff syndrome. This condition is mostly associated with neurologic complications.

    Carotenemia (**choice A**) results from excessive intake of vitamin A and leads to a yellowing of the skin, especially on the palms and soles. A deficiency of niacin can lead to pellagra (**choice C**), which is a disease typically associated with dermatitis, dementia, and diarrhea. Pernicious anemia (**choice D**) is a condition caused by a deficiency of vitamin B_{12}, or cyanocobalamin. Scurvy (**choice E**) is caused by a deficiency of vitamin C and can lead to perifollicular hemorrhage.

29. **The correct answer is A.** Unstable ventricular tachycardia should be cardioverted before the rhythm progresses to ventricular fibrillation.

    Ventricular fibrillation (**choice B**) should be defibrillated, not cardioverted.

    In atrial fibrillation that has an unknown onset or an onset greater than 48 hours (**choice C**), the patient must be anticoagulated first for at least 3 weeks before cardioversion is attempted. If the patient is symptomatic and needs to be urgently cardioverted, the patient must be heparinized and have a transesophageal echocardiography to exclude a clot. Only then can the patient be cardioverted.

    Multifocal atrial tachycardia (**choice D**) is treated with medications such as a beta-blocker, a calcium channel blocker, amiodarone, or diltiazem.

    Unstable bradycardia (**choice E**) is treated with an intervention sequence consisting of pharmaceutical interventions and transcutaneous pacing.

30. **The correct answer is C.** A pink vagina suggests a nonpregnant state. Cyanosis of the vagina and cervix occurs at about the seventh week of pregnancy.

    Choices A, B, D, and E are the signs and symptoms of pregnancy.

31. **The correct answer is E.** The sequence of the auditory pathway is as follows: organ of Corti → spiral ganglion in the cochlea → vestibulocochlear nerve (CN VIII) → cochlear nuclei (dorsal and ventral) → superior olivary nuclei → lateral lemniscus → inferior colliculus → medial geniculate nucleus of the thalamus (MGN) → primary auditory cortex (Heschl gyrus). Each ear projects to both sides of the brainstem and cortex via multiple commissures, including the trapezoid body (which contains fibers crossing contralateral to the superior olivary nucleus), the commissure of the inferior colliculus (connecting the right and left inferior colliculi), and another commissure that connects the right and left nuclei of the lateral lemniscus. Therefore, a lesion of any structure up until the superior olivary nuclei will produce an ipsilateral deafness. The only structure listed that is proximal to the superior olivary nuclei is the organ of Corti. The inferior colliculus (**choice A**), the lateral lemniscus (**choice B**), and the medial geniculate body (**choice C**) all receive information from both ears, and unilateral hearing loss could not result from a lesion of any of these structures.

    The medial lemniscus (**choice D**) is not a part of the auditory system. It is part of the somatosensory system, which conveys proprioception, discriminative touch, and vibration information. More specifically, neurons of the gracile and cuneate nuclei send projections that decussate as the internal arcuate fibers and ascend as the medial lemniscus to synapse in the ventroposterolateral nucleus (VPL) of the thalamus.

32. **The correct answer is A.** Digoxin is a cardiac glycoside. It increases the contractility of the heart, decreases the heart rate, and decreases the conduction velocity through the AV node.

    Diltiazem (**choice B**) is a calcium channel blocker. Lisinopril (**choice C**) is an ACE inhibitor. Metoprolol (**choice D**) is a beta-blocker. Terazosin (**choice E**) is an alpha-1-adrenergic blocker.

33. **The correct answer is D.** This patient has stable angina. A stress exercise test can detect ischemia that is not present at rest. The stress exercise test can evoke chest pain or show ST depression.

    A resting EKG (**choice A**) does not show how the heart responds under stress. It can be normal in up to 50% of patients with stable angina.

    Echocardiography (**choice B**) examines the morphology and function of the heart. It is not used as a diagnostic procedure for angina.

    Angiography (**choice C**) is the definitive diagnostic procedure for coronary artery disease. Angiography is invasive and costly, and is not the diagnostic test of choice for angina pectoris.

Holter monitoring (**choice E**) is used to document suspected rhythm disturbances.

34. **The correct answer is E.** "Painful bones," renal stones, "abdominal groans," and "psychic moans" characterize signs and symptoms of hyperparathyroidism. The laboratory findings are consistent with hyperparathyroidism.

    Laboratory findings of osteomalacia (**choice A**) show a low-to-normal level of serum calcium, a low level of phosphorus, an elevated-to-normal level of alkaline phosphatase, and an elevated level of parathyroid hormone.

    Laboratory findings of hyperthyroidism (**choice B**) show elevated levels of calcium and phosphorus, an elevated-to-normal level of alkaline phosphatase, and a low level of parathyroid hormone.

    Laboratory findings of osteoporosis (**choice C**) typically show normal levels of serum calcium, phosphorus, and alkaline phosphatase, and a normal-to-elevated level of parathyroid hormone.

    Laboratory findings of Paget disease (**choice D**) typically show a normal-to-elevated level of serum calcium, phosphorus, and parathyroid hormone, and an elevated level of alkaline phosphatase.

35. **The correct answer is C.** In a patient with lobar pneumonia, tactile fremitus is increased. There is also dullness on percussion, and transmitted voice sounds are increased as in egophony, bronchophony, and whispered pectoriloquy, and there are bronchial or bronchovesicular breath sounds over the involved area.

36. **The correct answer is D.** A fasting serum gastrin level should be obtained with the patient off his H2RA for 24 hours. More than 90% of patients with Zollinger-Ellison syndrome develop peptic ulcers. The frequency of this patient's ulcers suggests a gastrin-secreting tumor.

    Long-term treatment with H2RAs (**choice A**) and treating with omeprazole instead (**choice B**) is not indicated until further evaluation is obtained. A PPI could certainly be used, but this complicated history deserves consideration of a gastrinoma.

    Regarding **choice C**, if *H. pylori* testing is negative by appropriate laboratory method, it is unlikely that "triple" therapy for *H. pylori* will improve this patient's outcome.

    Antacid therapy (**choice E**) is useful for mild gastroesophageal reflux disease.

37. **The correct answer is B.** Pemphigus is an autoimmune disorder caused by disruption of desmosomes that link keratinocytes, which are responsible for the production of the family of keratin proteins that provide the barrier function of the epidermis. Desmosomes are most common in epithelial cells that are subject to wear and tear and are the spot-welds that hold cells together.

    Actin microfilaments (**choice A**) help maintain cell shape and interact with myosin in striated muscle cells. Actin microfilaments form the core of microvilli and stereocilia.

    Gap junctions (**choice C**) are junctional specializations between adjacent cells that allow the passage of small ions through connexin channels in the adjacent membranes. These junctions permit cell-to-cell communication.

    Microtubules (**choice D**) play a role in chromosomal movement by forming the mitotic spindle; they are the organelles used in intracellular transport and form pairs of tubules that convey motility to cilia and flagella.

    Tight junctions (**choice E**) are formed by the point-to-point fusion of opposed cell membranes near the luminal surfaces of epithelia. They form the anatomic component of many barriers in the body. In the epidermis, however, keratin proteins provide the necessary barrier function of keeping water and exogenous materials out of the body.

38. **The correct answer is E.** In SCID, both humoral and cellular immunity are impaired, leading to opportunistic infections that include all major categories of infectious agents.

39. **The correct answer is B.** Women with a normal BMI should gain 25 to 35 lb during pregnancy. Women who are underweight should gain 28 to 40 lb, while overweight women should gain only 15 to 25 lb. Women who are expecting twins should gain 35 to 45 lb during pregnancy.

40. **The correct answer is C.** Risk factors for the development of thromboembolus are hypercoagulability, endothelial injury, and disturbed blood flow. Laminar flow of blood (**choice A**) is normal flow, not disturbed flow. Decreased level of factor V (**choice D**) leads to hemorrhage. Hypocoagulability (**choice B**) and thrombocytopenia (**choice E**) do not lead to thromboembolus formation.

41. **The correct answer is A.** Plants do not contain cholesterol. Cholesterol comes from animal products, such as meat, dairy products, fish, and poultry (**choices B, C, and E**).

Some whole-wheat products (**choice D**) contain hydrogenated oils. Hydrogenated oils are a source of trans-fatty acids. Trans-fatty acids along with saturated fats are the primary dietary causes of high blood cholesterol.

42. **The correct answer is D.** Patients with selective IgA deficiency may have circulating antibodies to IgA. Fatal anaphylaxis may ensue if they are transfused with blood products with serum containing IgA, although many patients with selective IgA deficiency are asymptomatic and never diagnosed. Symptomatic patients may have recurrent sinopulmonary infections and diarrhea, and also have an increased incidence of autoimmune and allergic diseases.

AIDS (**choice A**) predisposes for infections and neoplasms, but not anaphylaxis. C1 esterase inhibitor deficiency (**choice B**) is an autosomal dominant disease characterized by recurrent attacks of colic and episodes of laryngeal edema, without pruritus or urticarial lesions. This disorder is also known as hereditary angioedema. DiGeorge syndrome (**choice C**) is characterized by thymic aplasia and, sometimes, hypoparathyroidism. The disorder is due to abnormal development of the third and fourth pharyngeal arches. Wiskott-Aldrich syndrome (**choice E**) is a form of immunodeficiency associated with thrombocytopenia and eczema.

43. **The correct answer is B.** Cholestyramine is a bile acid sequestrant. It binds intestinal bile acids to form insoluble complexes and is not systemically absorbed.

Atorvastatin (**choice A**) is a HMG-CoA reductase inhibitor. It is systemically absorbed.

Gemfibrozil (**choice C**) is a fibrinic acid that is systemically absorbed. Fenofibrate (**choice E**) is also classified as a fibrinic acid. They both inhibit peripheral lipolysis and decrease the hepatic extraction of free fatty acids.

Niacin (**choice D**) is systemically absorbed. It is classified as a nicotinic acid. The mechanism of action is not completely understood, but it is thought to inhibit lipolysis in adipose tissue and increase lipoprotein lipase activity.

44. **The correct answer is D.** This question tests your knowledge of how vitamin B_{12} is normally absorbed. In summary, parietal cells in the gastric lining secrete a glycoprotein called intrinsic factor into the gastric lumen. This protein binds to vitamin B_{12}, protecting it from degradation and allowing for its eventual absorption. At the level of the ileum, B_{12} bound to intrinsic factor is actively reabsorbed. Therefore, a loss of intrinsic factor or of its reabsorption site, the

ileum, would lead to the need for lifelong injection of vitamin B_{12}.

Megaloblastic anemia (**choice A**) refers to an anemia related to either folate deficiency or vitamin B_{12} deficiency. Many patients need only supplementation and changes to diet to correct this anemia. Lifelong vitamin B_{12} administration is needed in conditions that permanently affect B_{12} absorption and reabsorption. Removal of the colon, jejunum, or gallbladder (**choices B, C,** and **E**) would not affect reabsorption of intrinsic factor or B_{12}. A total absence of bile (which occurs with bile duct blockage, but not with cholecystectomy) may lead to malabsorption of fat-soluble vitamins such as A, D, E, and K but not of B_{12}.

45. **The correct answer is A.** Smoking, being overweight, a sedentary lifestyle, testosterone, and certain medications such as diuretics can lower HDL levels.

Losing weight, estrogen therapy, maintaining a physically active lifestyle, and insulin therapy (**choices B, C, D,** and **E**) can increase HDL levels.

46. **The correct answer is D.** This patient is in hypertensive crisis (also known as malignant hypertension) with signs of target organ dysfunction. Sodium nitroprusside is a rapid arterial and venous dilator. It is considered the drug of choice for hypertensive crisis.

Intravenous labetalol can be used for a hypertensive crisis. Oral labetalol (**choice A**) has a longer onset of action than the intravenous form and should not be used during a hypertensive crisis.

Sublingual nitroglycerin (**choice B**) is typically used in unstable angina, acute myocardial infarction, pulmonary edema, and treatment of left ventricular insufficiency. It is an agent used in treatment of hypertensive urgencies.

Clonidine (**choice C**) has an onset of action of 30 to 60 minutes with a peak effect in 2 to 4 hours. It sometimes requires a lengthy period, up to 6 hours, for an adequate response and therefore is not the most appropriate therapy.

Captopril (**choice E**) is not used in malignant hypertension. It can be use in hypertensive urgencies.

47. **The correct answer is C.** Venous insufficiency is caused by chronic obstruction or valvular incompetence of the deep lower veins. Patients complain of a generalized ache in the lower extremities made worse with prolonged standing and alleviated with elevation of the lower extremities. Typical physical findings include pitting edema and shiny, atrophic, brownish

skin. Ulcerations may develop at the side of the ankle, especially medially.

Chronic arterial insufficiency (**choice A**) is incorrect. It presents with intermittent claudication that progresses to pain at rest. Objective findings show decreased or absent pulses; absent or mild edema; shiny, atrophic skin; and loss of hair over the foot and toes.

Cellulitis (**choice B**) is characterized by erythema, warmth, and tenderness of the involved area.

Characteristics of lymphatic statis (**choice D**) are nonpitting edema, skin thickening, and lack of skin pigment changes. Ulceration is rare.

Orthostatic edema (**choice E**) is one cause of pitting edema. There is no skin ulceration, thickening, or pigment change.

48. **The correct answer is D.** Elevated unconjugated bilirubin is noted in conditions that result in a breakdown of red blood cells. Bile duct obstruction, bile duct disease, and intrahepatic disruption will elevate conjugated bilirubin.

49. **The correct answer is A.** Although it is hard to develop a deficiency in oil-soluble vitamins (A, D, E, K) because the liver stores these substances, deficiency states can be seen in chronic malnutrition (specifically chronic fat deprivation) and chronic malabsorption. Vitamin A is necessary for formation of retinal pigments (deficiency can cause night blindness) and for appropriate differentiation of epithelial tissues (including hair follicles, mucous membranes, skin, bone, and the adrenal cortex).

Vitamin C (**choice B**), which is water soluble rather than oil soluble, is necessary for collagen synthesis. Vitamin D (**choice C**) is important in calcium absorption and metabolism. Vitamin E (**choice D**) is a lipid antioxidant that is important in the stabilization of cell membranes. Vitamin K (**choice E**) is necessary for normal blood coagulation.

50. **The correct answer is B.** Psoriasis results from an increase in the number of proliferating cells in stratum basale plus stratum spinosum. This results in greater epidermal thickness and continuous turnover of the epidermis.

The dermal papillae (**choice A**) are projections of the dermis that extend into the overlying epidermis. They contain connective tissue, vascular loops, and specialized nerve endings.

The stratum corneum (**choice C**) is the superficial stratum consisting of several layers of flat, anucleated, and cornified (keratinized) cells.

Stratum granulosum (**choice D**) consists of flat polygonal cells filled with basophilic keratohyalin granules.

Stratum lucidum (**choice E**) is the transitional zone of flat eosinophilic or pale-staining anucleated cells found only in regions with thick stratum corneum. These strata do not contain dividing keratinocytes.

51. **The correct answer is C.** Sarcoidosis is an inflammatory disease that causes granulomatous inflammation of the lungs in most patients. Patients may be symptomatic or display a variety of symptoms depending on the organs affected. Patients with lung involvement will complain of persistent cough and shortness of breath on exertion. Generalized symptoms of fever, night sweats, loss of appetite, and/or weight loss are common. Bilateral hilar adenopathy supports the diagnosis of sarcoidosis. Histologic evidence of noncaseating granulomas further confirms the diagnosis.

Although tuberculosis (**choice B**) should be on the differential because it may present similarly, the bilateral hilar adenopathy is almost exclusive to sarcoidosis.

52. **The correct answer is A.** The high pH indicates alkalosis. A low P_{CO_2} and a normal HCO_3^- indicate the alkalosis is of respiratory nature.

53. **The correct answer is C.** Signs and symptoms of otitis externa include itching, ear pain, purulent and foul-smelling discharge, and hearing loss if the ear canal is filled with purulent discharge. Tenderness over the tragus is common.

Cerumen impaction (**choice A**) is visible on otoscopy and can cause decreased hearing.

Acute otitis media (**choice B**) is a middle ear infection. It occurs more frequently in children and often presents with ear pain, fever, and decreased hearing. Objective findings reveal an erythematous, bulging, and nonmobile tympanic membrane. Rarely, the tympanic membrane ruptures, which causes otorrhea. Mastoiditis (**choice E**) is a potential complication of untreated acute otitis media. Postauricular pain, erythema, and fever are usually present.

Serous otitis media (**choice D**) is caused by obstruction of the eustachian tubes, which causes a negative pressure and subsequently transudate fluid in the middle ear. Physical examination findings show a retracted tympanic membrane ranging in color from gray to amber, air fluid levels, and hearing loss.

54. **The correct answer is B.** Because the patient has latent, not active, tuberculosis and is younger than 35 years, the patient should be treated with isoniazid for 9 months. Treatment with isoniazid reduces the risk of developing active tuberculosis in the future.

55. **The correct answer is A.** Bleeding time is an important test of platelet function and vascular integrity. Vitamin C is a cofactor for lysyl hydroxylase, an enzyme involved in cross-linking of newly formed collagen chains, enhancing the stability and strength of the collagen molecule. Deficiency of vitamin C leads to fragile blood vessel walls that may bleed into the dermis, causing purpura.

    Fibrinogen levels (**choice B**) are not markedly affected by vitamin C deficiency. The platelet count (**choice C**) reflects bone marrow megakaryocytic activity and the stability of platelets in the circulation. The prothrombin time (**choice D**) measures the activity of factors of the extrinsic coagulation pathway, and the activated partial thromboplastin time (**choice E**) measures the activity of intrinsic pathway factors. Several factors (X,V, II, and I) are common to both pathways, so deficiency of any of these factors will affect both measures.

56. **The correct answer is B.** Entropion is an inward turning of the lid margin. Entropion occurs more commonly in the geriatric population.

    Ptosis causes drooping of the upper eyelid (**choice A**).

    Puffy eyelids secondary to herniated fat (**choice C**) are common in the elderly population.

    Exophthalmos causes protrusion of the eyeball forward (**choice D**). It may be seen in Graves disease.

    A retracted eyelid (**choice E**) may be caused by hyperthyroidism.

57. **The correct answer is C.** Erythromycin and clarithromycin are the first-line treatment for *Mycoplasma pneumonia*. Alternative therapy may include doxycycline or certain fluoroquinolones.

58. **The correct answer is B.** To make a definitive diagnosis of gout, the joint aspiration should show negatively birefringent crystals (i.e., needle-shaped crystals that are yellow when parallel to the axis of polarized light). The white cell count ranges from 5,000 to 75,000/mm^3, and the population is mostly PMNs. The aspirated fluid tends to have a decreased viscos-

ity and poor mucin clot formation due to decreased hyaluronate levels.

WBC count of 500/mm^3 (56% monocytes/40% lymphocytes) (**choice A**) is a normal joint aspiration because the white cell count is <1,000/mm^3.

Pseudogout/calcium pyrophosphate deposition disease (CPPD) (**choice C**) is characterized by the presence of positively birefringent crystals (i.e., rhomboid crystals that glow blue when parallel to the axis of polarized light).

WBC count of 20,000/mm^3 (74% PMNs) and thin fluid (**choice D**) is suggestive of rheumatoid arthritis with an inflammatory presentation (numerous white cells and PMN predominance).

Septic arthritis (**choice E**) tends to show a white cell count >50,000/mm^3.

59. **The correct answer is A.** This question is asking you to draw a parallel between a condition caused by increased carbon monoxide poisoning and one of the answer choices. When an individual is exposed to increased levels of carbon monoxide secondary to prolonged exposure to automobile exhaust fumes, the carbon monoxide will bind to the hemoglobin molecules. Therefore, the blood will have decreased oxygen-carrying capacity. Anemic hypoxia is also caused by a decreased oxygen-carrying capacity of the blood.

    Circulatory hypoxia (**choice B**) results when there is insufficient oxygen delivered to tissues secondary to diminished tissue blood flow, despite a normal Pao$_2$ and hemoglobin concentration. Histotoxic hypoxia (**choice C**) occurs when the tissue cannot use the oxygen delivered because of a toxic agent, such as cyanide. Hypoxic hypoxia (**choice D**) occurs when the Pao$_2$ is reduced, as in the case of lung disease or high altitude. Obstructive apnea (**choice E**) is a condition that results when obstructions in the nasal passage cause the development of apnea.

60. **The correct answer is C.** Acute angle closure glaucoma is considered an ocular emergency. Treatment must be started promptly to prevent visual loss.

    Macular degeneration (**choice A**), cataracts (**choice B**), and diabetic retinopathy (**choice D**) warrant evaluation, treatment, and follow-up but are not ocular emergencies.

    Pinguecula (**choice E**) is a benign neoplasm of the conjunctiva. It does not interfere with vision. No treatment is necessary.

Test 2

Block 1

1. A 27-year-old woman undergoes a routine pelvic exam that demonstrates an enlargement of the right adnexa. Ultrasound studies show a 6-cm cystic mass in the ovary. The ovary is resected and the gross examination of the pathologic specimen demonstrates a large, relatively thin-walled cystic space filled with hair and cheesy white debris. What is the most likely diagnosis?

   A. Dermoid cyst
   B. Endometrioid cyst
   C. Ovarian serous cystadenoma
   D. Dysgerminoma
   E. Tubo-ovarian abscess

2. A 15-year-old girl is taken to a physician because she has never had a menstrual period. Physical examination demonstrates short stature, a neck with thick folds attaching it to the shoulder, widely spaced nipples, and short fourth metacarpals. Genetics studies are ordered. Y-specific probe analysis is positive for a Y-bearing cell line. This patient is at greatest risk for developing which of the following tumors?

   A. Adenofibroma
   B. Dermoid cyst
   C. Gonadoblastoma
   D. Mucinous cystadenocarcinoma
   E. Serous cystadenocarcinoma

3. A 53-year-old man presents to an emergency department with pressing substernal pain. The pain has been present for about 4 hours. If the patient's disease process involves the inferior wall of the heart, which of the following groups of leads would likely show the most prominent ECG changes?

   A. I, aVL, V_4-V_6
   B. II, III, aVF
   C. V_1-V_3
   D. V_1-V_6
   E. RV_4, RV_5

4. A 62-year-old man with known severe atherosclerotic disease develops severe hypertension. Serial laboratory studies show increasing blood urea nitrogen and creatinine. Aortography is performed, which demonstrates that the opening into one renal artery is nearly occluded. The juxtaglomerular cell enzyme involved in the production of hypertension in this man acts upon which of the following substrates?

   A. Aldosterone
   B. Angiotensin I
   C. Angiotensin II
   D. Angiotensin III
   E. Angiotensinogen

5. A chest x-ray has been obtained on a patient with a cough and fever. A silhouette sign of the right atrial border is noted. This most likely represents which of the following?

   A. Left lower lobe pneumonia

   B. Lingular pneumonia

   C. Pneumothorax

   D. Right lower lobe pneumonia

   E. Right middle lobe pneumonia

6. A patient complains of burning retrosternal pain after eating a large meal. Bending over aggravates his symptoms. The history is consistent with which of the following diagnoses?

   A. Acute cholecystitis

   B. Angina pectoris

   C. Esophageal spasm

   D. Peptic ulcer

   E. Reflux esophagitis

7. Which of the following is the mechanism of action of paroxetine?

   A. It blocks reuptake of serotonin/norepinephrine.

   B. It blocks reuptake of serotonin.

   C. It blocks reuptake of dopamine/norepinephrine.

   D. It blocks both dopamine and serotonin receptors.

   E. It inhibits monoamine oxidase.

8. A 17-year-old boy is brought into the emergency room. He complains of pain and swelling of the scrotum that occurred suddenly. He has a history of undescended testes. On physical exam, a tender, nontransilluminable lesion is seen. Elevation of the scrotum above the pubic symphysis while the patient is supine does not relieve pain. He denies any recent sexual contact. Which of the following is the most likely diagnosis?

   A. Varicocele

   B. Testicular cancer

   C. Epididymitis

   D. Testicular torsion

   E. Orchitis

9. A 38-year-old man presents to the clinic complaining of an acute onset of fever accompanied by swelling and redness of his left eyelid. On examination, he is found to have proptosis of the left eye accompanied by restricted movement of the ipsilateral eye. What is the most likely diagnosis?

   A. Acute iritis

   B. Blepharitis

   C. Graves disease

   D. Orbital cellulitis

   E. Retrobulbar hemorrhage

10. Which of the following features comprise metabolic syndrome?

   A. Hypertension, elevated HDL, decreased LDL, and central obesity

   B. Low HDL, high LDL, insulin resistance, hypertension, and high triglycerides

   C. Obesity, diabetes, osteoporosis, and thrombocytopenia

   D. Insulin resistance, hypotension, hypouricemia, and diabetes insipidus

   E. Fasting blood glucose equal to or greater than 126 mL/dL on two separate occasions

11. A 25-year-old man falls while skateboarding and strikes the left side of his head against a concrete retaining wall. On physical examination, only a minor scalp abrasion is present at the site of the impact, with minimal bleeding that stops after several minutes. He was initially alert following the accident, but then became unconscious 30 minutes later. CT scan of the head is noted below. Which of the following is the most likely diagnosis?

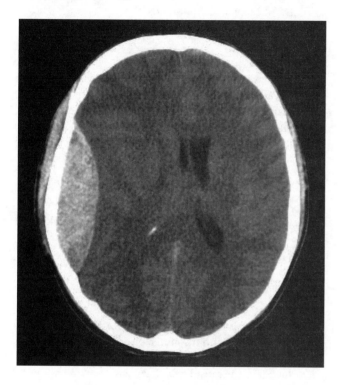

A. Acute subdural hematoma

B. Chronic subdural hematoma

C. Epidural hematoma

D. Subarachnoid hemorrhage

E. Lacunar infarct

12. A 4-year-old boy is brought in by his mother complaining of a severely pruritic rash for the past few weeks. There are excoriations on the boy's lower abdomen, buttocks, and hands, with red papules. A few small burrows are noted. What is the most likely diagnosis and treatment for his condition?

A. Seborrheic dermatitis; topical steroids, hydrocortisone cream

B. Dyshidrotic eczema; antiparasitics, Lindane

C. Seborrheic dermatitis; antihistamines

D. Pityriasis rosea; antihistamine, dry-clean all clothing and bedding

E. Scabies; antiparasitics, permethrin cream

13. Which of the following is the hallmark laboratory finding noted in acute myelogenous leukemia?

A. Auer rods

B. Heinz bodies

C. Hirano bodies

D. Howell-Jolly bodies

E. Philadelphia chromosome

14. A 27-year-old man presents with fever, dry cough, and pleuritic chest pain upon return from a hiking trip in the Ohio River Valley region. The physical examination is remarkable for cervical adenopathy and decreased breath sounds at both lung bases. Further history reveals that he was exposed to bat droppings while exploring caves during his trip. What is the most likely causative organism?

A. *Aspergillus fumigatus*

B. *Coccidioides immitis*

C. *Histoplasma capsulatum*

D. *Mycoplasma tuberculosis*

E. *Rickettsia rickettsii*

15. During an operation to remove an inflamed appendix, a surgeon notes the presence of a 6-cm long and 2-cm wide diverticulum located several feet proximal to the ileocecal junction. This diverticulum is most likely a remnant of which of the following embryonic structures?

    A. Bulbus cordis

    B. Ligamentum arteriosum

    C. Mesonephros

    D. Neural crest

    E. Vitelline duct

16. What is the drug of choice for a patient with both benign prostatic hyperplasia and hypertension?

    A. Alpha-blocker

    B. Beta-blocker

    C. Calcium channel blocker

    D. ACE inhibitor

    E. Hydrochlorothiazide

17. A 49-year-old woman presents to your clinic with a history of sudden onset of fever and productive cough for the last 48 hours. She had recovered from influenza about 10 days prior to the onset of fever. She has right pleuritic chest pain. Her pulse is 120/min, respirations are 20/min, temperature is 39.1°C (102.4°F), pulse oximetry is 90% on room air, and blood pressure is 120/70 mm Hg. Physical examination of her lungs should reveal which physical findings?

    A. Hyperresonance on percussion and bronchial breath sounds on the right

    B. Dullness to percussion, decreased breath sounds, and decreased tactile fremitus on the right

    C. Dullness to percussion, bronchial breath sounds, and egophony on the right

    D. Tympany on percussion, vesicular breath sounds, and increased tactile fremitus on the right

    E. Hyperresonance on percussion and tracheal deviation

18. A patient presents with abdominal cramping and foul-smelling diarrhea after returning from a camping trip. Stool exam reveals trophozoites and cysts. Which of the following medications would be the best treatment option for this patient?

    A. Chloramphenicol

    B. Clindamycin

    C. Metronidazole (Flagyl)

    D. Itraconazole (Sporanox)

    E. Lamivudine (Epivir)

19. You have a 45-year-old patient who is being treated for elevated LDL. She is taking nicotinic acid and complains of severe hot flashes and pruritus after ingestion. She would like to continue taking the medicine because it is less expensive than her other options. Which of the following would you recommend to this patient?

    A. Have her take her dosage with orange juice.

    B. Have her take her dosage every other day.

    C. Have her take an aspirin before she takes her dosage.

    D. Prescribe Benadryl after each dose.

    E. Stop the medication and start her on a statin.

20. A 19-year-old white woman, G1P2, presents 2 weeks postdelivery with insomnia, disorientation, and voices telling her that her baby is the devil. Which of the following is the most likely diagnosis?

    A. Postpartum depression

    B. Postpartum psychosis

    C. Conversion disorder

    D. Bipolar disorder

    E. Schizophrenia

21. A 34-year-old former rodeo rider comes into the emergency department complaining of right foot drop, severe exacerbation of lower back pain with some radiation into the right lateral calf, and urinary retention for the past 24 hours. There is no history of trauma within the past 3 weeks of the onset of symptoms. Which of the following should be immediately evaluated?

   A. Cauda equina syndrome

   B. Lumbar degenerative disk disease without herniation

   C. Lumbar spondylosis without myelopathy

   D. Myofascial back pain

   E. Right sacroiliitis

22. A 32-year-old bisexual man with a history of multiple sex partners is now in a monogamous relationship, feels well, and desires HIV screening. Which one of the following laboratory tests is the MOST appropriate screen for HIV?

   A. CBC and blood cultures

   B. HIV ELISA and CD4 count

   C. HIV ELISA, Western blot test if positive

   D. HIV ELISA, viral load if positive

   E. Viral load and CD4 count

23. A 75-year-old man with a 40-pack-year history of smoking and hypercholesterolemia is diagnosed with severe atherosclerosis. Atherosclerotic occlusion of which of the following arteries would result in insufficient perfusion of the urinary bladder?

   A. External iliac

   B. Inferior epigastric

   C. Internal iliac

   D. Internal pudendal

   E. Lateral sacral

24. A 78-year-old patient just had hip replacement surgery for a fracture. The nurse contacts you 28 hours after surgery to report that the patient has sudden onset of tachypnea and right-sided pleuritic chest pain. You suspect a pulmonary embolism. Which of the following findings would you expect on physical examination of the lungs?

   A. Bronchial breath sounds throughout

   B. Dullness to percussion

   C. Hyperresonance on percussion

   D. Normal physical examination

   E. Tactile fremitus

25. A patient is diagnosed with an early, simple small bowel obstruction. Which of the following objective findings would you expect to find?

   A. Bowel sounds consisting of clicks and gurgles occurring at a frequency of 20 per minute

   B. Peristaltic rushes and high-pitched tinkles

   C. No bowel sounds

   D. Radiographic evidence of air-fluid levels outside the bowel

   E. Radiographic evidence of dilated loops of bowel with haustral markings

26. A 30-year-old white woman is admitted to your medical unit for observation of abdominal pain. Twelve hours after admission she becomes nauseous, with vomiting, tremors, and agitation. She has a history of alcohol consumption (approximately a 12-pack of beer per day). What is the most appropriate initial treatment?

   A. Gentamicin

   B. Compazine

   C. Mucomyst

   D. Naloxone

   E. Lorazepam

27. The most common bone malignancy typically occurs in adolescents and presents with pain or swelling in the bone or joint, commonly the knee. It is which of the following conditions?

    A. Osteoid osteoma

    B. Ewing sarcoma

    C. Osteosarcoma

    D. Osgood-Schlatter

    E. Chondroblastoma

28. A 42-year-old man presents for a follow-up visit for hypertension. He does not take any medications and has a history of benign familial essential tremor. His blood pressure is 152/94 mm Hg. A symmetric fine tremor of both hands is noted on physical examination. What is the most appropriate pharmacologic agent for use in treatment?

    A. Alpha-blocker

    B. Beta-blocker

    C. Calcium channel blocker

    D. ACE inhibitor

    E. Thiazide diuretic

29. A 26-year-old type 1 diabetic on insulin TID presents with the following blood sugars: at bedtime, 94 mg/dL; at 3:00 A.M., 50 mg/dL; and at 7:00 A.M., 220 mg/dL. Which of the following is the most likely cause?

    A. Dawn phenomenon

    B. Waning of insulin plus dawn phenomenon

    C. Somogyi effect

    D. Primary hypoglycemia

    E. Insulin allergy

30. A 55-year-old white man complains of pimples on his nose that are aggravated by drinking coffee or alcohol. His skin is oily and he has diffuse erythema, telangiectasias with superimposed papules, and pustules on his nose. What is the most likely diagnosis?

    A. Miliaria

    B. Folliculitis

    C. Acne vulgaris

    D. Rosacea

    E. Milia

31. A 50-year-old man presents with a 3-month history of intermittent epigastric pain. He describes the pain as a dull ache, ranging in severity from 0 out of 10 to 8 out of 10. The pain is aggravated by coffee ingestion and improves after most meals. He is currently on no medications. On physical examination, sclerae are clear and epigastric tenderness is noted. Which of the following is the most likely diagnosis?

    A. Acute pancreatitis

    B. Cholelithiasis

    C. Duodenal ulcer

    D. Esophageal stricture

    E. Gastric carcinoma

32. A 67-year-old patient presents to the clinic with a history of productive cough for 3 months. He has a 60-pack-year smoking history. Which of the following chest x-ray findings is most consistent with chronic obstructive pulmonary disease?

    A. Hampton hump

    B. Hyperinflation of the lung

    C. Kerley B lines

    D. Pulmonary vascular congestion

    E. Reticular-nodular pattern

33. Two weeks ago, a patient was treated with a course of clindamycin for a medical complaint. Now the patient complains of abdominal pain and persistent, foul-smelling, watery diarrhea since she finished the course of antibiotics. Which of the following is the most likely pathogen responsible for the patient's symptoms?

    A. *Clostridium difficile*

    B. *Clostridium perfringens*

    C. *Cryptosporidium parvum*

    D. *Giardia lamblia*

    E. *Saccharomyces boulardii*

34. A patient complains of abdominal pain, low-grade fever, weight loss, nausea, vomiting, and diarrhea. The patient has had similar symptoms in the past, but the symptoms resolved spontaneously after a few weeks. A colonoscopy with biopsies is performed. Endoscopic evaluation shows skip lesions, a cobblestone appearance, and deep and longitudinal fissures. Which of the following diagnoses do you suspect?

    A. Crohn disease
    B. Diverticulitis
    C. Irritable bowel syndrome
    D. Ischemic colitis
    E. Ulcerative colitis

35. A 30-year-old white female presents with thickened skin, telangiectasias, loss of normal skin folds, and fingertip ulcerations. She denies any constitutional symptoms, fever, arthritis, muscle weakness, or other symptoms. Which of the following is the most likely diagnosis?

    A. Rheumatoid arthritis
    B. Polymyalgia rheumatica
    C. Wegener granulomatosis
    D. Scleroderma (systemic sclerosis)
    E. Reactive arthritis (Reiter syndrome)

36. A 58-year-old man arrives at the office for follow-up after routine urinalysis during a pre-employment physical reveals hematuria. The patient admits to having a 38-pack-year history of smoking. Which of the following will confirm the suspected diagnosis?

    A. CBC and blood chemistry
    B. Pelvic and abdominal CT scans
    C. Intravenous urogram
    D. Retrograde pyelography
    E. Cystoscopy and biopsy

37. Following thyroidectomy, hoarseness of the voice may occur. This condition is caused by damage to the

    A. internal laryngeal nerve
    B. recurrent laryngeal nerve
    C. thyroarytenoid muscle
    D. vestibular folds
    E. vocal folds

38. A 50-year-old male sheepherder presents with a painless ulcer on his right hand. The ulcer has a black necrotic scab with surrounding edema. The patient states it was initially red, elevated, and itchy. The patient is afebrile and denies any constitutional symptoms. Gram stain of the ulcer reveals gram-positive rods with a boxcar-like appearance. Which of the following is the most appropriate treatment?

    A. Rifampin
    B. Cefuroxime
    C. Doxycycline
    D. Vancomycin
    E. Erythromycin

39. What is the most common organism responsible for urinary tract infections?

    A. *Escherichia coli*
    B. *Helicobacter pylori*
    C. *Klebsiella pneumoniae*
    D. *Staphylococcus epidermidis*
    E. *Staphylococcus saprophyticus*

40. A 32-year-old man is accused of murdering four people. The man has a history of impulsivity and refusal to conform to social norms. On interview, you note a charming, intelligent man who seems to show no remorse. He denies any wrongdoing and appears self-centered and insincere. Which of the following diagnoses is supported by your interview?

    A. Avoidant personality disorder
    B. Antisocial personality disorder
    C. Dependent personality disorder
    D. Passive-aggressive personality disorder
    E. Obsessive-compulsive personality disorder

41. A 47-year-old obese man presents to you for follow-up on his type 2 diabetes. His most recent Hgb-A$_{1c}$ was 7.2 at his last visit 1 month ago. His systolic blood pressure has been in the 150s and his diastolic pressures have averaged in the 90s. Which of the following antihypertensive agents should be recommended?

    A. Alpha blocker

    B. Beta blocker

    C. Calcium channel blocker

    D. ACE inhibitor

    E. Hydrochlorothiazide

42. A patient is diagnosed with Barrett esophagus. The endoscopic examination showed which of the following?

    A. Columnar epithelium-lined lower esophagus

    B. Esophageal varices

    C. Peptic stricture

    D. Schatzki ring

    E. Squamous cell carcinoma

43. A 40-year-old man is brought to the emergency department after being found unconscious on the street. On exam, you note respiratory depression, pinpoint pupils, and pulmonary edema. You also find track marks along his arms and ankles. Which of the following is the most appropriate treatment?

    A. Activated charcoal nasogastric tube

    B. *N*-acetylcysteine

    C. Naloxone

    D. Lorazepam

    E. Labetalol

44. Which of the following is used to prevent isoniazid-induced peripheral neuropathy?

    A. Vitamin B$_1$ (thiamine)

    B. Vitamin B$_2$ (riboflavin)

    C. Vitamin B$_3$ (niacin)

    D. Vitamin B$_6$ (pyridoxine)

    E. Vitamin B$_{12}$ (cobalamin)

45. A 60-year-old man develops a chronic anemia. Initially, his blood smears show a normochromic, normocytic anemia with mild poikilocytosis, reticulosis, and polychromatophilia. After several years, many severely misshapen red cells, many of which have shapes resembling "teardrops," are seen in the smear. An attempt at bone marrow aspiration fails to aspirate any marrow. Which of the following processes is the most likely cause of this patient's anemia?

    A. Chronic low-level blood loss

    B. Hereditary disease

    C. Marrow fibrosis

    D. Mineral deficiency

    E. Vitamin deficiency

46. A 54-year-old man decides to have a colonoscopy because a good friend recently died of adenocarcinoma of the colon. A large, flat, polypoid lesion is found in his upper rectum. It is too large to be removed by scope but is biopsied. His physician calls him 2 days later to tell him that the pathology laboratory diagnosed a villous adenoma. The patient asks if he has cancer. His physician explains that the lesion is not malignant but that there is a chance that it could progress to an adenocarcinoma. Which of the following most closely approximates the chance of a malignant transformation of this polyp?

    A. 2%

    B. 10%

    C. 35%

    D. 65%

    E. Nearly 100%

47. A 26-year-old white woman presents with complaints of infertility for 2 years. She reports irregular menstrual cycles, fatigue, and weight gain. Her labs indicate an elevated testosterone. She is 5 feet, 3 inches tall and weighs 160 lb. She has some hirsutism and acne along the face and back. Which of the following would you recommend for treatment of her infertility?

    A. Weight loss

    B. Medroxyprogesterone acetate

    C. Spironolactone

    D. Finasteride

    E. Flutamide

48. Travelers visiting endemic areas may receive prophylaxis for malaria with any of the following medications **EXCEPT**?

    A. Quinine

    B. Chloroquine

    C. Doxycycline

    D. Mefloquine

    E. Atovaquone and proguanil

49. A healthy 71-year-old man describes visual loss in his right eye. Flashes of light and a curtain-like loss of lateral vision began when he awoke 8 hours ago, and the symptoms have persisted. Which of the following is the most likely diagnosis?

    A. Retinal vein occlusion

    B. Occipital lobe seizure

    C. Retinal detachment

    D. Amaurosis fugax

    E. Ocular migraine

50. A 78-year-old woman arrives at the emergency room from the nursing home facility where she lives. The patient has a fever of 101° F with accompanying shivering. Her past medical history includes type 2 diabetes mellitus. The attendant at the nursing home reports an increase in micturition. Family members report a change in the patient's demeanor. Physical exam reveals tachycardia during auscultation. The patient screams in pain during costovertebral palpation. Results from an ordered urinalysis show bacteriuria and pyuria. CBC reveals leukocytosis with a left shift. Which of the following is the most likely diagnosis?

    A. Glomerulonephritis

    B. Nephritic syndrome

    C. Cystitis

    D. Acute tubulointerstitial nephritis

    E. Pyelonephritis

51. A 65-year-old man with a 90-pack-year history of smoking presents with a 6-month history of shortness of breath and slowly progressive dyspnea on exertion. He has a productive cough of clear-to-white sputum that is daily and continuous. He has no fever, and there has been no change in his pattern of sputum production. Physical examination reveals normal vital signs, prolonged exhalation, scattered rhonchi, elevated jugular venous pressures, and moderate peripheral edema. His hematocrit is 50%. Which of the following medical therapies will most likely prolong his survival?

    A. Albuterol nebulizer treatments

    B. Enalapril

    C. Low prednisone therapy

    D. Oxygen

    E. Theophylline

52. Which of the following best describes the mechanism of action of cimetidine?

    A. A prostaglandin with mucosal protective and antisecretory properties

    B. Blocks the action of histamine by competitive antagonism of the H_1 receptor

    C. Blocks the action of histamine by competitive antagonism of the H_2 receptor

    D. Irreversibly inhibits H^+/K^+ ATPase

    E. Neutralizes gastric acids

53. An 80-year-old woman presents to the emergency department after having accidentally taken too many of her propranolol pills. She is confused but responds to your verbal commands. What of the following additional findings would you expect to note on her physical exam?

    A. Fever of 38.5° C (101.3° F), vomiting, and diarrhea

    B. Heart rate of 40/min, hypotension, and temperature of 35° C (95° F)

    C. Heart rate of 150/min, a prominent S_3 heart sound, and hyperreflexia

    D. Heart rate of 70/min, hypertension, diaphoresis, and myosis

    E. Heart rate of 60/min, hyperglycemia, hypotension, and combative behavior

54. Crohn disease is associated with which of the following laboratory findings?

    A. Hyperalbuminemia

    B. Hyperkalemia

    C. Hypernatremia

    D. Macrocytic anemia

    E. Thrombocytopenia

55. The development of extrapyramidal signs and symptoms is most likely to be experienced by a 67-year-old man receiving which of the following antiemetic preparations?

    A. Calcium carbonate

    B. Dimenhydrinate

    C. Dronabinol

    D. Ondansetron

    E. Prochlorperazine

56. Which of the following directly inhibits insulin secretion?

    A. Alpha-2-adrenergic agonist

    B. Beta-2-adrenergic agonist

    C. Cholecystokinin

    D. Glucagon

    E. Muscarinic agonists

57. A 58-year-old man presents to the emergency department with complaints of sudden-onset blindness in his right eye that has been present for 1 hour. He denies trauma or any other symptoms. He has no history of similar symptoms and does not wear contact lenses. The symptoms resolve during the 2 hours he spent in the emergency department. Which of the following cardiac conditions is a risk factor for a future cerebrovascular event, such as the possible transient ischemic attack presented by the patient?

    A. Aortic stenosis

    B. Atrial fibrillation

    C. Bradycardia

    D. Pericarditis

    E. Restrictive cardiomyopathy

58. A mother brings her 10-year-old son to the clinic because she noticed a rash on his arm. She also reports that her son has a fever and has been complaining of tiredness, headache, chills, and a backache. The mother states that her son returned from summer camp in the woods 2 weeks ago, where the boy told her he had been bitten by a tick. On physical examination, the physician assistant notices a rash with a red, raised border and central clearing. What is the drug of choice in this patient?

    A. Penicillin G

    B. Tetracycline

    C. Ceftriaxone

    D. Doxycycline

    E. Amoxicillin

59. Which of the following hormones is released from the posterior pituitary gland?

    A. Growth hormone

    B. Prolactin

    C. Vasopressin

    D. Adrenocorticotropic hormone

    E. Follicle-stimulating hormone

60. A 25-year-old man recovering from a bout of bronchitis suddenly develops a shaking chill followed by fever of 41° C (105.8° F), chest pain, and a productive cough. His sputum is streaked with brown. His respiratory rate is 32/min, and a chest x-ray shows consolidation in the right lower lobe. Which of the following is the most likely causative agent?

    A. *Staphylococcus aureus*

    B. *Klebsiella pneumonia*

    C. *Streptococcus pneumonia*

    D. *Bacillus anthracis*

    E. *Escherichia coli*

End of Block 1

Block 2

1. A diabetic patient with severe peripheral vascular disease undergoes amputation of his foot. The tissues of the surgically removed foot will most likely show which of the following?

   A. Carcinoma

   B. Caseous necrosis

   C. Enzymatic fat necrosis

   D. Gangrenous necrosis

   E. Hemosiderosis

2. A 43-year-old woman presents with excruciating pain near her nose and mouth. Which of the following is the most likely involved nerve?

   A. Facial

   B. Vagus

   C. Trigeminal

   D. Glossopharyngeal

   E. Recurrent laryngeal

3. Adrenocorticotropic hormone (ACTH) promotes the production of cortisol by stimulating which of the following reactions?

   A. 11-deoxycortisol to cortisol

   B. 17-hydroxyprogesterone to 11-deoxycortisol

   C. Cholesterol to pregnenolone

   D. Pregnenolone to progesterone

   E. Progesterone to 17-hydroxyprogesterone

4. Overstimulation of the parasympathetic nervous system would result in which of the following?

   A. Bradycardia

   B. Constriction of the peripheral blood vessels

   C. Decreased peristalsis in the small intestine

   D. Decreased secretions of the salivary glands

   E. Mydriasis

5. A 44-year-old man presents with fever, productive cough with brown sputum, rigors, and lethargy for 7 days. Chest x-ray reveals a right middle lobe infiltrate with a pleural effusion. You perform a thoracentesis to obtain pleural fluid for examination. The results yield a pH of 7.1, a glucose of 32 mg/dL, and a positive Gram stain. Which of the following is the most appropriate next step in management?

   A. Administration of oral antibiotics

   B. Chest CT scan

   C. Drainage of the pleural effusion

   D. Oncology consultation

   E. Repeat chest x-ray

6. A 50-year-old patient complains of change in bowel habits, alternating constipation, and increased frequency of defecation. An occult blood test is positive. A barium enema shows an "apple core" appearance in the descending colon. Which of the following is the most likely diagnosis?

   A. Benign polyp

   B. Colon cancer

   C. Diverticulosis

   D. Intussusception

   E. Sigmoid volvulus

7. A 25-year-old woman presents with her mother for being "out of control." The mother states that over the past few weeks, her daughter has not been sleeping and has been spending money recklessly and that she has been fired from four jobs over the past 6 months. On examination, you note the daughter's pressured speech, lack of focus, and distractibility. Her past medical history is unremarkable. Which of the following is the most likely diagnosis?

   A. Avoidant disorder

   B. Schizophrenia

   C. Generalized anxiety disorder

   D. Histrionic disorder

   E. Bipolar disorder

8. A 25-year-old woman with a history of occasionally painful migratory arthralgias presents with a tender, swollen, and warm left knee. On examination, you also note an erythematous papular rash on the knee. Synovial fluid shows >50,000/mm³ WBCs with >90% PMNs. She has no past medical history of strep infection or trauma. What is the most appropriate treatment?

   A. Compression, ice, and elevation

   B. Intra-articular cortisone

   C. Indomethacin

   D. Amoxicillin

   E. Ceftriaxone

9. An afebrile 45-year-old man comes to the emergency room complaining of pain in his lower back. He reports that he has an increase in both frequency and urgency for urinating. The patient denies any pain during urination. Urinalysis demonstrates hematuria but no bacteriuria or pyuria. KUB shows a ureteral stone proximal to the ureterovesical junction. Ultrasound shows the stone to be approximately 4 mm. What is the initial step in the management of this patient?

   A. Wait for the stone to pass spontaneously

   B. Administer fluids and analgesics

   C. Lithotripsy

   D. Ureteroscopy

   E. Pyelolithotomy

10. A 42-year-old woman comes to the physician because of intermittent spotting. She states that she first noticed this a few years ago, but that she has not had health insurance and, therefore, has not sought evaluation until now. She has no medical problems. Speculum examination reveals what seems to be a cervical cancer. Further evaluation demonstrates the patient to have advanced cervical cancer with obvious parametrial involvement. Which of the following is the most appropriate management of this patient?

   A. Cisplatin-based chemotherapy

   B. Cisplatin-based chemotherapy concurrent with radiation therapy

   C. Hydroxyurea

   D. Radiation therapy

   E. Radiation therapy combined with hydroxyurea

11. A 24-year-old developmentally disabled male patient presents to the clinic with his mother, who is concerned about his recent significant weight loss. He is able to offer no history. The mother states that he has seemed listless, but otherwise notes no specific complaints. On physical examination, you note that he has lost 22 lb since his last visit 12 weeks ago. His blood pressure is 90/64 mm Hg, pulse is 82/min, and respirations are 14/min. Heart and lung exam are within normal limits. There is sparse axillary and pubic hair distribution. Also noted is a gross peripheral field deficit on visual field exam by confrontation. What is the most likely etiology for these physical exam findings?

    A. Adrenal adenoma

    B. Cushing disease

    C. Pituitary macroadenoma

    D. Parathyroid adenoma

    E. Hypothyroidism

12. You suspect a radiculopathy involving the C5 nerve. Which of the following active-resistance, muscle-strength maneuvers tests the motor function of C5?

    A. Abduction of the fifth finger

    B. Elbow extension

    C. Forearm pronation

    D. Shoulder abduction

    E. Shoulder shrug

13. A 15-year-old African American boy presents with a macular rash with hypopigmentation and mild pruritus. He states that "it flares up every year" and usually goes away on its own. Which of the following would help to confirm the diagnosis?

    A. Skin biopsy

    B. Blood culture

    C. Oil immersion slide

    D. Fungal scraping

    E. Complete blood count

14. A 6-year-old girl presents to the clinic with a 1-week history of bruises on her lower legs. The child appears well, but the mother reports that the child had an upper respiratory infection 2 weeks ago. You note multiple petechiae scattered over the lower extremities. There are several small ecchymotic areas over the lower extremities and upper arms. There is no lymphadenopathy and no hepatosplenomegaly. Complete blood count result was normal with only a slightly decreased platelet count at 90,000/mm³. Which of the following is the best intervention at this time?

    A. No treatment is necessary at this time except for monitoring the platelet count.

    B. The child will need to be admitted to the hospital for a splenectomy.

    C. The child will need to begin long-term, low-dose corticosteroid therapy.

    D. High-dose immunoglobulin therapy is needed to raise the platelet count.

    E. The child should receive a platelet transfusion.

15. A 24-year-old man returns from a hiking trip in the western United States with a maculopapular rash at the ankles and wrists that is now becoming more generalized and petechial. He has early neurologic abnormalities and evidence of renal failure. The drug of choice in treating this patient is

    A. prednisone

    B. doxycycline

    C. trimethoprim/sulfamethoxazole

    D. amoxicillin/clavulanate

    E. acyclovir

Items 16–18: The response options for the next three items are the same. You'll be required to select one answer for each item in the set.

For the following conditions, select the appropriate pharmacologic cause (choices A–E).

    A. Bleomycin

    B. Clozapine

    C. Haloperidol

    D. Isoniazid

    E. Sulfonamides

16. Agranulocytosis

17. Pulmonary fibrosis

18. Stevens-Johnson syndrome

19. Accumulation of which of the following substances indicates aging at a cellular level?

    A. Beta-carotene

    B. Bilirubin

    C. Hemosiderin

    D. Lipofuscin

    E. Melanin

20. A 46-year-old African American woman presents with a history of night sweats, weight loss, cough, and shortness of breath progressing over the past 6 weeks. Her laboratory results reveal an elevated alkaline phosphatase and an elevated angiotensin-converting enzyme level. Bronchoscopy with biopsy reveals a noncaseating granuloma. The most likely diagnosis for this patient is

    A. asbestosis

    B. asthma

    C. emphysema

    D. sarcoidosis

    E. tuberculosis

21. Colonoscopic examination reveals hundreds of polyps varying in size and configuration throughout the colon and rectum. Which of the following is the most likely diagnosis?

    A. Benign lymphoid polyps

    B. Familial adenomatous polyposis

    C. Hyperplastic polyps

    D. Inflammatory polyps

    E. Lipomas

22. A 60-year-old female smoker complains of weight loss and progressive dysphasia. Which of the following diagnoses is the most consistent with the history?

    A. Achalasia

    B. Esophageal varices

    C. Esophageal cancer

    D. Mallory-Weiss tear

    E. Zenker diverticulum

23. A 28-year-old Caucasian man presents with his fiancee for evaluation of behavioral problems. His fiancee states that he has been defensive, overly sensitive, and secretive. He admits to not trusting his friends or family and to feeling that "everyone is out to hurt me." Which of the following is the most likely diagnosis?

    A. Schizoid personality disorder

    B. Conversion disorder

    C. Narcissistic personality disorder

    D. Paranoid personality disorder

    E. Major depressive disorder

24. A 56-year-old Caucasian woman presents with widespread musculoskeletal pain for the past 8 months, fatigue, insomnia, and tenderness to palpation in 15 of 18 specific points. What is the laboratory evaluation most likely to show?

    A. Positive rheumatoid factor and CRP

    B. Elevated ESR and WBC

    C. Decreased hemoglobin/hematocrit

    D. Normal lab test results

    E. Elevated CPK and LDH

25. A woman is brought to the emergency room by her family because they are concerned with her shallow breathing. The family states that the patient has been ill for the past 2 days with a stomach virus and has been vomiting excessively. An arterial blood gas ordered as part of the laboratory workup gave the following results:

pH	7.60
HCO_3^-	35 mEq/L
P_{O_2}	85 mm Hg
P_{CO_2}	40 mm Hg

    What is this condition?

    A. Uncompensated respiratory alkalosis

    B. Metabolic acidosis

    C. Compensated metabolic alkalosis

    D. Respiratory acidosis

    E. Uncompensated metabolic alkalosis

26. A 31-year-old woman presents to the emergency department with a 12-hour history of palpitations and dyspnea. The palpitations began suddenly, although the patient does report feeling "anxious and irritable" for the past few weeks. She also notes a 5-lb weight loss over the past 4 weeks in spite of a good appetite. On physical examination, you note that her skin is warm and moist and that she has a fine tremor of both hands. Cardiac exam reveals a hyperdynamic PMI with an irregularly irregular rhythm, and a pulse deficit of 40. No murmurs are noted. Lungs are clear. ECG reveals atrial fibrillation with a ventricular rate of 140 to 180 bpm. On the basis of her history and physical exam findings, what is the most likely etiology for her atrial fibrillation?

    A. Anorexia nervosa

    B. Thyrotoxicosis

    C. Panic disorder

    D. Hyperparathyroidism

    E. Hypothyroidism

27. A 58-year-old woman who had cervical spine fusion surgery 2 years ago presents with complaints of neck pain and feeling "off-balance" when ambulating for the past 2 months. Which of the following physical examination findings specifically indicates a myelopathy due to severe cervical spinal cord compression?

    A. Decreased grip

    B. Decreased patellar deep tendon reflex

    C. Limited flexion of the neck

    D. Positive Babinski sign unilaterally or bilaterally

    E. Unequal pupillary reaction to light and accommodation

28. A 30-year-old pregnant Caucasian woman presents with recurring episodes of vesicular eruptions along the labia. These episodes occur about eight to ten times per year and last approximately 2 weeks. Which of the following is correct about her condition?

    A. This patient would be a good candidate for prophylactic treatment to prevent recurrences

    B. Oral acyclovir taken 5 times a day for a week will be curative for her condition

    C. The risk of transmitting the lesions vaginally to her child is minimal

    D. Her condition is not considered a sexually transmitted disease

    E. Her condition is secondary to local irritation

29. A 24-year-old Mediterranean woman with a past history of anemia presents for her first antenatal pregnancy visit. She does not know her family history because she is adopted. A complete blood count and iron studies reveal:

Red blood cells	5 mL/kg
Hemoglobin	10 g/dL
Hematocrit	30%
Mean corpuscular volume	72 fl
Serum ferritin	140 µg/L
Total iron-binding capacity	normal

    What is the next step in management?

    A. Initiate oral iron replacement.

    B. Initiate parenteral iron replacement.

    C. Initiate vitamin B_{12} replacement.

    D. Obtain a peripheral smear.

    E. Perform a Schilling test.

30. Which of the following is a manifestation of secondary syphilis infection?

    A. A single, painless, indurated papule of the penis

    B. A painless ulcer on the cervix

    C. Aortic aneurysm rupture

    D. Painless bilateral inguinal lymphadenopathy

    E. Diffuse maculopapular rash

31. A patient who is being treated for a myocardial infarction that occurred 2 hours ago is medicated with IV nitroprusside. Which of the following is the expected action of this drug?

    A. Constriction of arterioles alone

    B. Constriction of both arterioles and venules

    C. Constriction of venules alone

    D. Dilatation of arterioles alone

    E. Dilatation of both arterioles and venules

32. A 12-year-old previously healthy girl presents with a 7-day history of a dry and nonproductive cough, low-grade fever, headache, and myalgias. Examination of the thorax reveals normal inspiration and expiration with a few widely scattered rhonchi. Chest x-ray reveals interstitial patchy infiltrates bilaterally. Cold agglutinins are negative. Which of the following is the most likely diagnosis?

    A. Cystic fibrosis

    B. Hyperreactive airway disease

    C. *Mycoplasma* pneumonia

    D. Pneumococcal pneumonia

    E. Viral pneumonia

33. A 46-year-old overweight woman complains of right upper quadrant pain and nausea and has vomited several times. She describes the pain as steady and severe. The patient also reports eating a large, fatty meal prior to the start of her symptoms. Which of the following is the most appropriate test to confirm the diagnosis?

    A. Complete blood count

    B. CT scan

    C. Radiograph

    D. Serum bilirubin

    E. Ultrasound

34. A 48-year-old Caucasian man presents for follow-up of a shoulder injury from a car accident that occurred 2 months ago. He complains of insomnia, anxiousness, and lack of focus. He has continual thoughts that he is going to crash his car into poles and barricades—so much so that he has stopped driving. Which of the following is the most likely diagnosis?

    A. Adjustment disorder

    B. Generalized anxiety disorder

    C. Post-traumatic stress disorder

    D. Obsessive-compulsive disorder

    E. Major depressive disorder

35. A 16-year-old boy presents with right knee pain after a fall while playing soccer. He states that he fell awkwardly and heard a "clicking" sound. On examination, you note a swollen knee and that he has pain with twisting and squatting. Which of the following tests will confirm the diagnosis?

    A. Lachman test

    B. Anterior drawer test

    C. McMurray test

    D. Homan test

    E. Murphy test

36. A 56-year-old man comes to the urgent care center because of a sudden onset of a 38.9°C (102.0°F) fever with associated pain in the lower back and perineum. He also complains of an urgent need to urinate, but when he urinates there is only a small amount of urine with associated pain. What should be avoided in this patient when doing the physical exam?

    A. Transillumination of the scrotum

    B. Palpating for costovertebral angle tenderness

    C. Digital rectal exam

    D. Vigorous prostatic massage

    E. Palpation of the testicles

37. A 47-year-old woman presents with a complaint of profound xerostomia. Which of the following chronic medications is most likely causing her symptoms?

    A. Amitriptyline

    B. Enalapril

    C. Fluoxetine

    D. Ibuprofen

    E. Medroxyprogesterone

38. A 24-year-old woman comes to the clinic at the urging of her friends. She denies feeling ill and states she has never felt better and is currently "at the top of her game." One of her friends accompanying her to this visit, however, tells the physician that she has been acting strangely. Over the last 2 weeks, the patient has been staying up to all hours of the night, has been bringing multiple strange men home, and has been running up incredible amounts of credit card debt from wild shopping sprees. Her past medical history is remarkable for depression, for which she has been treated for 4 months with paroxetine. Physical examination reveals a mildly agitated woman who cannot seem to sit still but otherwise appears normal. Neuropsychiatric examination is remarkable only for a virtually continuous flow of accelerated speech that is impossible to interrupt. Which of the following is the most appropriate management at this time?

    A. Add gabapentin to the patient's medical regimen

    B. Change paroxetine to amitriptyline or desipramine

    C. Discontinue paroxetine and follow closely

    D. Discontinue paroxetine and start lithium immediately

    E. Increase the dose of paroxetine and follow closely

39. A 29-year-old woman comes to the physician because of a 1-week history of a mucopurulent vaginal discharge. She is sexually active with two different men. Her last menstrual period was 2 weeks ago and was normal. Physical examination is unremarkable. A Pap smear result is normal, but a chlamydia probe is positive. Cultures for gonorrhea are negative. Which of the following is the most appropriate management?

   A. Prescribe a single oral dose of azithromycin; have her return if symptoms persist.

   B. Prescribe a single oral dose of azithromycin; have her return for a test of cure following treatment.

   C. Prescribe a 14-day course of oral doxycycline; have her return if symptoms persist.

   D. Prescribe a 14-day course of doxycycline; have her return for a test of cure following treatment.

   E. Prescribe a 7-day course of metronidazole; have her return if symptoms persist.

40. A 68-year-old man presents to the emergency room with severe right forearm pain after using the arm to rise from a chair. He felt a "snap" and immediate severe pain, and is now unable to pronate or supinate his right forearm. He is currently on a beta-blocker for hypertension, and on lovastatin for hyperlipidemia. He has no other significant past medical history, and has no history of previous fractures. His physical examination is significant only for some exaggerated kyphosis and bilateral bowing of his tibias. X-ray reveals a mid-metaphyseal fracture of the radius, which is nondisplaced. In addition, there are multiple bone "fissures" in both the radius and ulna with slightly increased bone density. Labs reveal a normal serum calcium, a normal serum phosphorus, and a normal serum 25-hydroxyvitamin-D. Alkaline phosphatase is markedly high. What is the most likely diagnosis?

   A. Osteoporosis

   B. Osteomalacia

   C. Hyperparathyroidism

   D. Paget disease of bone

   E. Vitamin D intoxication

41. A 34-year-old woman complains of severe headache and nausea 12 hours after a diagnostic lumbar puncture. The headache is exacerbated when the patient sits up and is relieved when she lies flat. On examination, she is afebrile and has no neurologic deficits. She is alert and oriented. Her lumbar puncture site has minimal clear discharge without erythema, increased warmth, palpable tenderness, and fluctuance in the area of the lumbar puncture. What is the etiology of the clear drainage?

   A. Dural leak

   B. Epidural abscess

   C. Epidural hematoma

   D. Lumbar puncture wound infection

   E. Meningitis

42. A 67-year-old Caucasian man presents for a general skin examination. He denies any problems. On exam, a 1-cm, smooth, pearly papule along his left nostril is noted. What is the preliminary diagnosis?

   A. Squamous cell carcinoma

   B. Basal cell carcinoma

   C. Malignant melanoma

   D. Epidermoid cyst

   E. Sebaceous adenoma

43. A 6-year-old female patient presents with low-grade fever and facial rash. Now the mother reports a faint pink rash on the child's trunk, arms, and legs. HEENT exam is within normal limits except for some clear rhinorrhea. You note on exam that the patient has a bilaterally flushed appearance of the cheeks and a lacy pink rash most noticeable on the arms and chest. There is no lymphadenopathy. The child's immunizations are up to date. What is the most likely diagnosis?

   A. Rubeola

   B. Rubella

   C. Erythema infectiosum

   D. Roseola

   E. Varicella

44. The primary pharmacologic action of nitroglycerin involves which of the following?

    A. Decreased heart rate

    B. Decreased production of angiotensin II

    C. Relaxation of vascular smooth muscle

    D. Increased inotropic effect of the heart

    E. Increased renal elimination of fluids

45. A 25-year-old man comes to the urgent care center complaining of blood in his urine. He also states that 4 weeks ago, he started having abdominal pain, dark-colored stools, and raised purplish lesions on his legs. He also stated that he has pain in his knees and ankles. What diagnostic test would confirm that the hematuria is related to the other symptoms?

    A. Renal ultrasound

    B. Renal biopsy

    C. Cystoscopy

    D. Urinalysis

    E. Intravenous urography

46. A 60-year-old Asian woman presents with episodes in which her heart races and she is jittery and cannot function. The episodes last from 5 to 15 minutes and occur two or three times per week. Which of the following is the most appropriate treatment?

    A. Long-acting benzodiazepines and cognitive therapy

    B. Selective serotonin reuptake inhibitors and cognitive therapy

    C. Inpatient intensive cognitive therapy

    D. Beta-blockers and dopamine antagonists

    E. Intravenous sodium lactate

47. Which of the following is thought to be a major contributor to the cachexia often experienced by patients with advanced cancer?

    A. Clathrin

    B. Histamine

    C. Interferon

    D. Interleukin-2

    E. Tumor necrosis factor

48. Amoxicillin exerts its antibacterial effect by which of the following mechanisms?

    A. Competitive inhibition of para-amino-benzoic acid

    B. Inhibition of bacterial cell wall synthesis

    C. Inhibition of DNA-gyrase

    D. Irreversible binding to the 30S subunit of bacterial ribosomes

    E. Irreversible binding to the 50S subunit of bacterial ribosomes

49. Warfarin exerts its anticoagulant properties by inhibiting the production of

    A. cyclooxygenase

    B. fibrinogen

    C. platelets

    D. thromboxane A_2

    E. vitamin K-dependent clotting factors

50. A 52-year-old man who has smoked for 32 years presents with a history of a persistent cough. The cough has not responded to two courses of antibiotics. His chest x-ray reveals a solitary right lung mass. His purified protein derivative test is negative. What is the next step in the evaluation of this patient's lung mass?

    A. Complete blood count

    B. CT scan of the chest

    C. Erythrocyte sedimentation rate

    D. PET scan

    E. Thoracentesis

51. A 66-year-old African American man has been a patient of the clinic for the past 15 years and presents today for a routine check-up. He has a long-standing history of controlled hypertension and a strong family history of coronary heart disease. His blood pressure today is 132/88 mm Hg. He denies dyspnea, diaphoresis, or lower extremity edema. Which of the following would most likely be present on his annual EKG?

    A. Global ST elevation

    B. Tall peaked T waves

    C. Right axis deviation

    D. Left bundle branch block

    E. Transient ST depression

52. An elderly patient is diagnosed with fecal impaction. What is the most appropriate next step in the management of this patient?

    A. Administration of methylcellulose

    B. Administration of a stool softener

    C. Bedside digital dislodgement

    D. Sigmoidoscopy

    E. Surgical intervention

53. The primary metabolic effect of the principal hormone secreted by alpha cells of the pancreas is

    A. augmentation of calcium deposition in bone

    B. increase of amino acid storage in the liver

    C. promotion of lipogenesis in liver and adipose tissue

    D. inhibition of gluconeogenesis

    E. stimulation of glycogenolysis

54. A patient is diagnosed with a hereditary disorder that results in the development of splenomegaly, spherocytes, and increased reticulocytes on peripheral blood smear. If his red cells are also microcytic and hyperchromic, which of the following would be the most appropriate pharmacotherapy?

    A. Azathioprine

    B. Cyanocobalamin

    C. Folic acid

    D. Iron sulfate

    E. Methotrexate

55. A patient with small cell carcinoma suffers from myasthenia gravis and, following electrophysiologic testing, is diagnosed with Lambert-Eaton syndrome. This patient would be most effectively managed by treatment with which of the following drugs?

    A. Azathioprine

    B. Baclofen

    C. Carbamazepine

    D. Pyridostigmine

    E. Verapamil

Items 56–58: The response options for the next three items are the same. You will be required to select one answer for each item in the set.

For the following conditions, select the appropriate pharmacologic cause (choices A–E).

    A. Cimetidine

    B. Trazodone

    C. Metoclopramide

    D. Isoniazid

    E. Sulfonamides

56. Priapism

57. Galactorrhea

58. Extrapyramidal symptoms

59. A 38-year-old attorney is taken to the emergency department by his wife. He has had a fever and headache for 3 days and recently has become disoriented and irritable. A lumbar puncture is performed. The opening pressure is 300 mm H_2O and the cerebrospinal fluid (CSF) contains 200 white blood cells (85% lymphocytes) and 100 erythrocytes. CSF glucose is 85 mg/dL, and protein is 65 mg/dL. Bacteriologic cultures are negative, as are all latex particle agglutination tests for fungi and bacteria. The drug of choice for this condition relies on activation by which viral enzyme?

    A. Adenosine kinase

    B. DNA polymerase

    C. Protease

    D. Reverse transcriptase

    E. Thymidine kinase

60. A physician assistant is testing the sensation on the foot in a diabetic man. The patient is unable to sense a pinprick on the undersurface of his smallest toe. This finding indicates pathology of which of the following nerves?

    A. Lateral plantar nerve

    B. Medial plantar nerve

    C. Saphenous nerve

    D. Sural nerve

    E. Tibial nerve

End of Block 2

Block 3

1. A 32-year-old woman presents to your clinic for advice prior to pregnancy. She has both hypertension and insulin-dependent diabetes mellitus (IDDM). Her hypertension is managed with an angiotensin-converting enzyme inhibitor (ACEI). After performing a complete history and physical examination, you advise her to

   A. stop the insulin and begin an oral hypoglycemic

   B. stop the ACEI and begin methyldopa

   C. continue both the insulin and ACEI

   D. add a diuretic to the ACEIs to prevent pregnancy-induced edema

   E. modify her diet

2. A 65-year-old woman presents with pain in the left lower quadrant for the past 3 days. She has had several similar episodes over the last 6 months. On physical examination, there is abdominal tenderness in the left lower quadrant with rebound tenderness. Her hemoglobin is 13.6 g/dL, and WBC count 15,400/mm^3 with 82% neutrophils and 18% lymphocytes. Urinalysis shows 5 to 6 white blood cells per high power field. Which of the following is the most likely diagnosis?

   A. Ischemic colitis

   B. Acute diverticulitis

   C. Acute pyelonephritis

   D. Irritable bowel syndrome

   E. Appendicitis

3. A 2-week-old newborn is brought to the emergency department by her mother. The mother reports projectile vomiting after breast feeding. Physical examination of the newborn's abdomen reveals an olive-shaped mass to the right of the midline. Which of the following is the most likely diagnosis?

   A. Appendicitis

   B. Intussusception

   C. Meckel diverticulum

   D. Pyloric stenosis

   E. Ventral hernia

4. A 20-year-old white female presents with a 5-year history of binging and purging. What supportive clinical findings would you expect to find on exam?

   A. Oral thrush

   B. Erosion of tooth enamel

   C. Hemorrhoids

   D. Decreased mini-mental status exam score

   E. Retinal hemorrhages

5. A 56-year-old woman with a history of diabetes mellitus presents with burning and tingling in the thumb, index finger, and middle finger of her left hand. She states the pain is worse at night. This patient's symptoms are most likely caused by entrapment of which nerve?

   A. Ulnar

   B. Median

   C. Radial

   D. Sciatic

   E. Peroneal

6. A patient with known Berger disease has a urine protein level of 2 g/d and a blood pressure of 150/100 mm Hg. A drug from what class of medications would reduce the proteinuria and hypertension?

   A. Angiotensin-converting enzyme inhibitors

   B. Beta-blockers

   C. Calcium channel blockers

   D. HMG-CoA reductase inhibitors

   E. Thiazide diuretics

7. Intramuscular injections should be given in the upper, outer quadrant of the buttocks to prevent damage to which of the following nerves?

   A. Common peroneal

   B. Lateral femoral cutaneous

   C. Obturator

   D. Sciatic

   E. Superior gluteal

8. A 35-year-old pregnant woman comes to the physician because of a "huge growth" behind her ear. She says that she began to notice it about 6 months ago, after she got her ears pierced. She wears silver-plated nickel earrings and is a seasonal agricultural worker. Physical examination shows a 4.5-cm, firm, exophytic, erythematous nodule on the posterior aspect of her left ear. She has mild acne on her face, back, and chest. A biopsy taken from the lesion shows many broad and irregular collagen bundles with an increased number of capillaries and fibroblasts. Which of the following is the most likely cause of the nodule?

   A. Blockage of a hair follicle with sebum and keratin

   B. Injury from ear piercing

   C. Nickel exposure from the earrings

   D. Pregnancy

   E. Sun exposure

9. Which of the following is the mechanism of action of acarbose?

   A. It increases body sensitivity to insulin.

   B. It increases insulin receptor activity.

   C. It increases insulin secretion.

   D. It delays digestion of carbohydrates.

   E. It decreases hepatic glucose production.

10. Café-au-lait lesions are associated with

   A. ependymomas

   B. metastatic tumors

   C. multiple myeloma

   D. neurofibromatosis

   E. staphylococcal infections

11. A 6-month-old white male infant presents for a check-up. He has a history of severe infantile eczema. Which of the following conditions would you expect to find in his family history?

   A. Varicella

   B. Mononucleosis

   C. Skin cancer

   D. Asthma

   E. Reye syndrome

12. A 40-year-old woman comes to the urgent care center because of a sudden onset of severe, watery diarrhea for the past 6 hours. She describes the stool as gray and murky. She states that it does not smell like stool and there is no blood or pus. She denies fever, nausea, vomiting, and abdominal pain. The patient states that she returned from a trip to Peru 1 week prior to her symptoms developing. On physical exam, the patient has decreased skin turgor and is slightly tachycardic. What is the most likely diagnosis?

   A. Cholera

   B. Shigellosis

   C. *Campylobacter* dysentery

   D. Giardiasis

   E. Salmonellosis

13. A 48-year-old African American man presents to the clinic for hypertension. Multiple readings have demonstrated elevated blood pressures. He has no significant past medical history and takes no medications. He has been on the DASH diet and exercising three times a week for the past 8 weeks with no improvement in his readings. What is the most effective first-line therapy for this patient?

   A. Captopril

   B. Hydrochlorothiazide

   C. Propranolol

   D. Clonidine

   E. Prazosin

14. A 61-year-old man is brought to the emergency department for chest pain. The patient has a long history of coronary artery disease and stable angina. The angina is usually precipitated by activity and relieved by rest. His provider recently prescribed him sildenafil and he has been using the drug with success. This morning, he developed acute-onset substernal chest pain that radiates to his left arm. Rest does not relieve this pain. You suspect that the patient is having a myocardial infarction. The patient last took sildenafil the night before. Which of the following treatments is *absolutely contraindicated* in this situation?

    A. Aspirin

    B. Metoprolol

    C. Morphine

    D. Nitroglycerin

    E. Oxygen at 2 to 5 L/min

15. A 14-year-old boy is experiencing a severe asthma attack. Although he is using accessory muscles to breathe, the auscultation of his chest reveals no audible wheezing. His heart rate is 160/min and respirations are 52/min. Which of the following arterial blood gas results represents the worst prognosis for this patient?

    A. pH 7.35; pCO_2 62 mm Hg; pO_2 60 mm Hg

    B. pH 7.44; pCO_2 38 mm Hg; pO_2 70 mm Hg

    C. pH 7.60; pCO_2 18 mm Hg; pO_2 60 mm Hg

    D. pH 7.52; pCO_2 28 mm Hg; pO_2 80 mm Hg

    E. pH 7.44; pCO_2 45 mm Hg; pO_2 88 mm Hg

16. A man presents with an abscess near the coccyx. He is diagnosed with pilonidal disease. Which of the following is the most appropriate next step?

    A. Antibiotic administration

    B. Excision of the pilonidal disease

    C. Incision and drainage

    D. Shaving of the natal cleft

    E. Warm sitz bath

17. A 56-year-old white woman presents for her physical exam. She states that her mother passed away suddenly 6 months ago and she is having difficulty moving on with her life. She is unable to get out of bed in the mornings and is not eating. She was fired from her job and her husband has filed for divorce. Which of the following best describes her situation?

    A. Uncomplicated grief

    B. Complicated grief

    C. Post-traumatic stress disorder

    D. Adjustment disorder

    E. Bipolar disorder

18. Which of the following tests may be used to confirm the diagnosis of Sjögren syndrome?

    A. Schilling test

    B. Serum protein electrophoresis

    C. Rheumatoid factor

    D. Schirmer test

    E. Antinuclear antibody

19. A 59-year-old man comes to the office reporting increased hesitancy during urination as well as increased frequency at night. After urination he still feels that his bladder is not quite empty. What finding should be expected from the digital rectal exam?

    A. Tender and boggy prostate

    B. A prostate with focal nodules and induration

    C. A firm, nontender prostate without nodules that is uniformly enlarged

    D. An increase in the tone of the anal sphincter

    E. Periprostatic tenderness

20. A person undergoes a routine pre-employment physical. During the physical, it is noted that the patient's uvula is deviated to one side. Additionally, when the back of the throat is touched with a cotton swab, no gag reflex is elicited. These findings suggest damage to which of the following cranial nerves?

    A. Facial

    B. Glossopharyngeal

    C. Hypoglossal

    D. Trigeminal

    E. Vagus

21. A 25-year-old woman gives birth to a baby with a low birth weight, microcephaly, and scattered bluish-purple spots over her trunk and abdomen. Which of the following is the most likely etiologic agent?

    A. Poxvirus

    B. Cytomegalovirus

    C. Orthomyxovirus

    D. Parvovirus B19

    E. Retrovirus

22. During the neurology component of a physical examination on a 26-year-old man, fibrillations of his tongue are seen. Which of the cranial nerves is possibly affected?

    A. Cranial nerve II (optic nerve)

    B. Cranial nerve V (trigeminal nerve)

    C. Cranial nerve VII (facial nerve)

    D. Cranial nerves IX and X (glossopharyngeal and vagus nerves)

    E. Cranial nerve XII (hypoglossal nerve)

23. Long-term topical steroid use for dermatologic conditions may result in which of the following?

    A. Hyperpigmentation

    B. Decreased skin infections

    C. Striae

    D. Thickening of the skin

    E. Decreased tolerance to the topical steroid

24. Which of the following laboratory studies are helpful in the diagnosis and treatment of xanthomas?

    A. Urinalysis, estrogen, alpha-fetoprotein, CBC

    B. Progesterone, DHEAS, prolactin levels

    C. Estrogen, CBC, TSH, DHEAS, HDL

    D. HDL, VLDL, LDL

    E. Serum testosterone, viral culture, RPR

25. A patient who has had a gastrectomy, bariatric surgery for obesity, or severe Crohn disease of the terminal ileum must be monitored for evidence of which hematologic abnormality?

    A. Aplastic anemia

    B. Folic acid deficiency

    C. Glucose-6-phosphate deficiency

    D. Iron deficiency

    E. Vitamin B_{12} deficiency

26. A 16-year-old girl comes to the adolescent clinic because she had sex for the first time 5 days ago. She says now she feels sick and has a low-grade fever. She is also feeling pain and a burning sensation in her genitals. She tells the physician assistant that she is afraid to look. Based on the clinical presentation, what should the physician assistant expect to see when she examines the patient's genitalia?

    A. Shallow ulcers with a red border and serous secretions

    B. A firm, punched-out lesion with rolled borders

    C. Soft, fleshy growths on the vulva forming "kissing lesions"

    D. Irregularly shaped lesions with red, undermined margins on a yellow-gray base

    E. Elevated lesions with rolled, elevated margins on a red, rough base

27. A 68-year-old woman presents to the emergency department with a 1-week history of a nonproductive cough and progressive shortness of breath. Her past medical history is significant for rheumatic heart disease, and chronic obstructive pulmonary disease. Her vital signs are: temperature 35.6° C (96.1° F), heart rate 110/min (irregular), respiratory rate 26/min, and blood pressure 70/40 mm Hg. On pulmonary examination, bilateral rhonchi with a prolonged expiratory phase are appreciated. Cardiovascular examination is significant for an irregular rhythm and a grade III/VI low-pitched decrescendo murmur with an opening snap. Bilateral lower extremity edema is noted as well. Which of the following would be the most likely finding on an electrocardiogram?

   A. Atrial fibrillation
   B. Ventricular tachycardia
   C. First-degree heart block
   D. Atrial flutter
   E. Left ventricular hypertrophy

28. A patient complains of fever, malaise, nausea, and vomiting. Physical examination reveals a tender and enlarged liver. Upon questioning, the patient states that he was vacationing in Mexico approximately 1 month ago. Which of the following is the most likely diagnosis?

   A. Hepatitis A
   B. Hepatitis B
   C. Hepatitis C
   D. Hepatitis D
   E. Hepatitis G

29. A 6-year-old boy presents with a 7-month history of inattentiveness, hyperactivity, and fidgeting. His teacher reports that he is easily distracted and has difficulty organizing tasks. What is the most likely diagnosis?

   A. Asperger disorder
   B. Attention deficit hyperactivity disorder (ADHD)
   C. Oppositional defiant disorder (ODD)
   D. Autistic disorder
   E. Rett disorder

30. A 12-year-old boy comes to the emergency room because of a sudden erection that persisted for 45 minutes. What information obtained in the history would be most useful in determining treatment of the patient?

   A. Sexual history
   B. History of cryptorchidism
   C. History of sickle cell disease
   D. History of drug abuse
   E. History of alcohol abuse

31. A 35-year-old pregnant patient presents with high blood pressure. The patient has a history of high blood pressure controlled with diet and exercise. On physical examination, blood pressure is 158/102 mm Hg, cardiac exam is unremarkable, and there is no peripheral edema. Electrolytes, renal function, CBC, and urinalysis are normal. Which of the following is the treatment of choice for this patient?

   A. Labetalol (Trandate)
   B. Aliskiren (Tekturna)
   C. Diltiazem (Cardizem)
   D. Valsartan (Diovan)
   E. Nitroprusside (Nitropress)

32. A 68-year-old woman consults a physician because she has been having chronic severe headaches, particularly involving the temporal and occipital regions. She has also had transient visual disturbances, including double vision, blurred vision, and difficulty reading. On questioning, she also reports having muscular pain on chewing hard substances. To confirm the suspected diagnosis, a biopsy of a blood vessel is taken from approximately 3 cm above and lateral to the lateral edge of her left eyebrow. Which of the following is the most likely diagnosis?

   A. Migraine headache
   B. Giant cell arteritis
   C. Trigeminal neuralgia
   D. Ophthalmic zoster
   E. Bell's palsy

33. A 78-year-old woman hospitalized for hip replacement surgery is discovered on admission labs to have a TSH of 18.0 μU/mL and a free T_4 level of 2 μg/dL. Her past medical history is significant for compensated congestive heart failure, for which she is on HCTZ 25 mg PO q d. Appropriate management for her hypothyroidism consists of

   A. Synthroid 0.15 mg PO q d; TSH recheck in 6 to 8 weeks

   B. Synthroid 0.025 mg PO q d increasing 0.025 mg q 4 weeks until euthyroid

   C. Synthroid 0.15 mg PO q d; TSH recheck in 1 week

   D. Synthroid 0.025 mg PO q d; TSH recheck in 6 to 8 weeks

   E. Synthroid should not be given to this patient

34. An 18-year-old patient presents with complaints consistent with intermittent visual auras for the past 6 months. Which of the following conditions are auras associated with?

   A. Epilepsy

   B. Huntington disease

   C. Parkinson disease

   D. Tardive dyskinesia

   E. Transient ischemic attacks

35. A 13-year-old girl presents with moderate cystic acne. She states that she has "tried everything available over-the-counter." Which of the following is the next step in the treatment of this patient?

   A. Oral contraceptive pills

   B. Topical hydrocortisone

   C. Clindamycin

   D. Isotretinoin

   E. Topical benzoyl peroxide

36. A 20-year-old woman comes to the gynecology clinic because of irregular, raised lesions on her vulva and anus. The bases of the lesions are white. There is no associated dysuria, itching, or discharge. Which of the following is the most likely diagnosis?

   A. Herpes simplex

   B. Molluscum contagiosum

   C. Adenovirus infection

   D. Human papillomavirus

   E. Erythema infectiosum

37. A mother brings her 1-month-old infant to the pediatric office for his DTaP vaccination because she will start taking him to the daycare center in 1 week. The physician assistant informs her that it is not yet time for this vaccine. At what age is the first DTaP vaccine administered?

   A. 2 months

   B. 4 months

   C. 6 months

   D. 12 months

   E. 15 months

38. A sharp instrument passing through the superior orbital fissure would most likely sever which of the following structures?

   A. Abducens nerve

   B. Facial nerve

   C. Mandibular nerve

   D. Maxillary nerve

   E. Middle meningeal artery

39. A parent brings her 8-year-old son to the pediatric office because of concern over the child's grades dropping over the past year. The mother states that at home, he must be reminded over and over again to complete tasks. In the classroom, according to the boy's teacher, he is not turning in homework and he moves quickly from one activity to another. Which of the following is the most likely diagnosis?

   A. Depression

   B. Conduct disorder

   C. Absence seizures

   D. Intellectual disability

   E. Attention deficit disorder

40. A 69-year-old woman with a history of type 2 diabetes, chronic renal insufficiency (baseline creatinine of 2.3 mg/dL), and hypertension presents with moderate dyspnea and right-sided pleuritic chest pain. She denies fevers, cough, or chills. Her temperature is 38.1°C (100.6°F), blood pressure is 130/70 mm Hg, pulse is 123/min, and respirations are 32/min. Physical examination shows a swollen and tender right calf. Lung examination is normal. Chest x-ray reveals no active disease. EKG shows sinus tachycardia with a S_1, Q3, and inverted T pattern in lead III. At this time, which of the following is the initial diagnostic test of choice for this patient?

   A. Magnetic resonance imaging

   B. Pulmonary arteriography

   C. D-dimer level

   D. Spiral chest CT scan

   E. Echocardiogram

41. A 17-year-old high school athlete with a history of intermittent wheezing with exercise presents to the emergency department with shortness of breath. She has obvious difficulty in breathing and has diffuse wheezes throughout both lung fields on auscultation. Her pulse oxygen on room air is 95%. The most effective treatment at this point is

   A. inhaled albuterol nebulizer

   B. intravenous hydrocortisone

   C. intravenous theophylline

   D. nasal canula oxygen

   E. subcutaneous epinephrine

42. A newborn is diagnosed with phenylketonuria. To promote maximal development and cognitive abilities throughout the newborn's life and into adulthood, which of the following foods should be restricted?

   A. Cereals

   B. Fruits

   C. Grains

   D. Soy products

   E. Vegetables

43. A 78-year-old man presents with gradual memory loss, orientation difficulties, and some mild language deficits. On mini-mental status exam, you note loss of visuospatial processing. The patient continues to work as a librarian, but is having some difficulty remembering tasks. The remainder of his examination and labs is normal. Which of the following is the most likely diagnosis?

   A. Parkinson disease

   B. Vitamin B_{12} deficiency

   C. Multiple sclerosis

   D. Alzheimer disease

   E. Alcoholism

44. Which of the following laboratory tests has a 99% sensitivity in the diagnosis of systemic lupus erythematosus (SLE)?

   A. Antinuclear antibody (ANA)

   B. Rheumatoid factor (RF)

   C. C-reactive protein (CRP)

   D. RPR/VRDL

   E. Erythrocyte sedimentation rate (ESR)

45. Which of the following portions of the mini-mental status examination tests attention and concentration?

   A. Indicate the year, season, month, day, and date

   B. Spell the word "world" backward

   C. Copy intersecting pentagons

   D. Repeat the phrase "No ifs, ands, or buts"

   E. Interpret the saying, "Don't cry over spilled milk"

46. A 25-year-old woman presents with recurring spontaneous abortions. Her past medical history includes four prior spontaneous abortions and deep venous thrombosis (DVT) 5 years ago. Which of the following is the most appropriate next step in establishing a diagnosis?

   A. Evaluation for in vitro fertilization

   B. Laboratory testing for antiphospholipid antibodies

   C. Progesterone challenge

   D. Laboratory testing of follicle-stimulating hormone/luteinizing hormone

   E. Duplex ultrasound of bilateral lower extremities

47. On physical examination, a bulging anterior fontanel with marked pulsations is noted in a 4-month-old. Which of the following is the most likely diagnosis?

    A. Mumps

    B. Acute sinusitis

    C. Normal development

    D. Shaken baby syndrome

    E. Congenital abnormality

48. A newly adopted 2-year-old boy is brought to the office for a well child exam. Because the parents do not have the boy's complete medical history, a complete physical is done. Upon palpation of the scrotum, no testes are felt. How should the patient be managed?

    A. An orchiopexy should be performed

    B. An orchiectomy should be performed

    C. Nothing should be done because the testes may descend spontaneously

    D. Human chorionic gonadotropin injections should be given

    E. An ultrasound should be performed to locate the missing testes

49. Which of the following is the treatment of choice for most tapeworm infections?

    A. Mebendazole (Vermox)

    B. Praziquantel (Biltricide)

    C. Niclosamide (Niclocide)

    D. Pyrantel pamoate (Antiminth)

    E. Metronidazole (Flagyl)

50. A 46-year-old man arrives for a routine physical examination. There is a family history of cancer and heart disease. Both his father and brother had myocardial infarctions prior to age 55. He exercises regularly and does not drink. Most of his diet is high in saturated fat and cholesterol. He smokes one pack of cigarettes per week. His examination is unremarkable. Which of the following is an appropriate screening test at this time?

    A. Fasting lipid profile

    B. Nonfasting total cholesterol level

    C. Oral glucose tolerance test

    D. Sigmoidoscopy

    E. Prostate specific antigen

51. A 24-year-old woman presents complaining of paroxysmal bilateral pallor and cyanosis of her finger tips, followed by rubor after her symptoms abate. The patient states that this "condition" is precipitated by cold or emotional upset and is relieved by warmth. Which of the following is the most appropriate pharmacotherapy?

    A. Atenolol

    B. Furosemide

    C. Gabapentin

    D. Nifedipine

    E. Vecuronium

52. What will injury to the lower division of the facial nerve during parotid surgery result in?

    A. Inability to furrow the brow (to frown) on the same side

    B. Numbness over the angle and mental region of the jaw on the same side

    C. Ptosis of the eye on the same side

    D. Weakness in closing the eye on the same side

    E. Weakness of the lower lip on the same side

53. An 18-year-old woman presents with malaise and icteric sclera. The patient states that two days ago she was diagnosed with a urinary tract infection and treated with trimethoprim-sulfamethoxazole. Laboratory testing reveals a two-day drop in hemoglobin from 13.5 g/dL to 11 g/dL and a reticulocyte count of 10%. Which of the following is the most likely diagnosis?

    A. Beta thalassemia

    B. Sickle cell anemia

    C. Vitamin B$_{12}$ deficiency

    D. Hereditary spherocytosis

    E. Glucose-6-phosphate dehydrogenase deficiency

54. A 10-year-old girl comes to the physician for an annual examination. She has been in good health for the past year, except for occasional asthma flares that she controls with an albuterol inhaler. She takes no other medications and has no medical problems. Physical examination is appropriate for age. The patient's mother wants to know when her daughter needs to begin having annual Pap smears. Which of the following represents the time at which this patient should begin having cervical cytology screening with Pap smears?

    A. Age 12 or with menarche

    B. Age 18 or with the onset of sexual activity

    C. Age 21 or 3 years after the onset of sexual activity

    D. Age 30 or 10 years after the onset of sexual activity

    E. Pap tests will not be necessary in this patient

55. Which of the following medications used in the treatment of Parkinson disease also possesses antiviral properties?

    A. Amantadine

    B. Bromocriptine

    C. Carbidopa

    D. Levodopa

    E. Selegiline

56. A 65-year-old woman seen in the emergency room complains of cramping and poorly localized mid-to-lower abdominal pain. She has vomited twice since the onset of pain. Past medical history is significant for diabetes mellitus. Her diabetes is controlled with oral medications. Past surgical history is significant for a hysterectomy. Physical examination reveals a tender and distended abdomen. Auscultation of the abdomen demonstrates high-pitched tinkles. Plain abdominal radiographs show a ladder-like pattern of dilated small bowel loops with air-fluid levels. Which of the following is the most likely etiology of the patient's condition?

    A. Adhesions

    B. Hernia

    C. Inflammatory bowel disease

    D. Neoplasm

    E. Volvulus

57. A 16-year-old Caucasian girl presents with her mother for assessment of her behavior. Her mother states that the girl is overly sensitive and reacts angrily if she is not included in everything the family does. The girl has made multiple suicide threats over seemingly minute issues. Which of the following is the most likely diagnosis?

    A. Narcissistic personality disorder

    B. Borderline personality disorder

    C. Avoidant personality disorder

    D. Passive-aggressive personality disorder

    E. Obsessive-compulsive personality disorder

58. A 35-year-old woman comes to the clinic for her yearly pelvic exam. Upon examination of the vagina, a bleeding ulceration is discovered. When asked if it is painful, the patient says no. A biopsy is done, and the ulcer is discovered to be a malignancy. Because this tumor was detected early, what is the recommended follow-up?

    A. Every 3 months for 5 years, then every 4 months for 2 years, and annually thereafter

    B. Every 3 months for 2 years, then every 6 months for 4 years, and annually thereafter

    C. Every 3 months for 2 years, then every 6 months for 3 years, and annually thereafter

    D. Every 3 months for 3 years, then every 4 months for 2 years, and annually thereafter

    E. Every 3 months for 4 years, then every 6 months for 3 years, and annually thereafter

59. Prostate cancer is inherited in an autosomal dominant manner. If the father is heterozygous and the mother is recessive, what is the probability that a male offspring will inherit the prostate cancer allele?

    A. 25%

    B. 50%

    C. 75%

    D. 100%

    E. 95%

60. A patient presents with severe angina and relates a history of angina, atherosclerosis, and documented coronary artery disease. On physical examination, he is noted to have carotid bruits bilaterally. His lab results reveal "borderline" serum troponin and an elevated CK-MB. The EKG shows ST elevation in leads V1 to V4. Which of the following would be the most likely site of this thromboembolic event?

    A. Left anterior descending artery

    B. Posterior descending branch of the right coronary artery

    C. Pulmonary artery

    D. Circumflex branch of the left coronary artery

    E. Aortic artery

End of Block 3

Block 4

1. A 25-year-old man comes to the clinic with chest pain at rest that is not always related to exercise. He reports two episodes of fainting during exercise, but has otherwise been healthy. There is a similar family history, and he relates that his father collapsed and died suddenly at age 50 while playing tennis. Physical examination reveals a systolic ejection murmur that is loudest along the left sternal border. Echocardiography shows asymmetric septal hypertrophy with outflow obstruction. Which of the following interventions would be most likely to decrease this patient's systolic murmur?

   A. Inhaling amyl nitrate

   B. Squatting

   C. Standing up

   D. Use of digoxin

   E. Valsalva maneuver

2. A 16-year-old girl presents with a 2-day history of cough that is productive of small quantities of white-yellow "phlegm." Her blood pressure is 114/78 mm Hg, heart rate is 84/min, respirations are 16/min, and temperature is 37.6° C (99.7° F). Her peak expiratory flow rate is 550 L/min. Her lungs are clear to auscultation. Which of the following is the most appropriate therapeutic recommendation?

   A. Albuterol metered dose inhaler as needed

   B. Amoxicillin for 7 days

   C. Fluids, rest, and acetaminophen as needed

   D. Oral prednisone for 5 days

   E. Penicillin V K for 7 to 10 days

3. Symptoms of diverticulitis include which of the following?

   A. Anal itching

   B. Bright red blood in the stool

   C. Fatty stools

   D. Left-sided abdominal pain

   E. Pain while having a bowel movement

4. Irresistible impulses to repeat a ritualistic act over and over again (i.e., handwashing) is known as a(n)

   A. obsession

   B. delusion

   C. compulsion

   D. hallucination

   E. phobia

5. A 40-year-old African American man presents with arthritis of the left knee and right ankle. He reports fever and weight loss over the past 2 weeks, and also complains of a few cold sores. Past medical history includes urethritis treated 3 weeks ago. Which of the following physical and laboratory findings would you expect to see in this patient?

   A. Telangiectasias, fibrotic skin, Raynaud syndrome, and HLA-B27 (–)

   B. Conjunctivitis, telangiectasias, and culture-positive joint fluid

   C. Urethritis, conjunctivitis, and HLA-B27 (+)

   D. Esophagitis, carditis, and erythema multiforme

   E. Rhinorrhea, lacrimation, and diaphoresis

6. A 10-year-old girl is brought to the office by her mother, who is concerned that the daughter may have "pink eye." The mother states that the girl has been rubbing her eyes constantly, sneezing, and generally appearing more tired than usual. She denies fever, discharge, or excessive lacrimation. Examination reveals bilateral injected sclera without discharge. The examination is otherwise unremarkable. Which of the following treatments is most appropriate?

    A. Nasal saline spray

    B. Nasal steroids

    C. Ocular antibiotics

    D. Ocular antihistamines

    E. Saline drops

7. A 20-year-old Italian gravida 2 para 1 woman who is at 20 weeks' gestation comes to the physician for her second prenatal visit. Her medical history is unremarkable, except that she has been taking phenobarbital for many years for a seizure disorder. Her lifestyle is free of risk from teratogens and unsafe practices. The laboratory studies from her first prenatal visit show: hemoglobin 9.9 g/dL, leukocyte count 12,000/mm³, platelets 224,000/mm³, MCV 84 fl, and red cell distribution width (RDW) 13. Which of the following is the most likely cause of these findings?

    A. Folate deficiency anemia

    B. Iron deficiency anemia

    C. Physiologic anemia

    D. Sickle cell trait

    E. Thalassemia

8. A typical presenting sign and/or symptom in a patient with hyperparathyroidism due to a parathyroid adenoma would include which of the following?

    A. A solitary thyroid nodule

    B. Hyperactivity or restlessness

    C. Tetany and muscle spasms

    D. Most patients are asymptomatic

    E. Weight gain, dry skin, and cold intolerance

9. Tumors of the spine originate most frequently from which area?

    A. Extradural space

    B. Intradural, extramedullary space

    C. Intradural, intramedullary space

    D. Peripheral nerves distal to the dorsal root ganglia

    E. Spinal column vasculature

10. A 56-year-old Caucasian woman presents with a rash on her face. She states that it is only on the right side and is painful. She has associated fevers and chills and denies use of any new detergents or soaps. On examination, you note a beefy red, diffusely swollen area along her right facies. The border is well demarcated and ends symmetrically in the middle of her nose. Which of the following pathogens is most likely involved?

    A. Group A beta-hemolytic strep

    B. *Neisseria gonorrhoeae*

    C. Varicella-zoster

    D. *Pseudomonas aeruginosa*

    E. *Rickettsia rickettsii*

11. In patients with known glucose-6-phosphate dehydrogenase deficiency, which of the following drugs can precipitate a hemolytic reaction?

    A. Amiodarone

    B. Amphotericin B

    C. Gentamicin

    D. Phenytoin

    E. Sulfonamides

12. An 18-year-old woman comes to the gynecology office complaining of vaginal itching. She also complains of a yellow-green discharge that has a smelly odor. Speculum examination reveals a red cervix with petechiae and diffuse vaginal erythema. The physician assistant prepares a saline slide of the vaginal secretions. Based on the patient's presentation, what should the physician assistant expect to see?

    A. Filaments and spores

    B. Epithelial cells covered with bacteria

    C. White, prominent papillae

    D. Motile, flagellated organisms

    E. Organisms forming a "spaghetti and meatballs" appearance

13. A 60-year-old man with a history of hypertension, hyperlipidemia, and peptic ulcer disease presents to the emergency department with 2 days of intermittent low substernal chest discomfort at rest. He had mild associated dyspnea, palpitations, and nausea. He denies diaphoresis, dizziness, or dyspepsia. The discomfort lasts anywhere from 25 to 40 minutes, with most episodes occurring in the early hours of the morning. His medications include lisinopril, digoxin, and aspirin. He does not smoke or drink. The physical examination is normal. An EKG was obtained, and a transient ST-segment elevation was noted. Which of the following is the most likely etiology of this patient's symptoms?

    A. Prinzmetal/variant angina

    B. Unstable angina

    C. Acute myocardial infarction

    D. Myocardial ischemia

    E. Stable angina pectoris

14. A patient reports a bulge in his groin when straining. He denies pain. Physical examination reveals a nonincarcerated, nonstrangulated inguinal hernia. Which of the following is the most appropriate treatment?

    A. Avoidance of activities that involve lifting or straining

    B. High-fiber diet

    C. No treatment is needed

    D. Surgical intervention

    E. Watchful waiting

15. You are treating a 36-year-old man who has schizophrenia, and you would like to start him on clozapine. Which of the following laboratory tests should you monitor?

    A. Liver function tests

    B. Complete blood count

    C. Urinalysis

    D. Renal function tests

    E. Thyroid function tests

16. A 12-year-old Caucasian boy presents with worsening right knee and hip pain for the last 2 weeks. On examination, you note loss of complete hip flexion and loss of ability to fully rotate the hip inward. The boy's mother states that he has been limping for the past few days. He denies trauma or previous injury. He is currently not participating in any sports or exercise. Which of the following is the most likely diagnosis?

    A. Osgood-Schlatter disease

    B. Knee bursitis

    C. Slipped capital femoral epiphysis

    D. Patellofemoral syndrome

    E. Osteomyelitis

17. A 50-year-old man with benign prostatic hyperplasia comes to the office because he is having urinary incontinence. What medication is best used for the treatment of this condition?

    A. Oxybutynin

    B. Imipramine

    C. Pseudoephedrine

    D. Bethanecol

    E. Prazosin

18. A patient is diagnosed with a 7 cm aortic aneurysm. Which of the following is the most appropriate management for this patient?

    A. Abdominal ultrasound every 6 months

    B. Refer to surgery for elective surgery

    C. Intensive blood pressure control

    D. Greenfield filter placement

    E. Begin anticoagulant

19. A 27-year-old primigravid woman at 18 weeks' gestation comes to the physician for a prenatal visit. She states that she is feeling well except for some fatigue. The pregnancy has been uncomplicated thus far. The patient has no medical problems. On examination, the patient's abdomen seems large for 18 weeks. An ultrasound is performed, which demonstrates twins, with a male and a female fetus. Which of the following is the type of twin pregnancy that this patient is most likely to have?

    A. Dichorionic/diamnionic

    B. Dichorionic/monoamnionic

    C. Monochorionic/diamnionic

    D. Monochorionic/monoamnionic

    E. Vanishing twin pregnancy

20. A 32-year-old woman presents with a 3-month history of galactorrhea and amenorrhea. Her serum hCG is negative and her serum prolactin is 220 ng/mL. The physical examination finding most likely to suggest mass effect and the need for surgical resection is

    A. visual field defects

    B. significant weight loss

    C. bilateral nipple discharge

    D. elevated blood pressure

    E. increased appetite

21. A 42-year-old man with a 30-year history of classic migraines presents to the emergency department with persistent, severe migraine headache for the past 5 days. His head CT scan is normal. The patient takes propranolol daily for migraine prophylaxis and uses sumatriptan for breakthrough headaches. Which of the following would be an appropriate medication to address this patient's condition?

    A. Calcium channel blocker

    B. Gabapentin

    C. Intramuscular or intravenous methylprednisolone

    D. Lithium carbonate

    E. Muscle relaxer

22. A 2-year-old girl is brought to the emergency room by her parents because she has developed wheezing and a low-grade fever. She is also hoarse and has a barking cough. History reveals that the patient is recovering from an upper respiratory tract infection. Lung auscultation reveals inspiratory and expiratory stridor. Neck radiographs reveal subglottic narrowing. What is the most likely diagnosis?

    A. Pharyngitis

    B. Epiglottitis

    C. Bronchiolitis

    D. Laryngotracheitis

    E. Pertussis

23. A patient recently admitted to the hospital for palpitations was diagnosed with atrial fibrillation. He was placed on digoxin, verapamil, and warfarin. He recently stopped taking his warfarin. His last dose was 2 weeks ago. He now presents to the office after an overseas flight, complaining of a warm, pale, and painful right leg that started an hour ago. Which of the following is the most likely explanation for his symptoms?

    A. Superficial vein thrombophlebitis

    B. Raynaud phenomenon

    C. Deep vein thrombosis

    D. Multiple sclerosis

    E. Varicose veins

24. A 58-year-old man presents with acute onset of left great toe pain. The patient denies any injury. Physical examination the toe is red and swollen. Examination of the synovial fluid reveals monosodium urate crystals. Which of the following most likely triggered this event?

    A. High NSAID intake

    B. Alcohol consumption

    C. Low-fat dairy products

    D. Elevated serum phosphate

    E. High-cholesterol diet

25. A 30-year-old motorcycle rider sustains head trauma in a traffic collision. His intracranial pressure is found to be elevated. In an effort to reduce this pressure, mannitol is administered. The mechanism of diuresis of mannitol is

    A. agonism at aldosterone receptors

    B. increase in osmotic pressure in the tubule

    C. inhibition of ADH release

    D. inhibition of carbonic anhydrase

    E. inhibition of the Na/K/2Cl megatransporter

26. A 40-year-old athletic woman presents to the emergency department complaining of substernal chest pain. She has had chest pain on exertion for the past 2 weeks. She describes a 40-minute episode of substernal tightness and numbness of the left arm that occurred during rest. Her father died suddenly at age 49. On physical examination, she appears comfortable and has a temperature of 36.8°C (98.2°F), a blood pressure of 155/98 mm Hg, a pulse of 90/min, and respirations of 22/min. Her heart has a normal-sounding S_1 and S_2. Her abdomen is modestly distended, and her ankles are edematous. EKG reveals normal sinus rhythm without significant ST abnormalities, but it does reveal left ventricular hypertrophy. A chest x-ray is obtained with results pending from radiology. She is given aspirin, low-molecular-weight heparin, and beta-blockers. Which of the following is the most appropriate next step in her management?

    A. Emergent cardiac catheterization

    B. Administration of thrombolytic therapy

    C. Obtain further serum cardiac markers

    D. Immediate exercise tolerance test

    E. Transthoracic echocardiogram

27. A 55-year-old alcoholic man presents to the emergency room with severe midepigastric abdominal pain with nausea and vomiting. He describes the pain as knife-like in quality and radiating to his back. The patient is mildly jaundiced, febrile, and tachycardic. The abdomen is soft, but the epigastrium is markedly tender. Which of the following is the most consistent with the history and physical examination?

    A. Acute pancreatitis

    B. Alcoholic hepatitis

    C. Cholecystitis

    D. Retrocecal appendicitis

    E. Small intestinal obstruction

28. A 25-year-old woman presents to your office for the tenth time over the course of 3 months. She complains of vague abdominal pain, urinary difficulties, and fevers on and off for the past 2 weeks. After an extensive workup, including a consultation with a gastrointestinal and genitourinary specialist, you have found no etiology for her complaints. Her past medical history includes generalized anxiety disorder, depression, and one failed suicide attempt 1 year ago. Which of the following is the most likely diagnosis?

    A. Munchausen syndrome by proxy

    B. Somatization disorder

    C. Conversion disorder

    D. Phobic disorder

    E. Panic disorder

29. A 40-year-old man presents with right wrist pain that is exacerbated by work and relieved with rest. He works as a gardener, and states that the pain began a few weeks ago and is slowly worsening. He denies any fever, chronic medical conditions, previous injury, or previous symptoms. On examination, there is no erythema, warmth, or swelling. He has tenderness on palpation of the radial aspect of the wrist and with passive range of motion. He also has a positive Finkelstein test. Which of the following is the most likely diagnosis?

    A. Gamekeeper's thumb

    B. de Quervain tenosynovitis

    C. Gonococcal tenosynovitis

    D. Volar flexor tenosynovitis

    E. Carpal tunnel syndrome

30. A 12-year-old boy comes to the emergency room with suspected testicular torsion. What is the gold standard test of diagnosis?

    A. Doppler ultrasound

    B. Radionucleotide scan

    C. Emergency surgical exploration

    D. Prehn sign

    E. Urinalysis

31. A patient with a family history of prostate carcinoma has his prostate-specific antigen (PSA) tested after an abnormal digital rectal exam revealed multiple nodules and areas of induration on the prostate. What PSA level suggests a high probability of bony metastasis?

    A. 2 ng/mL

    B. 4 ng/mL

    C. 8 ng/mL

    D. 9 ng/mL

    E. 15 ng/mL

32. A 58-year-old woman undergoes a chest x-ray for pneumonia. The chest film also includes the upper abdomen. A large, branching, partially opaque mass that resembles a deer antler is seen in the left upper abdomen. The patient has a long history of repeated urinary tract infections. Infection with which of the following organisms is most likely associated with the mass?

    A. *Escherichia*

    B. *Neisseria*

    C. *Proteus*

    D. *Staphylococcus*

    E. *Streptococcus*

33. A 36-year-old primigravid woman comes to labor and delivery because of contractions. Her prenatal course was complicated by hypertension but was otherwise uncomplicated. She is found to be 6 cm dilated, 100% effaced, and +1 station. Three hours later, at 3:00 P.M., she delivers a 9-pound, 6-ounce girl. By 3:15 P.M. her placenta has still not delivered, despite gentle cord traction and the administration of oxytocin. There is no evidence of active bleeding. Which of the following is the most appropriate next step in management?

    A. Dilation and curettage

    B. Expectant management

    C. Exploratory laparotomy

    D. Hysterectomy

    E. Manual removal of the placenta

34. Which of the following symptoms distinguishes sub-acute thyroiditis from Hashimoto thyroiditis?

    A. Pain with palpation of the thyroid gland

    B. Diffuse enlargement of the thyroid gland

    C. Insidious onset of symptoms

    D. Fullness in the neck

    E. Weight gain, cold intolerance, and dry skin

35. Carpal tunnel syndrome is diagnosed in a patient. Which of the following physical examination findings is consistent with this diagnosis?

    A. Weakness of the fifth digit

    B. Palpable tenderness over the lateral epicondyle

    C. Decreased sensation in the fifth digit

    D. Weakness of abduction and apposition of the thumb

    E. Wrist swelling and tenderness with increased warmth and erythema of the wrist

36. A 30-year-old man presents to the clinic complaining of severe poison ivy obtained while hiking in the mountains 2 days ago. On examination, you find weeping blisters and bullae along the ankles, shins, and upper extremities with some migration along the neck. Which of the following treatment options would you select?

    A. Sarna lotion

    B. Domeboro packs applied in the evening

    C. Prednisone × 2 weeks

    D. Amoxicillin × 1 week

    E. Hydrocortisone × 1 week

37. A 3-year-old is brought to the emergency room by his father because of a sudden-onset fever of 39.2 °C (102.5 °F), difficulty breathing, and a muffled voice. The child has no cough, but is drooling. Upon inspection, the child is sitting in the tripod position and leaning forward. What should immediately be done for this child?

    A. Endotracheal intubation

    B. Cool mist

    C. Racemic epinephrine aerosol

    D. Systemic steroids

    E. Aerosolized steroids

38. A 64-year-old man presents with acute epigastric pain, hematemesis, and lightheadedness. He was in his usual state of health when he suddenly experienced severe epigastric pain radiating through to his mid-back, along with lightheadedness and near syncope. Physical examination finds the patient normotensive and hemodynamically stable, and a pulsatile abdominal mass is noted. Which of the following would be the study of choice to confirm the diagnosis?

    A. Chest x-ray

    B. Abdominal angiography

    C. Abdominal ultrasound

    D. Contrast-enhanced CT scan

    E. Magnetic resonance imaging (MRI)

39. A 19-year-old nonsmoking woman developed a pulmonary embolism while on oral contraceptive pills. Which of the following is the most likely predisposing factor for her pulmonary embolism?

    A. Decreased protein C

    B. Decreased antithrombin III

    C. Factor V Leiden

    D. Hyperhomocysteinemia

    E. Increased protein S

40. A patient is diagnosed with Crohn disease and is currently asymptomatic. Which of the following would you recommend?

    A. Antibiotics

    B. Bed rest

    C. Corticosteroid

    D. High-residue diet

    E. Sulfasalazine

41. Positive symptoms of schizophrenia include which of the following?

    A. Emotional withdrawal

    B. Apathy

    C. Drug abuse

    D. Delusions

    E. Poverty of speech

42. A 3-year-old boy presents with left arm pain. His mother states that she did not see him fall, but yesterday he stopped using his left arm. On examination, you notice the left forearm is flexed 15 degrees at the elbow and the forearm is partially pronated. There is no erythema, warmth, or edema. Which of the following is the most likely explanation for these findings?

    A. Ulnar head dislocation

    B. Radial head dislocation

    C. Olecranon fracture

    D. Medial epicondylitis

    E. Lateral epicondylitis

43. A 50-year-old African American man comes to the clinic for the first time to be established as a patient. He requests a prostate-specific antigen (PSA) test be done because his father was diagnosed with prostate carcinoma. Given this patient's family history and ethnicity, what is the recommended age at which PSA testing should have begun?

    A. 25
    B. 30
    C. 35
    D. 40
    E. 45

44. A 52-year-old woman presents to the office for a routine visit. Her past obstetric history is significant for macrosomic infants. She is otherwise asymptomatic. Which of the following would be the most appropriate screening test to perform on this patient during this office visit?

    A. Oral glucose tolerance test
    B. Random blood glucose
    C. Fasting blood glucose
    D. Complete blood count
    E. Lipid profile

45. A 35-year-old woman with a family history of cerebral aneurysms is brought via emergency medical services to the emergency department. According to her husband, she experienced a sudden-onset and severe headache, followed by loss of consciousness. What part of the physical examination is best for determining the probability of a hemorrhage and her overall prognosis?

    A. Check the patient for ataxia
    B. Evaluate cranial nerve VII (facial nerve)
    C. Evaluate deep tendon reflexes
    D. Evaluate pronator drift
    E. Examine and categorize the patient using the Glasgow coma scale

46. While doing rounds in the long-term care unit, you examine an 80-year-old Caucasian woman with angular cheilitis. Which of the following statements is true regarding this condition?

    A. It is often due to vitamin C deficiency.
    B. The most common etiology in the elderly population is *Candida albicans.*
    C. It should be biopsied to rule out squamous cell carcinoma.
    D. It is caused by an underabundance of moisture in the mouth.
    E. It is often due to an overabundance of iron.

47. When does the use of MRI have an advantage over CT scanning?

    A. Helpful for patients with claustrophobia
    B. Patients with cardiac pacemakers
    C. Evaluation of soft tissue changes
    D. Evaluation of detailed bone structures
    E. Patients with permanent metallic implantable devices

48. A 24-year-old woman presents to the clinic with a 6-month history of oligomenorrhea and a 3-month history of bilateral nipple discharge. She has never been pregnant, and has never been sexually active. Her only significant past medical history is hospital admission for a psychiatric illness, the diagnosis of which is unclear. The patient's current medications include risperidone and a tricyclic antidepressant. Her serum hCG is negative. A serum prolactin level of 64 ng/mL would suggest what likely etiology?

    A. A pituitary macroadenoma
    B. A pituitary microadenoma
    C. Hypothyroidism
    D. Medication-induced hyperprolactinemia
    E. Hyperthyroidism

49. A fisherman is brought to the emergency room at 2:00 P.M. because he is vomiting, has dizziness, and is having difficulty breathing. His wife states that around midnight, her husband awoke complaining of dry mouth and difficulty swallowing. He also complains of double vision. The wife states that the last thing her husband ate was smoked herring, which he cooked himself from a catch he had vacuum-sealed. He ate at around 5:30 P.M. the previous evening. Physical examination reveals ptosis of the eyelids; fixed, dilated pupils; and cranial nerve palsies with impaired extraocular movements. What should be done immediately for this patient?

   A. Intubation and mechanical ventilation

   B. Gastric lavage

   C. Penicillin G

   D. Tetracycline

   E. Erythromycin

50. A 74-year-old woman presents with a 6-week history of severe bilateral, mainly left-sided headache associated with generalized weakness and weight loss. She has long-standing hypertension and hypercholesterolemia. She is febrile (40.0° C [104.0° F]) with blurred vision. Both temporal arteries are tender and nonpulsating, and her proximal muscles are weak and painful. Laboratory tests reveal a normochromic, normocytic anemia with a hemoglobin level of 10.5 g/L. ESR value is 105 mm/hour. Which of the following is the most likely diagnosis for this patient?

   A. Giant cell arteritis

   B. Polyarteritis nodosa

   C. Wegener granulomatosis

   D. Acute angle glaucoma

   E. Microscopic polyangiitis

51. A 50-year-old African American man presents with deep, aching pain in his left knee. He states that it worsens after playing tennis and is relieved with rest. He has some occasional stiffness in the morning, but it usually dissipates after a few minutes. On examination, you note some crepitus but no limitation of range of motion. He denies any chronic medical conditions and is on no medications. The most appropriate treatment is

   A. nonsteroidal anti-inflammatory drugs (NSAIDs)

   B. corticosteroids

   C. colchicine

   D. disease-modifying antirheumatic drugs (DMARDs)

   E. joint replacement surgery

52. A 35-year-old mother of five presents to your emergency department with complaints of worsening shortness of breath over the past week. On physical examination, she is noted to have generalized edema, pallor, tachypnea, and coughing. She also has a pansystolic murmur at the apex that radiates into the axilla, is loudest in the left lateral decubitus position, and increases in intensity with hand-gripping. Her chest examination reveals basilar rales. Her chest film shows moderate cardiac enlargement and pulmonary venous hypertension. An EKG shows low QRS voltage and nonspecific ST-segment changes when compared with her previous EKG performed 6 months ago. The patient's drug screen is positive for cocaine metabolites and ethanol. Which of the following is the most likely etiology of this patient's symptoms?

   A. Acute myocardial infarction

   B. Infectious myocarditis

   C. Hypertrophic cardiomyopathy

   D. Dilated cardiomyopathy

   E. Restrictive cardiomyopathy

Items 53–55: The response options for the next three items are the same. You will be required to select one answer for each item in the set.

For the following conditions, select the associated vitamin deficiency (choices A–G).

   A. Vitamin A

   B. Vitamin B_1

   C. Vitamin B_3

   D. Vitamin B_6

   E. Vitamin D

53. Rickets

54. Beriberi

55. Pellagra

56. A 36-year-old man presents to the urgent care center with nephrolithiasis. The physician assistant at that clinic notes that this is his third visit for renal stones in the past 8 months. Before that, the patient had never experienced a stone. Laboratory tests were performed during the last visit, and the patient was told to follow up for the results. A serum calcium level was elevated at 11.2 mg/dL. A PTH level is obtained and is also elevated. The most likely etiology for this patient's frequent calcium stone formation is

   A. secondary hyperparathyroidism

   B. hypoparathyroidism

   C. primary hyperparathyroidism

   D. Paget disease of bone

   E. vitamin D deficiency

57. A 50-year-old man presents to your office for an annual physical. He has a history of high blood pressure that is treated with antihypertensives. He currently has no complaints. During the physical examination, a digital rectal exam and a fecal occult blood test are performed. The fecal occult blood test is positive. The remainder of the physical examination is normal. Which of the following is the most appropriate next step?

   A. Colonoscopy

   B. Complete blood count

   C. Inform the patient that the consumption of meats can cause a false-positive result

   D. Recheck the patient in 3 months

   E. Refer the patient for surgical intervention

58. A 76-year-old man presents with low back pain with radiculopathy. He also states that he has some difficulty starting and stopping his urinary stream and has some numbness along both inner thighs. Which of the following is the most likely diagnosis?

   A. Scoliosis

   B. Spinal stenosis

   C. Cauda equina syndrome

   D. Spondylolisthesis

   E. Disk herniation

59. An 80-year-old woman presents with grimacing, tongue protrusion, lip-smacking, and rapid eye-blinking. Which of her medications is most likely the cause?

   A. Haloperidol

   B. Fluoxetine

   C. Metoprolol

   D. Ibuprofen

   E. Trazodone

60. A 45-year-old woman was found to have a 1.5-cm duodenal ulcer on endoscopy. Which of the following is the most appropriate next step in management of this patient?

A. Antacids

B. Fasting serum gastrin

C. Proton pump inhibitor and triple antibiotic therapy

D. Surgical intervention

E. Upper gastrointestinal series

End of Block 4

Block 5

1. A 19-year-old man comes to the clinic complaining of extreme pain while urinating. He also reports a yellow-green discharge from his penis. The physician assistant gives him 125 mg of ceftriaxone intramuscularly. For what common coinfection should this patient also be treated?

   A. *Treponema pallidum*

   B. *Gardnerella vaginosis*

   C. *Ureaplasma urealyticum*

   D. *Chlamydia trachomatis*

   E. *Chlamydia psittaci*

2. What is the most common type of thyroid cancer?

   A. Papillary carcinoma

   B. Medullary carcinoma

   C. Follicular carcinoma

   D. Anaplastic thyroid carcinoma

   E. Adenocarcinoma

3. A 22-year-old college student with a history of asthma presents to the student health department with worsening shortness of breath for the past 2 to 3 days. She has been using her albuterol inhaler every 4 to 6 hours without much relief. She denies fever, chills, or pleuritic chest pain. She has the sensation that she is "wheezing." Physical examination reveals diffuse wheezing throughout with prolonged exhalation. Otherwise, examination of the thorax is normal. Which of the following would be the most useful diagnostic test to perform before attempting nebulizer treatment?

   A. Arterial blood gases

   B. Helical CT scan of the chest

   C. Posteroanterior and lateral chest film

   D. Peak expiratory flows

   E. Pulmonary angiography

4. A 37-year-old male is diagnosed with Addison disease. Which of the following is the most appropriate management?

   A. Administer beta-blockers for blood pressure control

   B. Administer hydrocortisone with appropriate stress doses

   C. Surgical excision of the adrenal gland

   D. No therapy is required

   E. Administer dextrose IV daily

5. A 75-year-old woman presents with a history of rheumatoid arthritis and diabetes mellitus (noninsulin-dependent) for the past several years. She complains of a lack of balance, memory loss, and urinary incontinence for 9 months. Which of the following physical examination findings would be most indicative of idiopathic normal pressure hydrocephalus?

   A. Cranial nerve III (oculomotor nerve) palsy

   B. Gait ataxia

   C. Limited extension of the neck

   D. Loss of sharp/dull discrimination in a nondermatomal distribution in bilateral lower extremities

   E. Weakness of hand grip on the right

6. A 62-year-old patient complains of a severely pruritic patch of skin on the left ankle for 1 year. He states that he has tried over-the-counter hydrocortisone cream, which did not help. On examination, you note a 4- × 5-cm, brown, well-demarcated plaque with thickening and excoriation. Which of the following is the most likely diagnosis?

   A. Lichen simplex chronicus

   B. Psoriasis

   C. Cellulitis

   D. Scabies

   E. Ringworm

7. A 24-year-old IV drug user presents with fever, cough, and pleuritic chest pain. On examination, painful nodules of the fingers, red-brown streaks in the proximal nailbeds, and a loud murmur are observed. Blood cultures are likely to yield which of the following organisms?

   A. *Aspergillus fumigatus*

   B. *Coccidioides immitis*

   C. *Mycoplasma tuberculosis*

   D. *Staphylococcus aureus*

   E. *Streptococcus viridans*

8. A 32-year-old woman presents for reevaluation of her blood pressure readings. She takes no medications but does have a history of Raynaud phenomenon. The condition has seemed to worsen in intensity over the past two winters. Her systolic blood pressures are in the 150s. Her physical examination is unremarkable. What is the best drug therapy for this patient's blood pressure based on her history?

   A. Alpha-blocker

   B. Beta-blocker

   C. Calcium channel blocker

   D. ACE inhibitor

   E. Thiazide diuretic

9. A sexually active woman was recently treated for pelvic inflammatory disease. She now presents with right upper quadrant pain. An ultrasound of the right upper quadrant is normal. Which of the following diagnoses do you suspect?

   A. Appendicitis

   B. Cholecystitis

   C. Cholelithiasis

   D. Fitz-Hugh–Curtis syndrome

   E. Peptic ulcer

10. A 56-year-old obese woman presents with a 5-year history of borderline diabetes mellitus. She states that she no longer checks her blood sugars since she is asymptomatic. Laboratory testing on the day of her visit reveals a random blood sugar of 220 mg/dL and an $HgbA_{1c}$ of 10.6%. Which of the following is the key to prevention of long-term complications in this patient?

    A. Use an ACE inhibitor to prevent diabetic complications.

    B. Check feet daily to prevent ulcerations and gangrene.

    C. Undergo frequent eye examinations and urinalysis.

    D. Monitor daily fasting blood glucose level.

    E. Maintain $HgbA_{1c}$ at less than 7%.

11. A 25-year-old woman has been in labor for 5 hours and is experiencing strong, but erratic, contractions at intervals varying between 2 and 5 minutes. Due to the severity of her pain, nitrous oxide is made available and the obstetrician administers an opioid analgesic. The baby is delivered 90 minutes later and presents with respiratory depression and a low Apgar score. Which of the following is the most appropriate pharmacotherapy for the neonate?

    A. Aminophylline

    B. Dobutamine

    C. Epinephrine

    D. Flumazenil

    E. Naloxone

12. A 72-year-old man begins to notice resistance when he tries to raise his arms. He walks with a stooped posture, and his feet barely leave the floor when he walks. He seems to lack facial expression and has difficulty swallowing. A slight tremor is evident in his hands when he is sitting down. In which of the following areas would degenerating neuronal cell bodies most likely be found in this patient?

    A. Midbrain

    B. Motor cortex

    C. Spinal cord

    D. Striatum

    E. Thalamus

13. A 55-year-old man with hypertension and a past medical history of myocardial infarction is prescribed atenolol. This medication will lower his blood pressure by

    A. blocking catecholamine release

    B. blocking the conversion of angiotensin I to angiotensin II

    C. decreasing cardiac output

    D. decreasing intravascular volume

    E. increasing renin release from the kidney

14. A 60-year-old man with a 40 pack-year smoking history presents with increasing dysphagia to both solids and liquids for the past 2 months. He has also noted a 10-pound weight loss over this same time period. A barium swallow reveals a narrowing of the distal esophageal lumen with partial obstruction. Which of the following is the most likely diagnosis?

    A. Achalasia

    B. Esophageal cancer

    C. Lower esophageal web

    D. Plummer-Vinson syndrome

    E. Boerhaave syndrome

15. An 18-year-old woman presents to a physician because she has never begun menstruating. She is 152 cm (60 inches) tall, although her sisters are much taller. Physical examination reveals minimal breast development and widely spaced nipples. Delayed femoral pulses and an abdominal bruit are also noted. Which of the following is the most appropriate method for confirming her genetic disorder?

    A. Biochemical testing

    B. Cytogenetic analysis

    C. Linkage analysis

    D. DNA methylation analysis

    E. PCR multiplex deletion test

16. Which of the following is *NOT* precancerous?

    A. Adenomatous polyp

    B. Familial polyposis

    C. Villous adenoma

    D. Gardner syndrome

    E. Mucosal polyp

17. A previously healthy 17-year-old boy presents to the emergency room 10 hours after the onset of chest pain over the left trapezius muscle. He states he has had an upper respiratory tract infection for the past 9 days. On physical examination, a friction rub is heard over the precordium. He reports reduced pain after being given an aspirin. Which of the following is the most likely diagnosis?

    A. Acute pericarditis

    B. Pulmonary embolism

    C. Spontaneous pneumothorax

    D. Pericardial tamponade

    E. Tietze syndrome

18. Which of the following diuretics acts at the distal tubule of the nephron?

    A. Ethacrynic acid

    B. Furosemide

    C. Hydrochlorothiazide

    D. Mannitol

    E. Spironolactone

19. Reverse transcriptase activity is found in

    A. rabies virus

    B. hepatitis B virus

    C. HIV

    D. both HIV and hepatitis B virus

    E. both HIV and rabies virus

20. Carbon dioxide is transported in blood by a variety of mechanisms. Which of the following is quantitatively the *MOST* important method for transporting CO_2?

   A. As carbaminohemoglobin

   B. As CO_2 in gas bubbles

   C. As CO_2 in physical solution

   D. As sodium bicarbonate in red cells

   E. As sodium bicarbonate in serum

21. An unlabeled container of blood product is left in a laboratory. The technician must determine whether the sample is serum or plasma. An elevated level of which of the following substances would identify the specimen as plasma?

   A. Albumin

   B. Erythrocytes

   C. Fibrinogen

   D. Granulocytes

   E. Serotonin

22. A patient's carotid pulse has a quick upstroke associated with a wide pulse pressure. These findings are most suggestive of which of the following?

   A. Mitral stenosis

   B. Aortic regurgitation

   C. Pericardial tamponade

   D. Congestive heart failure

   E. Chordae tendineae rupture

23. A patient is diagnosed with celiac sprue. Which of the following grains can the patient have?

   A. Barley

   B. Oats

   C. Rice

   D. Rye

   E. Wheat

24. A 19-year-old man comes to the family clinic complaining of a fever and a rash that started at his wrists and ankles and is now spreading up his extremities. The rash is also on his palms and soles. He also states that he has a headache that will not go away regardless of what he tries. He states that his symptoms started 4 days after he returned from camping in the woods. He recalls being bitten by an insect but is unsure if it was a tick. Which of the following is the treatment of choice?

   A. Doxycycline

   B. Acyclovir

   C. Chloramphenicol

   D. Ciprofloxacin

   E. Trimethoprim and sulfamethoxazole

25. A 40-year-old patient with viral myocarditis has developed fatigue, progressively worsening shortness of breath, and lower extremity edema over the past 3 days. Chest x-ray shows no significant increase in heart size but reveals prominence of the superior pulmonary vessels. Which of the following is the most likely diagnosis?

   A. Congestive heart failure

   B. Coronary artery disease

   C. Pulmonary embolus

   D. Cor pulmonale

   E. Pneumonia

26. A patient presents with a narrow-complex tachycardia without chest pain. The blood pressure is 100/72 mm Hg and pulse is 116/minute. What is the next step in the treatment of this patient?

   A. Lanoxin (Digoxin)

   B. Verapamil (Isoptin)

   C. Vagal maneuver

   D. Pacemaker placement

   E. Laser ablation

27. An adult patient has a body mass index (BMI) of 28.0. According to the BMI, the patient is classified as which of the following?

   A. Muscular

   B. Normal

   C. Obese

   D. Overweight

   E. Underweight

28. A patient develops high fever, muscle rigidity, and change in mental status after starting a new medication. Laboratory testing reveals an elevated CPK. Which of the following medications is most likely associated with the development of these symptoms?

    A. Chlorpromazine (Thorazine)

    B. Chlordiazepoxide (Librium)

    C. Meperidine (Demerol)

    D. Selegiline (Eldepryl)

    E. Phenelzine (Nardil)

29. An 18-year-old woman comes to the physician assistant's office because a routine physical exam for college revealed that her blood pressure was 160/96 mm Hg. During this office visit, bruits are auscultated over the renal arteries. Based on the information already obtained, what is expected to happen with administration of an angiotensin-converting enzyme inhibitor?

    A. Abrupt deterioration of renal function

    B. Abrupt increase of renal function

    C. No change in renal function

    D. Abrupt decrease in blood pressure

    E. No change in blood pressure

30. A 24-year-old woman presents for a routine annual Pap and pelvic exam. She is asymptomatic. Her past medical history is unremarkable. Her only medication is oral contraceptives. On her physical exam, you discover a 1-cm nodule on the right superior lobe of her thyroid gland. Which of the following is the most appropriate next step?

    A. Have her return in 2 weeks to recheck the thyroid gland

    B. Order a thyroid scan

    C. Obtain thyroid function tests

    D. Begin propylthiouracil therapy

    E. Radioablation therapy

31. An 80-year-old man presents with a burning pain followed by numerous vesicles along the T6 dermatome. Which of the following is the preferred treatment for this patient?

    A. Acyclovir (Zovirax)

    B. Fluconazole (Diflucan)

    C. Beta interferon (Avonex)

    D. Tetracycline (Achromycin)

    E. Gabapentin (Neurontin)

32. A 28-year-old woman who has had neurologic symptoms for the past 12 months has been diagnosed with multiple sclerosis (MS). Which of the following findings would confirm the diagnosis?

    A. Elevated erythrocyte sedimentation rate

    B. Elevated serum white blood cell count

    C. Markedly decreased glucose levels in the cerebrospinal fluid

    D. Oligoclonal bands in the cerebrospinal fluid

    E. Positive antinuclear antibody titer

33. The area of auscultation for the aortic valve in the heart is performed at which of the following anatomic positions?

    A. Inferior border of the heart

    B. Left second intercostal space

    C. Left fifth intercostal space

    D. Right second intercostal space

    E. Xiphisternal junction

34. A 19-year-old patient presents with mild discomfort of the upper lateral left eyelid for the past 3 days. Physical examination reveals a red, swollen lid margin. Which of the following is the initial management of this patient?

    A. Oral antibiotic

    B. Warm compress

    C. Anesthetic eye drop

    D. Topical antihistamine

    E. Incision and drainage

35. An asymptomatic patient is diagnosed with diverticu-losis on a routine colonoscopic examination. Which of the following is recommended?

    A. Antibiotic therapy

    B. Decreased fluid intake

    C. High-residue diet

    D. Psyllium supplements

    E. Surgical intervention

36. A previously healthy 24-year-old woman presents to the emergency department with palpitations and dyspnea. On ECG, she is found to be in atrial fibrillation with a rapid ventricular response. What key physical examina-tion finding would suggest this patient's diagnosis?

    A. A loud systolic ejection murmur

    B. Exophthalmos

    C. A pericardial friction rub

    D. Dry, coarse hair and cool skin

    E. Weight gain

37. An 18-month-old presents with fever for the past 24 hours with temperatures to 101.5° F. The mother states that the child has had a runny nose for the past 10 days. On physical examination, tympanic mem-branes are found to be erythematous and bulging. Nasal turbinates are erythematous with clear drainage. Which of the following is the most likely diagnosis?

    A. Otitis media

    B. Viral rhinitis

    C. Otitis externa

    D. Allergic rhinitis

    E. Rhinitis medicamentosa

38. Which of the following antihypertensive medications is commonly used to preserve ventricular function in patients with congestive heart failure as well as pre-serve the function of the kidneys of diabetic patients?

    A. Atenolol

    B. Captopril

    C. Furosemide

    D. Methyldopa

    E. Verapamil

39. A patient diagnosed with appendicitis may have which of the following clinical manifestations?

    A. Asterixis

    B. Cullen sign

    C. Murphy sign

    D. Rovsing sign

    E. Shifting dullness

40. A 24-year-old man presents with a generalized erythe-matous, maculopapular rash involving the palms of the hands and soles of the feet. He also shows general-ized lymphadenopathy and flat, moist lesions in the genital area. The patient admits to having had a lesion on his penis a month or so before but says it did not bother him. Which of the following is the most appro-priate laboratory test to confirm the diagnosis?

    A. C-reactive protein

    B. Lyme titer

    C. FTA-ABS

    D. Gram stain

    E. Weil-Felix test

41. Which of the following is the most appropriate inter-vention for a patient suffering from a specific phobia, such as fear of animals?

    A. Lithium

    B. Benzodiazepine

    C. Exposure therapy

    D. Insight-oriented therapy

    E. Electroconvulsive therapy

42. A patient has received a large dose of epinephrine (α_1, β_1, β_2). What will be the blood pressure change after a dose of phentolamine (nonspecific alpha-blocker)?

    A. Decreased

    B. Increased

    C. No change

    D. Unpredictable

    E. Initial decrease followed by sharp increase

43. Which of the following is the therapy of choice in the patient with metabolic acidosis due to ingestion of methanol?

    A. Salicylates

    B. Paraldehyde

    C. Ethylene glycol

    D. Bicarbonate

    E. Ethanol

44. A 65-year-old homeless patient presents with fever, weight loss, anorexia, night sweats, and chronic cough. The cough has recently become productive with purulent sputum streaked with blood. On physical examination, the patient appears chronically ill and malnourished. Which of the following chest x-ray findings would most likely be noted?

    A. Eggshell calcification of hilar lymph nodes

    B. Hyperinflation with flattened diaphragms

    C. Pleural thickening and hyperinflation

    D. Cavitary lesions in the upper lobes

    E. Bilateral interstitial infiltrates

45. A 6-year-old boy presents with persistent vomiting and increased lethargy. The patient's mother states that yesterday the child had a fever, despite treatment with aspirin, and a severe sore throat. On physical examination, the patient is delirious and disoriented with hyperactive reflexes. The liver edge is 4 cm below the right costal margin. Which of the following is the most likely diagnosis?

    A. Reye syndrome

    B. Guillain-Barré syndrome

    C. Acute bacterial meningitis

    D. Phenylketonuria

    E. Lesch-Nyhan syndrome

46. A 65-year-old woman with a history of hypertension and diabetes mellitus and 30 pack-year smoking history presents to the emergency department with mild expressive aphasia, right facial weakness, and mild right arm weakness. Her husband states that she awakened 60 minutes ago and 15 minutes later starting having difficulty speaking and develops weakness. Physical examination reveals a blood pressure of 160/90 mm Hg. Head CT scan shows no intracranial hemorrhage. Which of the following is the most appropriate intervention?

    A. Aspirin

    B. Warfarin

    C. Clopidogrel

    D. Vena cava filter

    E. Tissue plasminogen activator

47. If a 58-year-old woman with an elevated total cholesterol and LDL cholesterol level is prescribed nicotinic acid (niacin), the patient is most likely to experience which of the following side effects?

    A. Bradycardia

    B. Facial flushing

    C. Hypoalbuminemia

    D. Hyperglycemia

    E. Renal dysfunction

48. A 34-year-old patient presents to the clinic with a 4 to 6-month history of generalized muscle weakness, fatigue, anorexia, bouts of diarrhea, and orthostatic light-headedness. On physical examination, the patient's BP is 96/60 mm Hg, heart rate is 114/min, and respirations are 16/min. The rest of the physical examination is relatively unremarkable except for hyperpigmentation of the buccal mucosa, and gingival and darkened creases of the palms of the hands. Which of the following is the most appropriate first laboratory test to obtain to confirm a diagnosis?

    A. 24-hour urine collection for cortisol

    B. Morning serum cortisol collection after 6 to 8 hours of sleep

    C. Dexamethasone suppression test

    D. CT scan of the adrenals

    E. Random cortisol level

49. All of the following are included in the management of constipation **EXCEPT**?

    A. Decreased fiber intake

    B. Docusate sodium

    C. Enemas

    D. Increased fluid intake

    E. Sorbitol

50. The oxygen-hemoglobin dissociation curve shifts to the left under which of the following circumstances?

    A. Carbon monoxide poisoning

    B. Decreased pH

    C. Increased 2,3-diphosphoglycerate (2,3-DPG)

    D. Increased P_{CO_2}

    E. Increased temperature

51. A 61-year-old previously healthy lawyer has had progressive symptoms of tremor with a stiff, shuffling gait for several months. At this point, what is an appropriate treatment for this patient?

    A. Anticonvulsant

    B. Beta-blocker

    C. Dopamine agonist

    D. Lithium carbonate

    E. Placement of a ventricular shunt

52. The most appropriate therapy in Graves disease for the cardiac manifestations of palpitations, tachycardia, and tremor is

    A. diltiazem

    B. propranolol

    C. propylthiouracil

    D. iodine

    E. radioablation

53. What is a fracture of the fifth metacarpal neck known as?

    A. Colles's fracture

    B. Salter-Harris' fracture

    C. Rolando's fracture

    D. Bennett's fracture

    E. Boxer's fracture

54. A physician assistant is counseling a 35-year-old patient on coronary artery disease risk factors during a routine physical examination. In addition to the usual risk factors (positive family history, obesity, hypertension, sedentary lifestyle, and hypercholesterolemia), hyperhomocysteinemia, which has recently been recognized as an independent risk factor for developing coronary artery disease, is discussed. Which of the following is recognized as a major factor leading to hyperhomocysteinemia?

    A. Decreased lipoprotein A

    B. Decreased folate levels

    C. Increased cholesterol levels

    D. Decreased fibrinolytic activity

    E. Hyperinsulinemia

55. An 82-year-old retired nurse presents to the office complaining of right upper extremity weakness for the past 6 hours. She has no other complaints. She is transported to the local hospital for a CT scan, which shows an intracerebral infarct with early hemorrhage in the area surrounding the infarct. What is an appropriate part of the management program for this patient?

    A. Anticoagulant therapy

    B. Follow-up serial CT scans and surgical evacuation if the hemorrhage worsens with clinical deterioration

    C. Immediate and rapid lowering of blood pressure via intravenous labetalol or nitroglycerine

    D. Placement of ventricular shunt

    E. Streptokinase thrombolytic therapy

56. A patient with type 2 diabetes had an elevated screening cholesterol done at a local health fair. You obtain a fasting lipid panel, and he returns to your office for results and management. His results are as follows:

    | Total cholesterol | 260 mg/dL |
    | LDL cholesterol | 150 mg/dL |
    | HDL cholesterol | 45 mg/dL |
    | Triglycerides | 195 mg/dL |

    What would the most appropriate treatment for this patient include?

    A. Begin a high-fiber diet.

    B. Begin niacin.

    C. Begin a fibrate.

    D. Begin a statin.

    E. Begin exercise and weight loss.

57. If a 68-year-old man has been receiving prednisone 10 mg daily for the past 6 months, the patient will most likely see which of the following side effects?

    A. Hypernatremia and hypoglycemia

    B. Hyperkalemia and hypercalcemia

    C. Hypocalcemia and hyperglycemia

    D. Hypokalemia and hypercalcemia

    E. Hyponatremia and hypoglycemia

58. A patient seen in the emergency room complains of intermittent cramping abdominal pain. Radiographs show a distended loop of bowel that rises up out of the pelvis. A barium enema shows an "ace of spades" deformity. Which of the following is the most appropriate intervention?

    A. Elective resection

    B. Emergent surgical intervention

    C. Gentle insertion of a flexible sigmoidoscope

    D. Percutaneous decompression

    E. Total abdominal colectomy

59. Which of the following anesthetics is primarily metabolized by plasma esterases?

    A. Bupivacaine

    B. Chloroprocaine

    C. Etidocaine

    D. Mepivacaine

    E. Prilocaine

60. A 57-year-old man is receiving cisplatin for treatment of a metastatic tumor. For the prevention of profound nausea and vomiting, he is administered an agent that selectively antagonizes the 5-hydroxytryptamine 3 (5-HT3) receptor. Based on this information, the patient is receiving

    A. diphenhydramine

    B. dronabinol

    C. granisetron

    D. metoclopramide

    E. prochlorperazine

End of Block 5

Test 2 Answers and Explanations

ANSWER KEY

Block 1

1. A
2. C
3. B
4. E
5. E
6. E
7. B
8. D
9. D
10. B
11. C
12. E
13. A
14. C
15. E
16. A
17. C
18. B
19. C
20. B
21. A
22. C
23. C
24. D
25. B
26. E
27. C
28. B
29. C
30. D
31. B
32. B
33. A
34. A
35. D
36. E
37. B
38. C
39. A
40. B
41. D
42. A
43. C
44. D
45. C
46. C
47. A
48. A
49. C
50. E
51. D
52. C
53. B
54. D
55. E
56. A
57. B
58. D
59. C
60. C

Block 2

1. D
2. C
3. C
4. A
5. C
6. B
7. E
8. E
9. B
10. B
11. C
12. D
13. D
14. A
15. B
16. B
17. A
18. E
19. D
20. D
21. B
22. C
23. D
24. D
25. E
26. B
27. D
28. A
29. D
30. E
31. E
32. E
33. E
34. C
35. C
36. D
37. A
38. D
39. A
40. D
41. A
42. B
43. C
44. C
45. B
46. B
47. E
48. B
49. E
50. B
51. D
52. C
53. E
54. C
55. A
56. B
57. A
58. C
59. E
60. A

Block 3

1. B
2. A
3. D
4. B
5. B
6. A
7. D
8. B
9. D
10. D
11. D
12. A
13. B
14. D
15. A
16. C
17. B
18. D
19. C
20. E
21. B
22. E
23. C
24. D
25. E
26. A
27. A
28. A
29. B
30. C
31. A
32. B
33. B
34. A
35. C
36. D
37. A
38. A
39. E
40. D
41. A
42. D
43. D
44. A
45. B
46. B
47. D
48. A
49. B
50. A
51. D
52. E
53. E
54. C
55. A
56. A
57. B
58. C
59. A
60. A

Block 4

1. B
2. C
3. D
4. C
5. C
6. D
7. C
8. D
9. A
10. A
11. E
12. D
13. A
14. D
15. B
16. C
17. E
18. B
19. A
20. A
21. C
22. D
23. C
24. B
25. B
26. C
27. A
28. B
29. B
30. B
31. C
32. C
33. B
34. A
35. D
36. C
37. A
38. D
39. C
40. E
41. D
42. B
43. D
44. A
45. E
46. B
47. C
48. D
49. A
50. A
51. A
52. D
53. E
54. B
55. C
56. C
57. A
58. C
59. A
60. C

Block 5

1. D
2. A
3. D
4. B
5. B
6. A
7. D
8. C
9. D
10. E
11. E
12. A
13. C
14. B
15. B
16. E
17. A
18. C
19. D
20. E
21. C
22. B
23. C
24. A
25. A
26. C
27. D
28. A
29. A
30. C
31. A
32. D
33. D
34. B
35. D
36. B
37. A
38. B
39. D
40. C
41. C
42. A
43. E
44. D
45. A
46. E
47. B
48. E
49. A
50. A
51. C
52. B
53. E
54. B
55. B
56. D
57. C
58. C
59. B
60. C

Block 1

1. **The correct answer is A.** The lesion described is a dermoid cyst, which is a common form of ovarian tumor. Ovarian dermoid cysts are formally classified as a subset of mature teratomas, but they are clinically separated from other teratomas because they are invariably benign (whereas other mature teratomas have at least some capacity of metastasizing). The wall of the lesion will show formation of tissue resembling skin and hair follicles.

2. **The correct answer is C.** The clinical description is typical for Turner syndrome. The presence of a Y-bearing cell line indicates that this patient is a mosaic 45,XO/46,XY. In these patients, the phenotype is usually female, but the intra-abdominal gonads are somewhat similar to undescended testes and have a predilection for developing gonadal malignancy, most characteristically gonadoblastoma. Screening for the presence of a Y chromosome-bearing cell line is consequently indicated in Turner syndrome patients, and patients so identified should have the intra-abdominal gonads removed prophylactically as soon as the diagnosis is made.

   Adenofibroma (**choice A**) is a tumor sometimes found in the tissues adjacent to the testes in normal males.

   Dermoid cyst (**choice B**) is a common benign tumor of the ovary.

   Mucinous and serous cystadenocarcinomas (**choices D and E**) are found in normal ovaries, but because they are derived from tissue resembling normal surface epithelium of the ovary, they do not occur more frequently in cryptorchid testes or the intra-abdominal gonads of 45,XO/46,XY mosaics.

3. **The correct answer is B.** This patient is having a heart attack. Involvement of the inferior wall of the heart is suggested by involvement of leads II, III, and aVF.

   Involvement of leads I, aVL, and V_4-V_6 (**choice A**) suggests lateral wall involvement.

   Involvement of leads V_1-V_3 (**choice C**) suggests anteroseptal involvement.

   Involvement of leads V_1-V_6 (**choice D**) suggests anterolateral involvement.

   Involvement of leads RV_4 and RV_5 (**choice E**) suggests right ventricular involvement.

   Posterior wall involvement is indicated by an R/S ratio >1 in V_1 and V_2 and T-wave changes (i.e., upright) in V_1, V_8, and V_9.

4. **The correct answer is E.** This patient has renal artery stenosis with renal hypertension due to activation of the renin-angiotensin system. When arteriolar pressure at the level of the juxtaglomerular cells near the glomeruli is low, the enzyme renin is secreted by the juxtaglomerular cells. Renin circulates in the blood, where it acts on angiotensinogen, which is synthesized by the liver, and circulates in the blood in the alpha-2 globulin fraction of the plasma. Renin cleaves angiotensinogen to form a 10-amino-acid-long, physiologically inactive peptide known as angiotensin I (**choice B**). Angiotensin-converting enzyme (located on endothelial cells in the lungs and elsewhere) then cleaves two amino acids off angiotensin I to form angiotensin II (**choice C**). Angiotensin II causes arteriolar constriction, leading to hypertension, and also stimulates the adrenal secretion of aldosterone (**choice A**), which induces renal sodium retention with resulting expansion of the vascular fluid space (and indirectly, total body water), also leading to increased blood pressure. Angiotensin II is degraded to angiotensin III (**choice D**), which still has some physiologic activity and a greater capacity to stimulate aldosterone secretion than to induce arteriolar constriction.

5. **The correct answer is E.** The silhouette sign refers to normal anatomy, which is obscured by an object on plain film of the chest. This could be infiltrate, blood, pus, or any kind of fluid. On a posteroanterior view of the chest, the right heart border corresponds to the right middle lobe of the lung.

   Left lower lobe pneumonia (**choice A**) is indicated by a loss of the left heart border or the left hemidiaphragm.

   The lingula is present only in the left chest. A loss of the left heart border suggests lingular pneumonia (**choice B**).

   A pneumothorax (**choice C**) does not demonstrate a silhouette sign on x-ray.

   Right lower lobe pneumonia (**choice D**) is indicated by a loss of the right hemidiaphragm.

6. **The correct answer is E.** Reflux esophagitis is caused by the reflux of gastric acid into the esophagus. There is inflammation of the esophageal mucosa. Symptoms include retrosternal pain that is described as burning or squeezing. The pain may radiate to the back. Large meals, bending over, and recumbency are aggravating factors. Antacids or proton pump inhibitors provide relief.

   The symptoms of acute cholecystitis (**choice A**) include right upper quadrant pain that may radiate to the scapular area. The patient may be nauseated and vomit. Large, fatty meals provoke the pain. Deep breathing aggravates the pain.

Typical symptoms of angina pectoris (**choice B**) include chest pain caused by physical exertion or emotional stress that is immediately relieved by rest or nitroglycerin.

Esophageal spasm (**choice C**) is incorrect. The pain of esophageal spasm is retrosternal and may radiate to the back, jaw, or arms. The pain is described as squeezing. Swallowing cold liquids or food is an aggravating factor.

A peptic ulcer (**choice D**) causes epigastric pain that may radiate to the back. The pain is gnawing or burning in quality and is intermittent. Food and antacids may provide relief.

7. **The correct answer is B.** Paroxetine and fluoxetine are both commonly used antidepressants, which selectively block serotonin reuptake.

The serotonin/norepinephrine reuptake inhibitors (**choice A**) include venlafaxine, which is useful for the treatment of refractory depression. Bupropion is a dopamine/norepinephrine reuptake inhibitor (**choice C**) that is used for the treatment of depression, adult ADHD, and smoking cessation.

Atypical antipsychotics such as clozapine and risperidone block both dopamine and serotonin receptors (**choice D**). They are associated with fewer side effects than are more "typical" antipsychotics.

Monoamine oxidase inhibitors (MAOIs; **choice E**) include phenelzine, tranylcypromine, and isocarboxazid. These agents prevent the inactivation of biogenic amines such as norepinephrine, serotonin, dopamine, and tyramine.

8. **The correct answer is D.** Testicular torsion usually occurs in patients who have a history of cryptorchidism. It usually has an acute onset and occurs in men aged 10 to 20 years. The associated clinical features include pain and scrotal swelling, with an acute, tender, nontransilluminable lesion seen.

A varicocele (**choice A**) also has an associated nontransilluminable lesion; however, this lesion is usually nontender. Also there is the "bag of worms" consistency usually felt with varicoceles.

Although testicular cancer (**choice B**) may be associated with a history of cryptorchidism, it usually involves painless, solid testicular swelling.

Epididymitis (**choice C**) is usually of gradual onset and occurs mostly from sexually transmitted diseases in this age group. Usually there are the associated

symptoms of fever and irritative voiding symptoms that lead the clinician to an infective process. Although not always diagnostic, Prehn sign was negative in this patient. Prehn sign is used to differentiate bacterial epididymitis and testicular torsion. Scrotal elevation relieves pain in epididymitis, but not in torsion.

Orchitis (**choice E**) in this age group is usually preceded by the mumps or may be caused by bacteria. Fever and tachycardia are usually present, indicating an infectious process.

9. **The correct answer is D.** This is a typical presentation of orbital cellulitis that originates from an infection of the paranasal sinuses.

Acute iritis (**choice A**) presents with acute onset of pain in the affected eye with photophobia, ciliary injection, and blurred vision. Conjunctival injection is minimal, if present at all.

Blepharitis (**choice B**), a superficial infection of the eyelid, generally presents without fever and is not accompanied by proptosis.

Graves disease (**choice C**), also known as hyperthyroidism, can present with mild proptosis and is usually accompanied by signs of thyrotoxicosis, including nervousness, restlessness, heat intolerance, increased sweating, fatigue, and weight loss. Fever is not usually part of the clinical picture.

Retrobulbar hemorrhage (**choice E**) presents with unilateral or bilateral proptosis, but is usually a direct result of localized trauma.

10. **The correct answer is B.** Metabolic syndrome is characterized by a group of metabolic disorders including insulin resistance, hypertension, prothrombic state, hyperuricemia, low HDL, high LDL, and high triglyceride levels and central obesity. People with metabolic syndrome are at increased risk of coronary heart disease, stroke, and type 2 diabetes.

Choices A, C, and D are incorrect because decreased LDL, increased HDL, osteoporosis, thrombocytopenia, and hypotension do not comprise the metabolic syndrome. A fasting blood glucose equal to or greater than 126 mL/dL on two separate occasions (**choice E**) is one of the diagnostic criteria for diabetes mellitus.

11. **The correct answer is C.** Epidural hematoma occurs following head trauma. The course that follows is immediate loss of consciousness, followed by a lucid period and then a short delay to altered mental status. CT scan shows a lens-shaped (convex) bleed protruding into the brain parenchyma due to the high arterial pressure bleeding that compresses the brain.

In acute subdural hematoma (**choice A**) after head trauma, there is immediate loss of consciousness and progressive deterioration due to tearing of the bridging veins. CT scan shows a crescent-shaped area due to the slow venous bleeding that follows the contour of the brain.

Chronic subdural hematoma (**choice B**) occurs most often in the elderly. Cerebral atrophy, normal in aging, causes the brain to be more mobile within the skull. Therefore, even minor trauma can tear venous channels, resulting in minor but accumulative bleeding. Also, symptoms can present subacutely far after the minor head trauma.

Subarachnoid hemorrhage (**choice D**) is heralded by the onset of severe, rapidly spreading pain. CT scan confirms blood in the subarachnoid space. The most common cause is not trauma, but rather a cerebral arteriovenous malformation or a berry aneurysm that spontaneously ruptures.

Lacunar infarcts (**choice E**) are not a result of trauma.

12. **The correct answer is E.** Scabies classically presents with intense pruritus and burrowing in the axillary folds, hands, and groin. The treatment of choice in a child is permethrin 5% applied in the evening, left on overnight, and rinsed off in the morning. The patient should also be advised to launder all linens to prevent spread and reinfection. The infection is caused by *Sarcoptes scabiei* and is highly contagious.

Seborrheic dermatitis (**choice A**) presents as scaly, greasy areas along the eyebrows, nasolabial folds, and scalp. Treatment usually includes antifungal shampoos and lotions; refractory cases may require steroid therapy.

Dyshidrotic eczema (**choice B**) is a recurrent or chronic relapsing form of vesicular palmoplantar dermatitis of unknown etiology. It presents with symmetric crops of clear vesicles and bullae on the palms and lateral aspects of the fingers.

Pityriasis rosea (**choice D**) presents with diffuse involvement of the trunk ("Christmas tree pattern") and has characteristic patches with fine collarette scales.

13. **The correct answer is A.** Auer rods are small blue rods found in the cytoplasm of the lymphocyte in acute myelogenous leukemia (AML).

Heinz bodies (**choice B**) are aggregates of denatured, precipitated hemoglobin within red blood cells and are found in peripheral smears of patients with glucose-6 phosphate dehydrogenase deficiency.

Hirano bodies (**choice C**) are eosinophilic, highly refractile, rod-like structures that are found adjacent to pyramidal neurons in the hippocampal formation in Alzheimer disease, Pick disease, and other neurodegenerative disorders.

Howell-Jolly bodies (**choice D**) are spherical, blue-black inclusions of red blood cells seen on Wright-stained smears. They are 1- to 2-μm-diameter nuclear fragments of condensed DNA normally removed by the spleen. They are seen in severe hemolytic anemias in patients with dysfunctional spleens or in patients after a splenectomy.

Philadelphia chromosome (**choice E**) is found in many patients with chronic myelogenous leukemia (CML).

14. **The correct answer is C.** A history of pulmonary symptoms following cave exploration and exposure to bat/bird droppings while in the Ohio River Valley is a classic presentation for *Histoplasma capsulatum*.

Aspergillus fumigatus (**choice A**) may present with pulmonary or allergic symptoms; however, there is no correlation with the Ohio River Valley. Antifungal treatment choices depend on the severity of the disease.

Coccidioides immitis (**choice B**) is found in the Southwestern United States. It often presents as flu-like symptoms and occasional arthralgias.

Mycoplasma tuberculosis (**choice D**) is incorrect because there are no risk factors presented for the acquisition of *M. tuberculosis*. The disease is often found among disadvantaged populations. Furthermore, primary tuberculosis is usually asymptomatic.

Finally, *Rickettsia rickettsii* (**choice E**) is an incorrect answer because the typical presentation of Rocky Mountain spotted fever would include the characteristic maculopapular rash.

15. **The correct answer is E.** The vitelline duct typically undergoes total obliteration in the seventh week of fetal life, but in rare cases its proximal part persists as a diverticulum from the small intestine. This is known as Meckel diverticulum and is located approximately 3 or 4 feet above the ileocolic junction.

The bulbus cordis (**choice A**) is a part of the primitive heart tube that will become part of the aorta and the pulmonary trunk.

The ligamentum arteriosum (**choice B**) is the postnatal remnant of the ductus arteriosis and not a diverticulum of the gut tube.

The mesonephros (**choice C**) is the primordial filtration apparatus that is replaced eventually by the metanephric kidney later in development. It has no role in the gastrointestinal development or attachment to the gut tube.

The neural crest (**choice D**) cells mainly give rise to neurons in ganglia, Schwann cells, pia and arachnoid, adrenal medulla, parafollicular cells, and the aorticopulmonary septum, but not gut diverticula.

16. **The correct choice is A.** Prazosin or doxazosin are therapies used successfully to treat benign prostatic hypertrophy and thus is a reasonable class of drugs for the management of hypertension in this patient.

    Beta-blockers (**choice B**), calcium channel blockers (**choice C**), ACE inhibitors (**choice D**), and hydrochlorothiazide (**choice E**) are all antihypertensive agents; however, they are not the treatment of choice for patients with concurrent benign prostatic hyperplasia.

17. **The correct answer is C.** This patient has a bacterial pneumonia and examination may reveal findings of a lobar, consolidated pneumonia. Percussion would be slightly dull, with bronchial breath sounds and egophony, whispered pectoriloquy, or increased tactile or vocal fremitus.

    Hyperresonance (**choice A**) is more likely with a pneumothorax, where there is air in the pleural space.

    Dullness to percussion with decreased breath sounds and decreased tactile fremitus (**choice B**) suggest a pleural effusion.

    Choice D is incorrect. Tympany and vesicular breath sounds are normal findings; increased tactile fremitus would occur in a consolidated pneumonia.

    Hyperresonance on percussion and tracheal deviation (**choice E**) are seen with a tension pneumothorax.

18. **The correct answer is C.** This patient presents with the classic signs and symptoms of infection with *Giardia*, a flagellate protozoan. The treatment of choice for *Giardia* is metronidazole (Flagyl).

    Chloramphenicol (**choice A**) and clindamycin (**choice B**) are used in the treatment of bacterial infections. Itraconazole (**choice D**) is used in the treatment of fungal infections. Lamivudine (**choice D**) is used in the treatment of viral infections.

19. **The correct answer is C.** Niacin may cause a prostaglandin-mediated flushing and pruritus, which may be reduced by pretreatment with aspirin or NSAIDs.

Lowering the dose and switching to extended-release tablets may also reduce side effects.

Taking iron with orange juice (**choice A**) may increase its absorption, but the link between niacin and orange juice has not been extensively studied. Taking her dosage every other day (**choice B**) would not be therapeutic. Because this is a prostaglandin-mediated reaction, an antihistamine (**choice D**) would not relieve all symptoms. At the patient's request, other measures such as reducing the side effect are preferable over beginning a new, more expensive drug (**choice E**).

20. **The correct answer is B.** Postpartum psychosis has a dramatic onset, occurring as early as 48 to 72 hours after delivery. The condition resembles a rapidly evolving manic or mixed episode with symptoms such as restlessness, insomnia, irritability, rapidly shifting depressed or elevated mood, and disorganized behavior. The mother may have delusional beliefs that relate to the infant or she may have auditory hallucinations that instruct her to harm herself or her infant.

    Typically, postpartum depression (**choice A**) develops insidiously over the first 3 months postpartum. Postpartum depression is more persistent and debilitating than the postpartum blues but does not involve delusional beliefs or hallucinations.

    Conversion disorder (**choice C**) involves a loss of neurologic function in the absence of organic disease. Bipolar disorder (**choice D**) consists of bouts of depression followed by mania.

    Schizophrenia (**choice E**) is characterized by abnormalities in thinking, emotion, and behavior. Two or more of the diagnostic criteria must be present for at least 1 month.

21. **The correct answer is A.** The symptom of urinary retention points to frank lumbar spine impingement, possibly from a disk herniation that is causing undue pressure in the cauda equina area of the spinal canal (below the L1 level). The right foot drop and right lateral calf pain point to a probable L5 nerve dysfunction, most specifically from an L4 to L5 disk herniation. The L5 nerve root compression symptoms of foot drop and urinary retention merit immediate evaluation for cauda equina syndrome before permanent nerve damage ensues. Even without specific spine trauma or recent trauma, a patient with a history of repetitive minor spine trauma is at risk for disk herniation, which leads to cauda equina syndrome. Disk herniation can occur spontaneously; those with probable degenerative disk disease also can herniate spontaneously.

In lumbar degenerative disk disease, a nonherniated disk (**choice B**) is unlikely to cause pressure on the nerve roots and/or lead to cauda equina syndrome.

Lumbar spondylosis without myelopathy (**choice C**) would be common with a history of repetitive minor lumbar trauma (such as in rodeo riding), but degenerative, arthritic changes in the lumbar spine are unlikely to cause urinary retention without the manifestation of myelopathy.

Myofascial back pain (**choice D**) generally presents as axial back pain that usually does not cause radicular pain. It is also not accompanied by neurologic symptoms and/or findings of right foot paresis.

Right sacroiliitis (**choice E**) is usually associated with fairly localized pain in the right lumbar area without neurologic symptoms/findings and without radicular pain.

22. **The correct choice is C.** Patients who are being screened for chronic HIV infection should have an ELISA antibody test. All positive test results must be confirmed with the highly specific Western blot test.

CBC and blood cultures (**choice A**) are generally useful in the diagnosis of an acute infection, but are neither sensitive nor specific as a screening tool for HIV infection. A CD4 count (**choice B**) is useful in the management of HIV infection. CD4 count and viral load testing (**choice E**) can be used to estimate a patient's risk of developing AIDS over the next decade. Viral load testing (**choice D**) and p24 antigen tests are useful in acute HIV infection (prior to seroconversion); however, viral load is not an appropriate screening tool.

23. **The correct answer is C.** The bladder is supplied by the vesicular branches of the internal iliac arteries. The internal iliacs arise from the common iliac artery.

The external iliac (**choice A**) also arises from the common iliac artery. It makes no contribution to the blood supply of the bladder.

The inferior epigastric (**choice B**) is a branch of the external iliac artery. It serves as a landmark in the inguinal region. Indirect inguinal hernias lie laterally to the inferior epigastric arteries, whereas direct inguinal hernias lie medially to these vessels.

The internal pudendal (**choice D**) is a branch of the anterior division of the internal iliac artery. It gives rise to the inferior rectal artery, perineal artery, artery of the bulb in men, urethral artery, deep artery of the penis or clitoris, and dorsal artery of the penis or clitoris.

The lateral sacral (**choice E**) is a branch of the posterior division of the internal iliac artery. It supplies sacral structures.

24. **The correct answer is D.** Many times, physical examination of the lungs in a pulmonary embolism is completely normal, as is the chest x-ray. It is important to remember that normal physical examination does not rule out a pulmonary embolism.

Dullness to percussion (**choice B**) suggests a pleural effusion or consolidation of lung tissue. Hyperresonance (**choice C**) suggests a pneumothorax. Bronchial breath sounds (**choice A**) suggest a consolidated area of lung. Tactile fremitus (**choice E**) suggests an infectious process as well.

25. **The correct answer is B.**

Choice A describes the characteristics of normal bowel sounds.

Choice C is incorrect. Bowel sounds may be heard in an early small bowel obstruction.

Choice D describes radiographic evidence of a perforation.

Choice E describes radiographic evidence of a large bowel obstruction.

26. **The correct answer is E.** Many alcoholics experience "the shakes" approximately 12 to 24 hours after their last consumption. Tremors may be accompanied by tachycardia, diaphoresis, anorexia, and insomnia. After 24 to 72 hours, the alcoholic may have generalized seizures. Delirium tremens (DT) begins 3 to 5 days later. Commonly used medications for alcohol withdrawal are lorazepam, diazepam, and chlordiazepoxide.

Gentamicin (**choice A**) is an antibiotic. Compazine (**choice B**) is an antiemetic, which may be an adjunctive therapy. Mucomyst (**choice C**) is used in APAP overdose. Naloxone (**choice D**) is used in opioid overdose.

27. **The correct answer is C.** Osteosarcoma is the most common malignancy of the bone and typically affects adolescents. The symptoms often occur after a sports-related injury, which can delay diagnosis.

Osteoid osteoma (**choice A**) presents with benign tumors found in children and adolescents. Ewing sarcoma (**choice B**) is a giant cell tumor that affects children but is not the most common malignancy of bone. Osgood-Schlatter (**choice D**) is a benign condition that affects adolescents. Chondroblastomas (**choice E**) are less common and are considered benign in most cases.

28. **The correct choice is B.** Propranolol, a potent beta-blocker, is the drug of choice for patients with familial essential benign tremor.

All the remaining choices are potential treatments for hypertension; however, only beta-blockers are indicated for patients with benign familial essential tremor.

29. **The correct answer is C.** Somogyi effect is prebreakfast hyperglycemia due to the surge of counterregulatory hormones in response to nocturnal hypoglycemia. Treatment includes eliminating the dose of intermediate insulin at dinnertime and giving it at a lower dosage at bedtime or increasing food at bedtime.

Dawn phenomenon (**choice A**) is reduced tissue sensitivity to insulin between 5:00 and 8:00 A.M.

Waning of insulin dose plus dawn phenomenon (**choice B**) presents with elevated blood glucose levels at 3:00 and 7:00 A.M.

Primary hypoglycemia (**choice D**) is incorrect because the elevated 7:00 A.M. glucose would not be present.

Insulin allergy (**choice E**) is an immediate-type hypersensitivity resulting in urticaria, and occasionally, anaphylaxis.

30. **The correct answer is D.** Rosacea is a chronic acneiform disorder of the pilosebaceous glands with associated increased reactivity of capillaries to heat, leading to flushing and telangiectasia. The skin lesions are papulopustular and primarily found symmetrically along the face.

Miliaria (**choice A**), also known as prickly heat or heat rash, is often found in newborns. It presents pinpoint sweat blisters with no redness.

Folliculitis (**choice B**) is an infection and inflammation of the hair follicles. This results in erythema and often pus-filled lesions. It would not be exacerbated by alcohol and would not be associated with telangiectasias.

Milia (**choice E**) are yellow, keratin-filled epidermal cysts and usually are not associated with erythema or telangiectasias.

31. **The correct answer is C.** Duodenal ulcer presents with epigastric pain that is commonly described as dull and aching. The pain may be aggravated by caffeine, smoking, alcohol, and NSAIDs. Symptoms are initially relieved by food, and then pain develops about 2 to 3 hours after the meal. Acute pancreatitis (**choice A**) presents with epigastric pain that radiates through to the back and is made worse with consumption of food. Cholelithiasis (**choice B**) is typically asymptomatic or may present with right upper quadrant pain. Esophageal stricture (**choice D**) presents with heartburn, regurgitation, and dysphagia. Gastric carcinoma (**choice E**) is typically asymptomatic. When symptoms do appear, they consist of heartburn, abdominal discomfort, loss of appetite, and weight loss.

32. **The correct answer is B.** This patient has chronic obstructive pulmonary disease with chronic bronchitis. His chest film would most likely appear hyperinflated. Lung fields should appear darker, as more air is present.

Hampton hump (**choice A**) is a classic radiographic finding for pulmonary embolism. It is a zone of homogeneous, wedge-shaped consolidation in the lung periphery. Its base is contiguous to a visceral pleural surface, and its rounded convex apex is directed toward the hilum.

Pulmonary vascular congestion and Kerley B lines (**choices D and C**) are both manifestations of congestive heart failure on chest radiograph.

The so-called reticular-nodular pattern (**choice E**) is observed in interstitial lung disease and with pneumonic infiltrates that display an interstitial pattern (*Mycoplasma*, viral disease, and *Pneumocystis*).

33. **The correct answer is A.** The patient has classic symptoms of pseudomembranous colitis. Pseudomembranous colitis is an antibiotic-associated colitis. The most common organism causing pseudomembranous colitis is *Clostridium difficile*.

Clostridium perfringens (**choice B**) is a rare cause of pseudomembranous colitis.

Choices D and C are incorrect because *Giardia lamblia* and *Cryptosporidium* are enteric parasites.

Saccharomyces boulardii (**choice E**) is a nonpathogenic yeast and has been used in experimental settings to treat chronic pseudomembranous colitis.

34. **The correct answer is A.** Crohn disease is an inflammatory disease that may affect any part of the gastrointestinal tract. It can be distinguished from other bowel diseases by radiographic and endoscopic results. Skip lesions, a cobblestone appearance, and deep longitudinal fissures are characteristic of Crohn disease.

Diverticulitis (**choice B**) is an inflammatory disease or local perforation of a diverticulum. Patients have abdominal pain in the left lower quadrant and fever. Diagnosis can be confirmed with a barium enema but should not be performed in the acute stages. A barium enema may show stricture formation, fistula, or pericolonic mass.

Characteristics of irritable bowel syndrome (**choice C**) include abdominal pain and alteration in bowel habits. Physical examination, laboratory findings, and diagnostic tests, such as barium enema and colonoscopy, are normal.

Ischemic colitis (**choice D**) can be differentiated from other gastrointestinal disorders by the abrupt onset of abdominal pain. The patient may experience bloody diarrhea and systemic symptoms.

Ulcerative colitis (**choice E**) is incorrect. Endoscopic results show friable mucosa, pseudopolyps, and rectal involvement, which can help distinguish ulcerative colitis from Crohn disease.

35. **The correct answer is D.** Scleroderma is a chronic condition characterized by generalized fibrosis of the skin and organs.

Rheumatoid arthritis (**choice A**) presents with arthritis and inflammation and is not usually associated with skin changes. Polymyalgia rheumatica (**choice B**) is a syndrome characterized by severe stiffness in the neck, shoulder girdle, and pelvic girdle. Wegener granulomatosis (**choice C**) is a rare disease characterized by vasculitis of the arteries and is accompanied by upper or lower respiratory tract symptoms in 90% of cases.

Reactive arthritis (Reiter syndrome; **choice E**) is a form of arthritis, or joint inflammation, that occurs as a "reaction" to an infection elsewhere in the body. It is a triad of urethritis, conjunctivitis, and aseptic arthritis. It commonly follows a dysenteric infection or sexually transmitted infection.

36. **The correct answer is E.** Cystoscopy is nearly 100% accurate in diagnosing bladder carcinoma. Histologic diagnosis is provided and confirmed with biopsy. Bladder carcinoma is more common in men and usually occurs during the fourth to seventh decades of life. Hematuria is the most common presenting symptom. Cigarette smoking is one of the risk factors and accounts for approximately 60% of new cases.

CBC and blood chemistry (**choice A**) are used to evaluate for infection and renal function. Pelvic and abdominal CT scans (**choice B**), intravenous urogram (**choice C**), and retrograde pyelography (**choice D**) are all used for staging of tumors.

37. **The correct answer is B.** The recurrent laryngeal nerves are branches of the vagus (CN X), and supply all intrinsic muscles of the larynx except the cricothyroid. The right recurrent laryngeal nerve recurs around the right subclavian artery. The left recurrent laryngeal nerve recurs in the thorax around the arch of the aorta and ligamentum arteriosum. Both nerves ascend to the larynx by passing between the trachea and esophagus, close to the thyroid gland.

The internal laryngeal (**choice A**) nerve is a purely sensory branch of the superior laryngeal nerve. The thyroarytenoid (**choice C**) is an intrinsic muscle of the larynx; its inner fibers are specialized as the vocalis muscle, which is related to the vocal ligament. It is not usually at risk during thyroid surgery. The vestibular folds (**choice D**), or false vocal folds, are located superior to the true vocal folds inside the larynx. They are not concerned with phonation. The vocal folds (**choice E**) form the boundaries of the rima glottidis inside the larynx and are not vulnerable during thyroidectomy.

38. **The correct answer is C.** Cutaneous anthrax, due to *Bacillus anthracis*, a gram-positive rod, is spread by contact with anthrax spores on the hides of animals, such as sheep. Cutaneous disease presents as a painless, boil-like lesion that forms an ulcer with a black eschar. The treatment of choice is doxycycline, ciprofloxacin, or clindamycin. The other antibiotics (**choices A, B, D, and E**) are utilized in the treatment of cutaneous anthrax.

39. **The correct answer is A.** *Escherichia coli* is the most common cause of urinary tract infections and is responsible for 80% of infections. *Proteus, Klebsiella, Enterobacter,* and *Staphylococcus saprophyticus* are also causative organisms.

Helicobacter pylori (**choice B**) is associated with gastritis and peptic ulcer disease. *Klebsiella pneumoniae* (**choice C**) can cause pneumonia, urinary tract infections, and sepsis, but still remains a secondary cause of urinary tract infections.

Staphylococcus epidermidis (**choice D**) is a common member of the normal florae of skin and mucous membranes. It is an important cause of nosocomial infections.

Staphylococcus saprophyticus (**choice E**) can cause urinary tract infections in young females.

40. **The correct answer is B.** Antisocial personality disorder (sociopathy) is behavior outside the usual ethical and legal codes without the presence of delusions, anxiety, or irrational thinking. These patients tend to be charming and above average in intelligence, but display untruthfulness, a lack of remorse, and antisocial behaviors.

41. **The correct choice is D.** Although all of the drug classes could be used to control blood pressure, ACE inhibitors are indicated in patients with type 2 diabetes mellitus. The goal of therapy should be to keep blood pressure below 130/80 mm Hg.

42. **The correct answer is A.** Barrett esophagus is caused by chronic severe gastrointestinal reflux disease. The squamous epithelium of the esophagus is replaced by metaplastic columnar epithelium.

   Esophageal varices (**choice B**) are caused by portal hypertension. Cirrhosis is the most common cause of portal hypertension.

   Peptic stricture (**choice C**) is a complication of esophagitis.

   Schatzki ring (**choice D**) is a thin ring of tissue in the distal esophagus.

43. **The correct answer is C.** Opioid overdose is consistent with the patient's findings of miosis, respiratory depression, and pulmonary edema. Naloxone is an opioid antagonist used to treat overdose.

   Activated charcoal (**choice A**) is not indicated as an initial treatment. N-acetylcysteine (**choice B**) is used in APAP overdose. Benzodiazepines (such as lorazepam, **choice D**) may be used in a variety of instances, including for alcohol withdrawal and conscious sedation. Labetalol (**choice E**) can be used for hypertensive crisis.

44. **The correct answer is D.** Isoniazid is used in the treatment of tuberculosis. Complications include peripheral neuropathy and elevated liver function tests. Peripheral neuropathy is typically noted with high-dose isoniazid and can be prevented by the use of vitamin B_6 (pyridoxine).

45. **The correct answer is C.** This patient's presentation is typical for myelofibrosis, which may occur either as an idiopathic condition or as a complication of clonal marrow disorders, including chronic myelogenous leukemia and polycythemia vera. In myelofibrosis, the marrow space becomes replaced by fibrosis, leading to an anemia secondary to loss of marrow blood-forming cells. Erythrocytes can be deformed as they squeeze through the altered marrow, leading to the presence of obviously abnormally shaped cells in the smear.

   Chronic blood loss (**choice A**) and iron deficiency (**choice D**) both cause a microcytic hypochromic anemia.

   Hereditary disease (**choice B**), such as sickle cell anemia or the various thalassemias, can cause abnormally shaped blood cells but would be expected to present at an early age, not in an older adult.

   Vitamin B_{12} and folate deficiencies (**choice E**) cause a macrocytic anemia.

46. **The correct answer is C.** About 35% of villous adenomas become malignant. This type of lesion is characterized by 80% or more of the glands being villous (elongated) as opposed to adenomatous polyps, in which most of the glands are tubular (circular). In villoglandular polyps, about one half is of each type. Both adenomatous polyps and villoglandular polyps have a risk of malignancy of only about 2%: much lower than that of villous adenomas.

47. **The correct answer is A.** Polycystic ovary syndrome (PCOS) presents with chronic anovulation, insulin resistance, obesity, and virilization. These patients have steady elevated states of estrogen, androgen, and LH levels instead of the fluctuating levels seen in unaffected women. Treatment in women who wish to become pregnant should begin with weight reduction. A decrease in body fat will lower the conversion of androgens to estrone and may help restore ovulation.

   Medroxyprogesterone acetate (**choice B**), spironolactone (**choice C**), finasteride (**choice D**), and flutamide (**choice E**) are not indicated—spironolactone, flutamide, and finasteride are potentially teratogenic.

48. **The correct answer is A.** Quinine may be used to treat active infection, but is not used in prevention.

   Chloroquine (**choice B**) may be used in areas where there is no reported resistance. Doxycycline (**choice C**) is an alternative to mefloquine; however, there is sun sensitivity reported with its use. Mefloquine (**choice D**) is the drug of choice in most areas, particularly those that report malaria drug resistance.

   Atovaquone/proguanil (**choice E**), also called Malarone, is a daily medication that can be started 1–2 days prior to travel and is available in pediatric dosing.

49. **The correct answer is C.** Retinal detachment is commonly preceded by photopsia and an increased number of floaters. With detachment, the patient will note persistent vision loss and describe the impression of a curtain being drawn down over the visual field. Retinal vein occlusion (**choice A**) presents with painless, acute onset of blurry vision. Occipital lobe seizure (**choice B**) presents with visual phenomena such as flashing white or colored lights or visual hallucinations. Amaurosis fugax (**choice D**) presents with transient incomplete loss of vision in one or both eyes, with no

history of floaters or flashes of light prior to the vision loss. Ocular migraine (**choice E**) presents with transient monocular visual loss lasting less than one hour.

50. **The correct answer is E.** The risk factors for pyelonephritis include diabetes mellitus as well as being an elderly institutionalized woman. Clinical features include fever, shaking chills, flank pain, and CVA tenderness. Tachycardia may be present. Urinalysis yields bacteriuria and pyuria, but not necessarily hematuria. CBC usually shows a leukocytosis with a left shift to confirm infection.

Glomerulonephritis (**choice A**) can occur in people with diabetes; however, it does not present with septic symptoms such as fever, chills, and tachycardia. Clinical features of glomerulonephritis include hematuria, oliguria or anuria, facial edema in the morning, and pedal edema in the evening. Hypertension is also common. Urinalysis usually reveals red blood cell casts, WBCs, and proteinuria.

Nephritic syndrome (**choice B**) is a glomerulonephropathy. Nephritic syndrome presents with facial edema, hematuria, and hypertension.

Cystitis (**choice C**) would not present with fever, CVA tenderness, or an elevated white blood cell count with a left shift.

Acute tubulointerstitial nephritis (**choice D**) usually occurs as a reaction to a new medication, but can be a reaction to systemic infection by bacteria and viruses. Clinical features include a sudden decrease in renal function, fever, and flank pain. There also can be a maculopapular rash if the cause is an allergen. Urinalysis usually reveals hematuria, pyuria, proteinuria, and WBC casts.

51. **The correct answer is D.** Oxygen therapy is the only medical therapy shown to improve survival in patients with chronic obstructive pulmonary disease.

All the other treatments listed may provide the patient relief from symptoms but do not alter the progression of the disease and have not been found to improve survival.

52. **The correct answer is C.** Cimetidine is an H_2 receptor antagonist.

Choice A describes misoprostol. **Choice B** describes an H_1 receptor antagonist, such as diphenhydramine. **Choice D** describes proton pump inhibitors, such as omeprazole, and **choice E** describes the mechanism of action of calcium carbonate, an antacid.

53. **The correct answer is B.** A heart rate of 40/min, cool extremities, and a temperature of 35°C (95°F) are all common signs and symptoms of beta-blocker overdose. Consider beta-blocker overdose in the differential diagnosis of a comatose or confused patient if clinical findings of bradycardia, hypotension, decreased body temperature, and hypoglycemia are present and no definite history of drug overdose exists.

A fever of 38.5°C (101.3°F), vomiting, and diarrhea (**choice A**) is a less likely choice in the setting of an elevated temperature. Vomiting and diarrhea are not associated with beta-blocker overdose.

A heart rate of 150/min, a prominent S_3 heart sound, and hyperreflexia (**choice C**) would be more likely associated with a stimulant or SSRI overdose.

Beta-blocker toxicity is not associated with diaphoresis or myosis (**choice D**). Bradycardia is more commonly seen.

A heart rate of 60/min, hyperglycemia, hypotension, and combative behavior (**choice E**) is not associated with beta-blocker overdose. Hypoglycemia, not hyperglycemia, is more common.

54. **The correct answer is D.** Vitamin B_{12} deficiency may occur in Crohn disease due to terminal ileum inflammation or resection. Vitamin B_{12} deficiency causes a macrocytic anemia. Crohn patients may have hypoalbuminemia due to malabsorption or intestinal protein loss.

55. **The correct answer is E.** Extrapyramidal signs and symptoms, such as pseudoparkinsonism, are commonly seen in patients receiving medications that block the dopamine receptor. Pseudoparkinsonism, as the name implies, is a condition in which patients experience signs and symptoms similar to the symptomatology associated with Parkinson disease. These symptoms include mask-like facies, drooling, tremors, pill-rolling motion, cogwheel rigidity, and shuffling gait. Pseudoparkinsonism symptoms are commonly seen in individuals taking antipsychotic medications and other phenothiazines such as prochlorperazine. None of the other answer choices are associated with the development of these symptoms.

Calcium carbonate (**choice A**) is an antacid. Dimenhydrinate (**choice B**) is an antihistamine commonly used in the treatment of motion sickness. Dronabinol (**choice C**) is a class II narcotic used in the treatment of severe nausea and vomiting; this agent is the psychoactive substance found in marijuana.

Ondansetron (**choice D**) is a 5-HT₃-receptor blocking agent and is used in the treatment of severe nausea and vomiting, especially in patients receiving emetogenic cancer chemotherapy.

56. **The correct answer is A.** Alpha-2-receptor agonists directly inhibit pancreatic insulin secretion. Beta-2-adrenergic agonists (**choice B**) stimulate insulin secretion. Cholecystokinin (**choice C**) is a hormone that causes not only gallbladder contraction, but also insulin secretion from the pancreas. Pancreatic glucagon release (**choice D**) acts as a paracrine stimulus for insulin secretion. Muscarinic activity (**choice E**) in the gastrointestinal tract enhances secretion of insulin from the pancreas.

57. **The correct answer is B.** Atrial fibrillation causes pooling of the blood in the atria. The accumulation of the blood can cause thrombi to form, which can be disseminated into the peripheral vasculature. This poses a significant risk factor for cerebrovascular events.

Aortic stenosis (**choice A**) can lead to congestive heart failure. The stenosis is usually caused by thickening and calcification of the aortic valve cusps that lead to a decreased ejection fraction.

Bradycardia (**choice C**) does not lead to thrombus formation or atrial fibrillation.

Pericarditis (**choice D**) can lead to cardiac tamponade and decreased cardiac output, but it is not a significant risk factor for thrombus formation in the heart.

Restrictive cardiomyopathy (**choice E**) mainly leads to right-sided heart failure.

58. **The correct answer is D.** This patient exhibits stage 1 Lyme disease. He has been bitten by a tick, which is the carrier of the spirochete *Borrelia burgdorferi*, which causes Lyme disease. The patient has the characteristic erythema migrans, or "bull's-eye" lesion—a flat or slightly raised red lesion that progresses with a central clearing. Other symptoms include fatigue, headache, fever, chills, and myalgias. Symptoms usually occur on an average of 7 to 10 days after the initial infection but may occur 3 to 30 days after the tick bite. The recommended drug for patients over the age of 8 with Lyme disease is doxycycline.

Penicillin G (**choice A**) and ampicillin are alternate drug choices for both adult and pediatric patients with Lyme disease. Ceftriaxone (**choice C**) is second-line treatment option in patients over the age of 8 with stage 1 Lyme disease. Amoxicillin (**choice E**) is recommended for pregnant and lactating women. Tetracycline (**choice B**) is recommended for the treatment of Rocky Mountain spotted fever, another disease caused by tick bites.

59. **The correct answer is C.** Vasopressin is produced in the hypothalamus and released by the posterior pituitary gland. Oxytocin is produced and released by the posterior pituitary as well.

All of the other choices, as well as LH and TSH, are produced by the anterior pituitary gland.

60. **The correct answer is C.** *Streptococcus pneumoniae* is the most common cause of bacterial pneumonia. It also causes otitis media, sinusitis, bronchitis, bacteremia, and meningitis.

Block 2

1. **The correct answer is D.** Gangrenous necrosis is a commonly used term for a pattern of a widespread coagulative necrosis (often with superimposed bacterial infection) that is commonly seen in surgical clinical practice. The most common clinical setting is severe vascular disease associated with diabetes mellitus. This condition occludes the arteries of the leg, causing ischemia that is initially most severe in the toes. Unfortunately, many diabetics undergo a series of amputations for gangrenous necrosis, losing first their toes, then their distal feet, then their ankles, and finally most of their legs either below or above the knee. The affected tissue may be black in color; liquefactive necrosis with abscess formation may also be present if bacterial infection is superimposed.

2. **The correct answer is C.** The clinical history suggests trigeminal neuralgia, which is characterized by extreme pain along the distribution of the maxillary and mandibular subdivisions of the fifth cranial nerve. The facial nerve (**choice A**) controls the muscles of facial expression. The vagus nerve (**choice B**) controls most pharyngeal constrictor muscles. The glossopharyngeal (**choice D**), the ninth cranial nerve, innervates the stylopharyngeus muscle. The recurrent laryngeal nerve (**choice E**) controls the laryngeal musculature.

3. **The correct answer is C.** All of the choices listed are reactions that occur in the synthetic pathway from cholesterol to cortisol. ACTH stimulates the first reaction in the pathway: cholesterol to pregnenolone. This reaction is catalyzed by the enzyme cholesterol desmolase. The next step in the pathway is pregnenolone to progesterone (**choice D**); progesterone is then converted to 17-hydroxyprogesterone (**choice E**); 17-hydroxyprogesterone is converted to 11-deoxycortisol (**choice B**) by the enzyme 21 beta-hydroxylase; and the 11-deoxycortisol is then converted to cortisol (**choice A**).

4. **The correct answer is A.** Stimulation of the parasympathetic nervous system will result in a decreased heart rate or bradycardia, dilation (not constriction) of the peripheral blood vessels (**choice B**), increased (not decreased) peristalsis in the small intestine (**choice C**), increased (not decreased) secretions of the salivary glands (**choice D**), and constriction of the pupils, not mydriasis (**choice E**). The sympathetic nervous system, as a general rule, opposes the parasympathetic nervous system. During periods of intense stress, the sympathetic nervous system will help the body handle the stressor by promoting a series of physiologic changes, such as dilation of the pupils, secretion of the sweat glands, increased heart rate, constriction of the blood vessels to nonessential organs, bronchodilation, and decreased peristalsis in the intestinal tract.

5. **The correct answer is C.** Drainage of a pleural effusion is indicated if the pH is below 7.2, glucose is under 40 mg/dL, or if the Gram stain is positive.

   Although the administration of intravenous antibiotics (**choice A**) may be necessary to eradicate the infection, the first priority for the management of this patient is drainage of the effusion.

   A chest CT scan (**choice B**) is unnecessary at this time because the results of the thoracentesis indicate that drainage of the effusion is in order.

   Oncology consultation (**choice D**) is not indicated because the pleural fluid is infected. If the pleural fluid had greater than 50% lymphocytes, an oncologic workup would have been considered.

   The repeat chest x-ray (**choice E**) is unlikely to yield any further information.

6. **The correct answer is B.** Patients with colon cancer may be asymptomatic for years. A change in bowel habits is typical of cancer in the left colon. The "apple core" appearance of the descending colon is indicative of colon cancer.

   A benign polyp (**choice A**) is incorrect. A barium enema would show a round filling defect with smooth edges.

   Patients with diverticulosis (**choice C**) may complain of abdominal pain, diarrhea, and constipation. Barium enema shows the presence of multiple diverticula.

   Intussusception (**choice D**) is a telescoping segment of the colon. It is typically seen in the pediatric population, in children under the age of 2.

   Intermittent cramping abdominal pain increasing in severity is typical of a sigmoid volvulus (**choice E**). A barium enema performed on a patient with a sigmoid volvulus would show a "bird's beak" deformity.

7. **The correct answer is E.** Bipolar disorder is a condition of extreme highs often followed by debilitating lows. It is often termed as manic depression. A manic episode is classified as symptoms lasting at least 1 week. Such patients feel euphoric, high, and often irritable. They require little sleep, yet have high amounts of energy. They also perform reckless acts without concern for consequences, as in this case.

Avoidant personality disorder (**choice A**) is characterized by extreme social anxiety. Patients often feel inadequate, avoid social situations, and seek out jobs that require little contact with others.

Schizophrenia (**choice B**) is a chronic psychotic disorder with fluctuating disturbances in thinking, behavior, and perception. These disturbances include the presence of "positive" symptoms, such as delusions, hallucinations, and disorganized speech and behavior, and "negative" symptoms, such as poverty of speech.

Generalized anxiety disorder (**choice C**) is characterized by chronic anxiety, exaggerated worry, and tension, even when there is little or nothing to provoke it. Histrionic personality disorder (**choice D**) is characterized as a person who always calls attention to himself or herself and is overly dramatic.

8. **The correct answer is E.** This patient is presenting with gonococcal arthritis. Most patients with suspected acute infectious arthritis should be hospitalized to establish a diagnosis and to monitor for improvement. Daily synovial fluid drainage has also been recommended for purulent effusions associated with gonococcal arthritis. The initial treatment of choice for gonococcal arthritis is a third-generation beta-lactamase–resistant cephalosporin, such as ceftriaxone.

Compressions, ice, and elevation (**choice A**) are appropriate treatment options for a mild trauma but not for a septic arthritis. Intra-articular cortisone (**choice B**) and indomethacin (**choice C**) are not appropriate treatments for gonococcal arthritis. Amoxicillin (**choice D**) does not provide enough coverage for gonococcal arthritis.

9. **The correct answer is B.** The stone is only 4 mm, so it does have the potential to pass spontaneously (**choice A**), but the patient should be kept hydrated and because he is in pain, he should be given analgesics.

Lithotripsy (**choice C**), ureteroscopy (**choice D**), and pyelolithotomy (**choice E**) are usually done to extract stones 5 mm and larger.

10. **The correct answer is B.** This patient has locally advanced cervical cancer, stage IIb, with obvious parametrial involvement. The traditional way of treating patients with this stage of cervical cancer was with primary radiation therapy. This radiation would be delivered with external beam radiation and with brachytherapy. Brachytherapy for cervical cancer involves the placement of radiation into the cervix to allow for maximal dose delivery to the tumor. Recently, however, several studies have shown

that concurrent cisplatin-based chemotherapy should be used together with radiation therapy for cervical cancer stage IIb or later. These trials showed a significant survival advantage for the patients who received the cisplatin-based chemotherapy together with the radiation therapy.

To treat this patient with only cisplatin-based chemotherapy (**choice A**) would not be correct. The trials showed the greatest survival advantage with the use of this chemotherapy together with radiation therapy.

Hydroxyurea (**choice C**) had been used together with radiation to improve the treatment of cervical cancer. Hydroxyurea alone would not be used, and the combination of cisplatin-based chemotherapy with concurrent radiation therapy has been shown to be superior to radiation therapy combined with hydroxyurea (**choice E**).

Radiation therapy (**choice D**) alone was the standard approach to the treatment of late-stage cervical cancer. As described, however, the results of several recent trials show that the treatment of late-stage carcinoma should involve the use of radiation and concurrent cisplatin-based chemotherapy.

11. **The correct answer is C.** A pituitary macroadenoma may obliterate the anterior pituitary gland and cause a deficiency of all pituitary hormones (FSH/LH/TSH/ACTH). This patient has lost secondary sex characteristics and is exhibiting evidence of adrenal insufficiency and hypothyroidism. In addition, the visual field defects point to the fact that the tumor is impinging on the optic chiasm.

An adrenal adenoma (**choice A**) usually causes cortisol excess. Even if the tumor were to eliminate cortisol secretion, the other signs and symptoms would not be present.

Cushing's disease (**choice B**) is caused by an ACTH-secreting pituitary adenoma. The clinical scenario is not consistent with a cushingoid appearance (buffalo hump, hirsutism, moon facies, and striae).

A parathyroid adenoma (**choice D**) would cause primary hyperparathyroidism. Increased parathyroid hormone secretion can cause a constellation of physiologic changes that can be remembered as "bones, groans, stones, and psychiatric overtones." These changes include increased bone turnover, abdominal pain, nephrolithiasis, and mental status changes. Hypothyroidism (**choice E**) results in weight gain, cold intolerance, and hypoactivity. Myxedema, dry skin, and coarse hair may be noted.

12. **The correct answer is D.** The deltoid muscle, which allows abduction of the shoulder, is innervated by C5.

    Abduction of the fifth finger (**choice A**) tests the motor function of the abductor digiti minimi, which is innervated by the ulnar nerve (C8 and T1).

    Elbow extension (**choice B**) tests the motor function of the triceps brachii, which is innervated by the radial nerve (C7 and C8).

    Forearm pronation (**choice C**) tests the motor function of the pronator teres, which is innervated by the median nerve (C6 and C7).

    Shoulder shrug (**choice E**) is a test for cranial nerve XI function.

13. **The correct answer is D.** Tinea versicolor (pityriasis versicolor) is a common fungal infection of the skin. It is caused by the fungus *Pityrosporum ovale*. Tinea versicolor usually affects the back, chest, and upper arms. It may cause mild pruritus. The diagnosis is confirmed with a fungal scraping to identify the hyphae and budding spores, or "spaghetti and meatball" appearance, of the fungus. Treatment includes the administration of topical selenium sulfide lotion or a single oral dose of ketoconazole.

    Skin biopsy (**choice A**), blood culture (**choice B**), and oil immersion slide (**choice C**) are not generally used to diagnose fungal conditions.

    Although a complete blood count (**choice E**) is useful to indicate the presence of infection, it will not be useful in the establishment of a definitive diagnosis.

14. **The correct answer is A.** Because this patient with idiopathic thrombocytopenia purpura is asymptomatic and platelet count is within reasonable range, no clinical intervention is necessary beyond continuing to monitor the platelet count.

    Choice B is only necessary if the platelet count were to continue to decline and were at dangerous levels (<50,000/mm^3 or lower).

    Long-term corticosteroid therapy (**choice C**) has many associated risks, including osteoporosis, cataract formation, avascular necrosis, gastric ulcers, immunosuppression, and adrenal suppression. It should be avoided, particularly in this asymptomatic pediatric patient.

    Intravenous immunoglobulin therapy (**choice D**) is used as a treatment option but is not needed with this patient.

    A platelet transfusion (**choice E**) is not indicated because the platelet level is above 20,000/mm^3 and no active bleeding is observed.

15. **The correct choice is B.** Doxycycline is the drug of choice in children and adults for Rocky Mountain spotted fever. Serologic testing does not become positive early enough to prevent infection and potential death, so empiric therapy is warranted with a suspicion of *Rickettsia rickettsii* infection.

    Prednisone (**choice A**) is frequently used to manage autoimmune or idiopathic vasculitis, but does not treat the infection.

    Bactrim is not indicated. Sulfa (trimethoprim/sulfamethoxazole, **choice C**) may worsen the clinical course.

    Augmentin (**choice D**) does not effectively treat rickettsial infection. Acyclovir (**choice E**) is an antiviral and would not be effective against Rocky Mountain spotted fever.

16. **The correct answer is B.** Agranulocytosis is a common side effect of clozapine. Other drugs that may cause agranulocytosis include carbamazepine and colchicine.

17. **The correct answer is A.** Bleomycin is utilized in the treatment of Hodgkin disease and testicular cancer. The most severe complication of bleomycin is pulmonary fibrosis. Both amiodarone and busulfan can cause pulmonary fibrosis as well.

18. **The correct answer is E.** Stevens-Johnson syndrome is also referred to as erythema multiforme major. The condition is serious and has a mortality rate of up to 10%. Often, the disease presents with mucous membrane involvement of the oral cavity and the conjunctivae. Causative agents include sulfonamides, ethosuximide, penicillins, phenytoin, carbamazepine, and barbiturates.

19. **The correct answer is D.** Lipofuscin is a brown pigment that accumulates with aging. It is believed to be produced from the peroxidation of lipids. Lipofuscin accumulation does not necessarily impair the ability of the cell to function and can be found in the hearts and livers of healthy elderly patients.

    Beta-carotene (**choice A**) is a carotenoid ingested in the diet (found in yellow vegetables such as squash, pumpkins, and carrots) and converted to vitamin A.

    Bilirubin (**choice B**) is a pigment derived from the metabolism of the heme group of hemoglobin. The conjugated form (also called the direct reacting portion) accumulates in biliary obstructions. The unconjugated form of bilirubin (indirect-reacting) accumulates in hemolytic processes.

    Hemosiderin (**choice C**) is the storage form of iron and stains blue with Prussian blue.

Melanin (**choice E**) is a brown-black pigment made by melanocytes in the skin. Melanin is also found in the iris, giving the eye its color.

20. **The correct answer is D.** This is a classic presentation of sarcoidosis. Patients may have relatively mild symptoms or those presented in this case. Angiotensin-converting enzyme activity is present, suggesting macrophage activation, serum alkaline phosphatase, and gamma-glutamyl transferase levels may be elevated with liver involvement. The key to this diagnosis is the biopsy of "noncaseating" granulomas. They present most commonly in the mediastinum, peripheral nodes, lungs, liver, eyes, and skin.

    Asbestosis (**choice A**) presents as a mild, restrictive airway disease and typically has pleural involvement.

    Clinical manifestations of asthma (**choice B**) include episodic shortness of breath, cough, chest tightness, and wheezing. Asthma can be triggered by a variety of factors, including inhaled allergens, upper respiratory infections, exercise, or gastroesophageal reflux.

    Emphysema (**choice C**) would not have noncaseating granulomas or an elevated alkaline phosphatase level.

    Although tuberculosis (**choice E**) is certainly in the differential diagnosis of a patient presentation such as this one, granulomas from tuberculosis are caseated.

21. **The correct answer is B.** Familial adenomatous polyposis (FAP) is a rare autosomal dominant disease. It is characterized by several hundred polyps varying in size and configuration throughout the colon and rectum.

    The sheer number of polyps should make you suspect the diagnosis of familial adenomatous polyposis, thus superseding all the other answer choices.

22. **The correct answer is C.** Esophageal cancer has a peak incidence between 50 and 60 years of age. Smoking increases the risk of esophageal cancer. Dysphagia and weight loss are two common symptoms.

    Patients with achalasia (**choice A**) complain of dysphagia, but weight loss usually is not significant.

    Esophageal varices (**choice B**) are caused by portal hypertension. Cirrhosis is the most common cause of portal hypertension. Patient will exhibit signs and symptoms of cirrhosis, as well as spontaneous hematemesis if there are bleeding varices.

    Patients diagnosed with Mallory-Weiss tears (**choice D**) present with retching, vomiting, and hematemesis.

    Patients diagnosed with Zenker diverticulum (**choice E**) complain of dysphagia and regurgitation of undigested food into the mouth. They may also report gurgling noises after eating, swelling of the neck, and halitosis.

23. **The correct answer is D.** Paranoid personality disorder is a pervasive distrust and suspiciousness of others such that their motives are interpreted as malevolent. The patients often hold unjustified doubts about the loyalty or trustworthiness of friends or associates.

    Schizoid personality disorder (**choice A**) is characterized by a lack of interest in social relationships, a tendency toward a solitary lifestyle, and emotional coldness. Conversion disorder (**choice B**) involves a loss of neurologic function in the absence of organic disease. Narcissistic personality disorder (**choice C**) is characterized by extreme feelings of self-importance, a high need for admiration, and a lack of empathy.

    Major depressive disorder (**choice E**) is characterized by the presence of five of the following symptoms: sleep disturbances, loss of interest or pleasure in activities, inappropriate guilt, decreased energy, decreased concentration, increased or decreased appetite, psychomotor retardation or agitation, and suicidal ideation. The symptoms must have persisted for at least 2 weeks.

24. **The correct answer is D.** Fibromyalgia is a chronic illness that causes pain in the muscles and ligaments. It may also cause fatigue, sleep problems, and depression. It does not manifest in lab or x-ray abnormalities, but is diagnosed clinically by history and evaluation of 18 tender points.

    Because this patient's lab test results would be normal, **choices A, B, C, and E** are incorrect.

25. **The correct answer is E.** This ABG suggests uncompensated metabolic alkalosis. A natural physiologic response is for the body to compensate. Her breathing is shallow in an attempt to hypoventilate to retain carbon dioxide. The patient has a history of vomiting, which leads to chloride depletion, which in turn leads to an increase in bicarbonate. Additionally, the arterial blood gas shows classic metabolic acidosis. The arterial pH and bicarbonate are both increased and the partial pressure of carbon dioxide is not increased, so the condition is not compensated.

    Respiratory alkalosis (**choice A**) shows a decrease in the partial pressure of carbon dioxide and an increase in pH. The bicarbonate usually decreases to compensate.

    Metabolic acidosis (**choice B**) shows a decrease in bicarbonate and a decrease in the pH.

    In compensated metabolic alkalosis (**choice C**), the partial pressure of carbon dioxide would be increased to compensate for the metabolic alkalosis.

Respiratory acidosis (**choice D**) shows a decreased pH and increased partial pressure of carbon dioxide.

26. **The correct answer is B.** Thyrotoxicosis may manifest in a young, healthy woman as atrial fibrillation. Other cardiac manifestations of thyrotoxicosis include sinus tachycardia, increased blood pressure, and a sensation of palpitations. This patient has classic historic and physical exam findings for thyrotoxicosis.

Anorexia nervosa (**choice A**) may manifest with weight loss, although there is usually a history of decreased appetite as well. Although arrhythmias may present as a result of electrolyte disturbances, the short-term nature of this patient's signs and symptoms are more consistent with thyrotoxicosis.

Panic disorder (**choice C**) is certainly in the differential diagnosis of this patient. Although her history could suggest panic attacks, her physical examination findings are most consistent with thyrotoxicosis. For that reason, a TSH would be warranted in the workup of all patients with a diagnosis of panic disorder.

Hyperparathyroidism (**choice D**) is typically asymptomatic when diagnosed. The mnemonic "bones, stones, groans, moans" describes the major manifestations of osteopenia, renal stones, abdominal discomfort and constipation, and disorders of mood.

Hypothyroidism (**choice E**) results in *weight gain*, cold intolerance, and hypoactivity. Myxedema, dry skin, and coarse hair may also be noted.

27. **The correct answer is D.** A positive Babinski sign indicates an upper motor neuron lesion, which is a characteristic finding in myelopathy.

Decreased grip (**choice A**) indicates C7 or C8 nerve dysfunction, but is not specific for myelopathy.

Decreased patellar deep tendon reflex (**choice B**) is found with dysfunction of the L2, L3, or L4 nerve roots.

Limited neck flexion (**choice C**) can be due to muscle spasm, prior neck fusion, or arthritis/spondylosis of the cervical spine. It is not specific for myelopathy.

Unequal papillary reaction to light and accommodation (**choice E**) manifests with abnormalities of cranial nerve II (the optic nerve) or intracranial dysfunction (e.g., in head trauma). It is not found specifically with myelopathy.

28. **The correct answer is A.** This patient has recurring outbreaks of genital herpes. In herpes simplex (HSV) infections, prophylaxis is indicated if the patient has six or more recurrences per year. Prophylactic or suppres-

sive treatment can reduce outbreaks by 85% and may reduce viral shedding by 90%.

Antiviral therapy such as oral acyclovir (**choice B**) may decrease the clinical manifestations of the disease but does not cure HSV. HSV may be transmitted vaginally (**choice C**), and all measures should be taken to prevent neonatal infection. HSV-2 is considered a sexually transmitted disease (**choice D**) and prevention of the spread of the disease should be addressed.

Although local irritation (**choice E**) may cause discomfort or erythema, it should not result in a vesicular rash.

29. **The correct answer is D.** The low mean corpuscular volume indicates that the anemia is microcytic. The differential should include: iron deficiency anemia, anemia of chronic disease, lead toxicity, and thalassemia. Iron deficiency anemia is excluded because the ferritin level is normal. Because no history of lead exposure is noted, lead toxicity can be excluded as a cause of the anemia. The normal total iron-binding capacity excludes anemia of chronic disease. Therefore, thalassemia is the most likely diagnosis. The peripheral smear in β-thalassemia will show microcytosis, hypochromia, and basophilic stippling.

Iron supplementation (**choices A and B**) should not be given to this patient because her iron level is within normal limits. Also, parenteral iron administration is associated with a high risk of anaphylaxis and thus reserved for those with complete intolerance to oral iron supplementation.

Vitamin B_{12} replacement therapy (**choice C**) should be initiated for megaloblastic anemia resulting from dietary deficiency, pernicious anemia, gastrectomy, or tapeworm infestation.

The Schilling test (**choice E**) can assist in establishing a cause for vitamin B_{12} deficiency. However, it is not useful in this patient because she has a microcytic anemia.

30. **The correct answer is E.** The diffuse maculopapular rash is a clinical manifestation of secondary syphilis. This should be differentiated with the chancre formation and regional lymphadenopathy of primary disease and the neurologic manifestations of tertiary disease.

Aortic aneurysm rupture (**choice C**) is a manifestation of tertiary syphilis.

Choices A, B, and D are all manifestations of chancre formation, which is typically painless and causes nontender symmetric inguinal lymphadenopathy. With or without treatment, the lesion heals within 4 to 6 weeks. The chancre is a presentation of primary syphilis.

31. **The correct answer is E.** Nitroprusside is a very useful IV agent that causes dilatation of both arterioles and venules. It has a very rapid onset of action and is typically used in an emergency department or intensive care unit situation. The typical setting is a patient with acute or chronic low cardiac output and high ventricular filling pressures due to poor systolic left ventricular function. Underlying causes for the poor ventricular function may be diverse: dilated cardiomyopathy, acute myocardial infarction, chronic coronary heart disease, or aortic or mitral incompetence. Nitroprusside can improve perfusion of vital organs and reduce the workload of the heart. Problems sometimes encountered with this drug include hypotension (best avoided by starting with a low dose and continuously monitoring systemic arterial and pulmonary capillary wedge pressures) and accumulation of toxic metabolites of cyanide in patients with liver or renal failure. Many physicians prefer to use IV nitrate, rather than nitroprusside, because of its lesser toxicity.

32. **The correct answer is E.** This patient has signs and symptoms of a viral infection. Viral pneumonias most frequently present as diffuse, patchy infiltrates.

    Cystic fibrosis (**choice A**) is unlikely, as the manifestations would have been more chronic in nature. The patient may have presented with poor growth, steatorrhea, and recurrent pulmonary infections.

    Hyperreactive airway disease (**choice B**) may certainly coexist in a patient with a viral pneumonia, but it would not, by itself, cause the signs and symptoms in this patient, nor would there be findings of bilateral patchy infiltrates with reactive airway disease.

    Mycoplasma pneumonia (**choice C**) may present as illustrated in this case, but cold agglutinins would be positive.

    Pneumococcal pneumonia (**choice D**) is bacterial and usually presents as a lobar pneumonia. The cough is usually productive, and physical examination findings usually suggest the pneumonia.

33. **The correct answer is E.** The patient has classic symptoms of an acute cholecystitis. An ultrasound usually is the only test needed to confirm the diagnosis.

    Choices A, B, C, and D are incorrect. An abdominal radiograph will occasionally show an enlarged gallbladder shadow or gallstones, but it is not the most appropriate diagnostic test. Increases in the serum bilirubin count and leukocyte count are common but not specific to acute cholecystitis.

34. **The correct answer is C.** Post-traumatic stress disorder (PTSD) develops after a person experiences a traumatic event. Patients suffer from flashbacks, panic attacks, nightmares, and feelings of isolation, guilt, and paranoia. PTSD can be terrifying and even disabling for some people. Other common symptoms of PTSD include recurring, intrusive, and distressing memories of the event. The diagnostic criteria must be present for longer than 1 month to qualify as post-traumatic stress disorder; any time period of less than 1 month is classified as an acute stress disorder.

    A person with adjustment disorder (**choice A**) often experiences feelings of depression, anxiety, or combined depression and anxiety. As a result, that person may act out behaviorally to family, work, or society.

    Generalized anxiety disorder (**choice B**) is characterized by chronic anxiety, exaggerated worry, and tension even when there is little or nothing to provoke it.

    Obsessive-compulsive disorder (OCD) (**choice D**) is characterized by the patient having intrusive and unwanted thoughts and repeatedly performing tasks to get rid of the thoughts.

    Major depressive disorder (**choice E**) is characterized by the presence of five of the following symptoms: sleep disturbances, loss of interest or pleasure in activities, inappropriate guilt, decreased energy, decreased concentration, increased or decreased appetite, psychomotor retardation or agitation, and suicidal ideation. The symptoms must have persisted for at least 2 weeks.

35. **The correct answer is C.** In a meniscal injury, a McMurray test will elicit a palpable (and sometimes audible) clicking sound.

    The Lachman (**choice A**) and anterior drawer (**choice B**) tests are used to confirm anterior cruciate ligament tears. ACL injuries may also present with pain and swelling, but a characteristic "pop" is heard at the time of injury, as opposed to the clicking sound consistently heard in the knee following a meniscal tear. Homan sign (**choice D**) is calf pain on foot dorsiflexion and is used to aid in the diagnosis of deep vein thrombosis. Murphy test (**choice E**) is used to diagnose acute cholecystitis.

36. **The correct answer is D.** The differential for this diagnosis does include acute bacterial prostatitis, which is the correct diagnosis. Although prostatic secretions are necessary to discover the causative organism, vigorously massaging the prostate may cause bacteremia and should be avoided.

Transillumination of the scrotum (**choice A**) is used to differentiate between hydrocele and varicocele. It would be of no assistance in the diagnosis of acute bacterial prostatitis.

The patient has urinary symptoms and pain in the back so it will not be wrong to test for CVA tenderness (**choice B**). Pyelonephritis can be on the differential list.

Because prostatitis should be on the differential diagnosis, the patient must undergo a digital rectal exam (**choice C**) to test for a tender, boggy prostate.

Palpation of the testicles (**choice E**) is important if epididymitis is suspected.

37. **The correct answer is A.** Xerostomia is a condition associated with a dryness of the mouth resulting from diminished or arrested secretion. Dry mouth is a very common side effect in medications that possess anticholinergic properties because there is a generalized drying of the mucous membranes. Of the medications listed, only amitriptyline has anticholinergic properties.

Amitriptyline (**choice A**) is a tricyclic antidepressant primarily used in the treatment of clinical depression. It is also used in the treatment of psychoneurotic anxiety or depressive reactions, as well as mixed symptoms of anxiety and depression.

Enalapril (**choice B**) is an angiotensin-converting enzyme (ACE) inhibitor used in the treatment of hypertension and congestive heart failure. Although it is not associated with the development of xerostomia, it is known to cause angioedema.

Fluoxetine (**choice C**) is a selective serotonin reuptake inhibitor (SSRI) indicated for the treatment of clinical depression. It is commonly associated with generalized anxiety symptoms.

Ibuprofen (**choice D**) is a nonsteroidal anti-inflammatory drug indicated for the treatment of mild to moderate pain and relief of fever. The most common side effect of ibuprofen is gastrointestinal irritation effects.

Medroxyprogesterone (**choice E**) is a progestin used in conjunction with estrogens to help prevent endometrial hyperplasia. Its most common side effects are nausea and vomiting.

38. **The correct answer is D.** This patient has bipolar disorder, manifesting with classic symptoms such as decreased need for sleep, pressured speech, sexual promiscuity, shopping sprees, and delusions of grandeur. The treatment of choice in acute mania is lithium or valproate plus an antipsychotic. Antidepressants, which can induce or worsen mania, need to be stopped imme-

diately and certainly should not be increased (**choice E**). When depression is present, an antidepressant such as paroxetine is appropriate but should not be continued once symptoms resolve.

Gabapentin (**choice A**) is unproven in the treatment of bipolar disorder and should absolutely not be used in place of conventional treatment. This is a serious condition with a high risk for suicide.

Changing the antidepressant to a tricyclic antidepressant such as amitriptyline or desipramine (**choice B**) is not appropriate. This patient is having a manic episode and should not be on antidepressants.

Although paroxetine should be stopped (**choice C**), this patient needs additional medical treatment. She will benefit from a mood stabilizer such as lithium or valproic acid, without which her bipolar disorder is likely to continue unabated.

39. **The correct answer is A.** Chlamydia is the one of the most common STDs in the United States, accounting for approximately half of all reports of STDs. The recommended treatment is either a single oral dose of azithromycin or a 7-day course of oral doxycycline, not a 14-day course of doxycycline (**choice C**). To prevent reinfection of the patient, guidelines state that it is necessary to treat all partners within 60 days of infectious signs and symptoms or positive probe. Patients do not need to be routinely retested for chlamydia following treatment unless the symptoms persist or reinfection is suspected, so **choices B and D** are incorrect.

Metronidazole (**choice E**) is the treatment for bacterial vaginosis and trichomoniasis. Routine follow-up testing after treatment is unnecessary in these conditions unless symptoms persist or reinfection is suspected.

40. **The correct answer is D.** Paget disease of bone is an idiopathic disease that affects both sexes equally. Symptoms include pain, fractures, and bony deformity. The most significant laboratory finding is a markedly elevated alkaline phosphatase. Diagnostic modalities include plain radiography and bone scans. Bisphosphonates are the treatment of choice.

Osteoporosis (**choice A**) is the most common metabolic bone disorder in the United States. Osteoporosis involves mainly trabecular bone, not cortical bone (as in this patient), and lab findings will all be within normal limits.

Osteomalacia (**choice B**) may manifest in overall cortical bone loss, and usually results from a lack of calcium in the diet, a lack of vitamin D, or an inability to metabolize vitamin D to its active form. Osteomalacia is most commonly found in patients with chronic renal failure or in those with a nutritional deficiency of calcium in the diet.

Hyperparathyroidism (**choice C**) would manifest on x-ray as a generalized loss of bone, but more importantly as an elevated serum calcium level as well as a low serum phosphorus level. Vitamin D levels would be normal. Alkaline phosphatase levels may be elevated in this patient secondary to his fracture, but should not be markedly elevated.

Vitamin D intoxication (**choice E**) would have an increased calcium level, an increased phosphorus level, and a normal-to-elevated alkaline phosphatase level.

41. **The correct answer is A.** Dural leaks are a common complication of spinal puncture. Dural leaks lead to decreased cerebrospinal fluid volume, decreasing the brain's supporting cushion. This is exacerbated when the patient sits upright or stands up due to increased tension on the brain's supporting structures. This tension is decreased if the patient lies flat.

Epidural abscess (**choice B**) usually manifests with increasingly severe and localized back pain in the area of the puncture, with possible onset of focal neurologic impairment due to pressure on the spinal cord and/or spinal nerve roots. There usually is no drainage present. The patient is also febrile. Symptoms usually present at least 24 to 48 hours after the spinal procedure.

Epidural hematoma (**choice C**), which will usually manifest with increasingly severe localized back pain in the area of the lumbar puncture, is an unusual complication of lumbar puncture. If present, there may be focal neurologic impairment due to pressure on the spinal cord and/or spinal nerve roots from the accumulation of blood. Drainage usually is not present, and signs/symptoms of infection are absent.

Lumbar puncture wound infection (**choice D**) usually presents at least 24 to 48 hours after the procedure. There usually is pus-like drainage from the area that is often accompanied by increasing peri-incisional erythema, as well as increased warmth. Fever often is also present.

Meningitis (**choice E**) can result from spinal invasive procedures but usually develops at least 24 to 48 hours post-procedure. The patient usually presents with fever and chills; sepsis is possible.

42. **The correct answer is B.** Basal cell carcinoma (BCC) is the most common skin malignancy. BCC typically presents as a translucent telangiectatic papule or nod-

ule occurring on a sun-exposed surface. The nose is a frequent site of involvement.

Squamous cell carcinoma (**choice A**) is the second-most common type of skin cancer. It usually develops on the skin and mucous lining of the body cavities (epithelium) but may occur anywhere. The area is typically red, elevated, and nodular, with crusted and/or bloody margins.

Malignant melanoma (**choice C**) is a lesion that has irregular borders and irregular pigmentation, and may be ulcerative. Epidermoid cysts (**choice D**) appear as firm, round, mobile, flesh-colored to yellow or white subcutaneous nodules of variable size.

Sebaceous adenoma (**choice E**) is a rare but benign tumor of sebaceous cells. It commonly presents as a smooth, round, yellow, firm nodule or polyp on the face or scalp.

43. **The correct answer is C.** This is the classic clinical presentation of erythema infectiosum (fifth disease), caused by parvovirus B19.

Rubeola (**choice A**) is measles. In this case the presentation is with conjunctivitis, high fever, ill appearance, macular red rash, and Koplik spots in the mouth. An immunization history should be checked.

Rubella (**choice B**) is German measles, but the child usually has occipital adenopathy and varying degrees of lymphadenopathy. An immunization history for MMR should always be checked.

Roseola (**choice D**) causes a high fever for 5 days with abrupt cessation of fever and onset of macular rash.

Varicella (**choice E**) presents as multiple vesicles with an erythematous base at different stages of development.

44. **The correct answer is C.** Nitroglycerin is a "nitrate vasodilator" primarily used in the prophylaxis, treatment, and management of angina pectoris. Nitroglycerin relaxes vascular smooth muscle by an unknown mechanism, which results in a dose-related dilation of both venous and arterial blood vessels. It promotes a peripheral pooling of blood and reduces venous return to the heart. Beta-receptor blocking agents, for example, exert their pharmacologic action by decreasing heart rate (**choice A**). Angiotensin-converting enzyme inhibitors decrease the production of angiotensin II (**choice B**) by inhibiting the enzyme responsible for its production. Cardiac glycosides, such as digoxin, increase the inotropic effect of the heart (**choice D**). Diuretics, such as furosemide and hydrochlorothiazide, increase the renal elimination of fluids (**choice E**).

45. **The correct answer is B.** The patient, although he is an adult, has Henoch-Schönlein purpura. Renal biopsy would reveal a focal glomerulonephritis with diffuse mesangial IgA deposits and proliferation of mesangial cells.

Renal ultrasonography (**choice A**) is useful in evaluating the size of kidneys, detecting masses, and evaluating polycystic disease, but an ultrasound cannot detect the presence of IgA deposits in glomerular tissue.

Cystoscopy (**choice C**) is useful in diagnosing bladder carcinoma. Urinalysis (**choice D**) will confirm hematuria but not show the IgA of Henoch-Schönlein purpura as the cause. Intravenous urography (**choice E**) is not useful for detecting IgA in glomerular tissue.

46. **The correct answer is B.** Panic disorder is characterized by the spontaneous and unexpected occurrence of panic attacks. The frequency can range from several attacks a day to only a few attacks a year. Selective serotonin reuptake inhibitors and cognitive therapy are generally used as first-line agents, followed by tricyclics. Benzodiazepines can achieve long-term control but should be reserved for refractory cases.

Benzodiazepines with cognitive therapy (**choice A**) and inpatient intensive cognitive therapy (**choice C**) may be used as second-line treatments. Beta-blockers and dopamine antagonists (**choice D**) are not indicated for panic disorder. Intravenous sodium lactate (**choice E**) has been shown to induce panic attacks.

47. **The correct answer is E.** Weight loss of more than 5% of body weight is considered a very adverse prognostic feature in cancer because it usually indicates the presence of widespread disease. (Uncommonly, a relatively small primary lesion that has not yet metastasized can cause cachexia.) Both tumor necrosis factor (TNF) and interleukin 1-beta have been implicated in the production of cachexia with weight loss, loss of appetite, and alteration in taste. Large tumor burdens may additionally alter protein and energy balance, often with negative nitrogen balance. Therapy, in whatever form (surgery, radiation, chemotherapy), may also contribute to cachexia late in the course secondary to effects on the digestive system.

Clathrin (**choice A**) is a protein that helps to form pinocytotic vesicles. Histamine (**choice B**) is released by mast cells and basophils and contributes to allergic responses. Interferon (**choice C**) is important in the body's response to viral infection. Interleukin 1-beta, not interleukin-2 (**choice D**), is produced by activated monocytes and macrophages and has been implicated in cachexia. Interleukin-2 is released by helper T cells and augments B-cell growth, as well as antibody production.

48. **The correct answer is B.** Amoxicillin is a penicillin antibiotic commonly used in the treatment of upper respiratory and ear infections and as a prophylactic antibiotic for infective endocarditis prior to a dental procedure. Penicillins, such as amoxicillin, are believed to exert their antibacterial effect through the inhibition of bacterial cell wall synthesis. These agents bind to one or more of the penicillin-binding proteins located on the cell walls of susceptible organisms. This action results in the inhibition of the third and final stage of bacterial cell wall synthesis. This effect accounts for the bactericidal effect of both penicillins and cephalosporins.

Sulfonamide antibiotics exert their antibacterial effect through the competitive inhibition of para-amino-benzoic acid (PABA; **choice A**), thereby inhibiting folic acid biosynthesis required for bacterial growth. Quinolone antibiotics inhibit DNA-gyrase (**choice C**), which is an enzyme necessary for bacterial DNA replication and repair.

Aminoglycosides, such as gentamicin, irreversibly bind to the 30S subunit of bacterial ribosomes (**choice D**) and therefore inhibit bacterial protein synthesis. Lincosamides, such as clindamycin, irreversibly bind to the 50S subunit of bacterial ribosomes (**choice E**) and therefore also suppress bacterial protein synthesis.

Note that macrolides, such as erythromycin, reversibly bind to the 50S subunit of bacterial ribosomes and suppress bacterial protein synthesis.

49. **The correct answer is E.** Warfarin is an anticoagulant that exerts its mechanism of action by interfering with the synthesis of the vitamin K–dependent clotting factors (II, VII, IX, X). Its antithrombotic effects are not fully seen until 2 to 5 days (mean of 3 to 4 days) after the first dose. It is indicated for the prophylaxis and treatment of atrial fibrillation with embolism, adjunctive treatment of coronary occlusion, and prophylaxis of systemic embolism (after MI) as well as various other indications.

Cyclooxygenase (**choice A**) is an enzyme that is inhibited by aspirin and the nonsteroidal anti-inflammatory drugs (NSAIDs); its production is not affected by warfarin. Fibrinogen (**choice B**) is a precursor of fibrin, which is an elastic filamentous protein that promotes coagulation; fibrinogen production is not affected by warfarin. The production of platelets (**choice C**) is not decreased in patients taking warfarin therapy. Aspirin and the NSAIDs are able to prolong bleeding time by the acetylation of platelet cyclooxygenase, which decreases the synthesis of thromboxane A$_2$ (**choice D**). Thromboxane A$_2$, a prostaglandin derivative, is a potent vasoconstrictor and inducer of platelet aggregation.

50. **The correct answer is B.** The next step in evaluation of a solitary pulmonary nodule is CT scan of the chest. Such a scan will offer additional information regarding the size and growth pattern of the nodule. Furthermore, in a patient who is classified as high risk for the development of lung cancer (age greater than 35, history of smoking, and nodule size greater than 2 cm), resection of the lesion should be considered.

Although a complete blood count (**choice A**) may be warranted, this patient does not have symptoms of an acute infection.

An erythrocyte sedimentation rate (**choice C**) is a non-specific marker of inflammation and would add little information to this clinical picture.

The PET scan (**choice D**) can serve to provide staging information for lung cancer.

Thoracentesis (**choice E**) would be warranted if the patient had a pleural effusion.

51. **The correct answer is D.** As many as 70 to 80% of patients with left bundle branch block have long-standing hypertension. There may also be yet another underlying cardiac disease.

Global ST elevation (**choice A**) is more commonly seen in pericarditis, although acute myocardial injury/ infarction must always be considered in the setting of ST elevation.

Tall peaked T waves (**choice B**) occur due to hyperkalemia. If the tall T waves are seen throughout the ECG, general hyperkalemia is present. P waves will be small, PR intervals short.

Right axis deviation (**choice C**) is typically seen with COPD, pulmonary emboli, valvular disease, and septal defects.

Transient ST depression (**choice E**) is almost always due to acute myocardial ischemia. The ECG signs of ischemia may come and go fairly quickly, even over a matter of minutes.

52. **The correct answer is C.** Bedside digital dislodgement is recommended as the initial treatment of a fecal impaction. If it is unsuccessful or if the pain cannot be controlled, treatment in the operating room (**choice E**) with local or regional anesthesia may be necessary.

Methylcellulose (**choice A**) is a fiber supplement. Fiber supplementations and stool softeners (**choice B**) are recommended for patients at risk for fecal impaction.

A sigmoidoscopy (**choice D**) should be performed after dislodgement to rule out an obstructing mass, such as a malignancy.

53. **The correct answer is E.** Glucagon is released from the alpha cells of the pancreas in response to hypoglycemia and stimulates glycogenolysis to increase serum glucose.

Augmented calcium deposition in bone (**choice A**) is achieved by calcitonin, which is secreted by the C cells in the thyroid gland. Glucagon plays no role in calcium metabolism.

Glucagon favors the conversion of amino acids to glucose (gluconeogenesis) rather than their storage in the liver (**choice B**).

Insulin (which generally has the opposite effects of glucagon) promotes lipogenesis in the liver and in adipose tissue (**choice C**).

Glucagon stimulates gluconeogenesis (**choice D**).

54. **The correct answer is C.** This patient has hereditary spherocytosis. In these patients, folic acid is given to sustain erythropoiesis. They are instructed to take supplementary folic acid for life to prevent a megaloblastic crisis.

Azathioprine (**choice A**) is an immunosuppressive agent used in autoimmune diseases such as systemic lupus erythematosus and rheumatoid arthritis and for immunosuppression in renal homografts.

Cyanocobalamin (**choice B**) or vitamin B$_{12}$ is used for naturally occurring pernicious anemia and for anemia produced by gastric resection.

Iron sulfate (**choice D**) is used for iron-deficiency anemia.

Methotrexate (**choice E**) inhibits dihydrofolate reductase. It is useful in acute leukemias, choriocarcinomas, non-Hodgkin lymphoma, cutaneous T-cell lymphoma, breast cancer, rheumatoid arthritis, psoriasis, and is also an abortifacient.

55. **The correct answer is A.** Lambert-Eaton syndrome or myasthenic syndrome may be associated with small cell carcinoma, sometimes developing before the tumor is diagnosed. Treatment with plasmapheresis and immunosuppressive agents such as prednisone

and azathioprine may lead to clinical and electro-physiologic improvement. Azathioprine is an agent that has an immuno-inflammatory response. It also is indicated for the treatment of rheumatoid arthritis (restricted to patients with severe, active, erosive disease not responsive to conventional therapy) and renal homotransplantation.

Baclofen (**choice B**) is a skeletal muscle-relaxing agent that acts by stimulating GABA-B receptors.

Carbamazepine (**choice C**) is an antiepileptic agent used for the treatment of grand mal and psychomotor seizures and for the treatment of trigeminal neuralgia.

Pyridostigmine (**choice D**) is an inhibitor of AChE; hence, it increases the action of ACh.

Verapamil (**choice E**) is a calcium channel block-ing agent indicated for the treatment of hyperten-sion, supraventricular tachycardia, Prinzmetal angina, chronic stable angina, supraventricular tachycardia, and atrial fibrillation.

56. **The correct answer is B.** Priapism is a common side effect of trazodone.

57. **The correct answer is A.** Cimetidine is an H$_2$ receptor antagonist used in the treatment of gastric reflux and peptic ulcers. A side effect of this medication can be galactorrhea in females and gynecomastia in males.

58. **The correct answer is C.** Extrapyramidal symptoms are disorders of movement, such as pseudoparkinsonism, acute dystonia, or akathisia. Metoclopramide has been found to cause EPS. It is an antiemetic and prokinetic agent.

59. **The correct answer is E.** Herpes encephalitis is the lead-ing cause of sporadic necrotizing encephalitis. It can occur during the primary infection or during recurrent infection. Without therapy, the mortality rate is 70%. Herpes encephalitis is treated with the antiviral acyclo-vir. Acyclovir is an acyclic analogue of the natural nucle-oside guanosine. Acyclovir is efficiently phosphorylated at a rapid rate by virus-specific thymidine kinase (TdK), but is slowly phosphorylated by the host TdK. The affinity of acyclovir for thymidine kinase produced by

normal host cells is approximately 250 times less than for the thymidine kinase induced by herpes simplex virus. This selective affinity results in the activation and concentration of acyclovir in virus-infected cells. Once acyclovir is converted into acyclovir monophosphate by the viral thymidine kinase, it is further converted to acyclovir triphosphate by other cellular enzymes. Acyclovir triphosphate competes with deoxyguanosine triphosphate for binding to the HSV DNA polymerase. When it is incorporated into the viral DNA, it prevents further elongation of the chain.

Adenosine kinase (**choice A**) is an abundant enzyme in mammalian tissues that catalyzes the transfer of the gamma-phosphate from ATP to adenosine. It is not a target of antiviral drugs.

DNA polymerase (**choice B**) can use acyclovir triphos-phate as a substrate.

Protease (**choice C**) of HIV cleaves viral polyprotein precursors needed to generate functional proteins and for the maturation of HIV-infected cells. Protease inhibitors such as saquinavir, indinavir, and amprenavir inhibit its function.

Reverse transcriptase (**choice D**) is an enzyme made by retroviruses that converts RNA to DNA. Zidovudine (AZT) interferes with retroviral reverse transcriptase and inhibits viral replication.

60. **The correct answer is A.** The lateral plantar nerve pro-vides sensory innervation to the lateral plantar aspect of the foot, including half of the fourth and the fifth digits of the foot.

The medial plantar nerve (**choice B**) provides sensory innervation to the medial plantar aspect of the foot, including the first three digits and half of the fourth digit.

The saphenous nerve (**choice C**) provides sensory innervation along the medial aspect of the leg.

The sural nerve (**choice D**) provides sensory innervation to the posterior leg and a small part of the lateral foot.

The tibial nerve (**choice E**) provides sensory innerva-tion to the entire plantar foot because the medial and lateral plantar nerves are branches of the tibial nerve.

Block 3

1. **The correct choice is B.** The appropriate management of a pregnant patient with IDDM is to continue insulin therapy. The management of hypertension in pregnancy should include methyldopa or hydralazine.

   Oral hypoglycemics (**choice A**) should not be used in pregnancy. ACEIs (**choice C**) are contraindicated in pregnancy. Diuretics (**choice D**) should not be used to treat hypertension in pregnancy, and dietary modification (**choice E**), although helpful, is not an adequate substitute for insulin therapy.

2. **The correct answer is B.** Acute diverticulitis presents with pain and tenderness in the left lower quadrant. White blood cell count will be elevated, with increased neutrophils and bands. Ischemic colitis (**choice A**) presents with abdominal pain, lower GI bleeding, diarrhea, fever, and abdominal tenderness on examination. Acute pyelonephritis (**choice C**) presents with CVA tenderness, elevated white blood cell count with left shift, and numerous white blood cells and bacteria in the urine. Irritable bowel syndrome (**choice D**) presents with chronic abdominal pain, bloating, and alteration in bowel habits, diarrhea, and constipation. Appendicitis (**choice E**) presents with pain in the right lower quadrant.

3. **The correct answer is D.** Symptoms of pyloric stenosis typically begin between the second and fourth week of life. Projectile vomiting and palpation of an olive-shaped mass to the right of the midline are classic characteristics of pyloric stenosis.

   Intussusception (**choice B**) typically occurs between 6 and 18 months of age. Classic characteristics include intermittent abdominal pain (which causes the infant to cry and vomit) and palpation of a sausage-shaped mass in the upper abdomen.

   Patients diagnosed with Meckel diverticulum (**choice C**) can present with painless rectal bleeding, painful diverticulitis, and intussusception.

   There is no sign of infection; therefore, **choice A** is incorrect.

   A ventral hernia (**choice E**) does not present with an olive-shaped mass. It presents, rather, with a bulging abdominal mass.

4. **The correct answer is B.** Bulimia nervosa is an eating disorder characterized by eating binges typically fol-lowed by efforts to purge calories through self-induced vomiting, laxative and/or diuretic abuse, prolonged fasting, or excessive exercise. Physical examination may reveal signs of dehydration, including enlarged parotid glands or tonsils, and dental caries and erosion of tooth enamel (perimolysis). Calluses on the hand from repeated self-induced vomiting, along with alopecia, xerosis, and nail fragility, may also be present.

   Oral thrush (**choice A**), hemorrhoids (**choice C**), a decreased mini-mental status exam score (**choice D**), and retinal hemorrhages (**choice E**) are not supportive findings of bulimia nervosa.

5. **The correct answer is B.** Carpal tunnel syndrome is an entrapment syndrome of the median nerve. Symptoms include burning, numbness, and tingling along the innervation of the median nerve (the thumb, index finger, and middle finger).

   Ulnar nerve entrapment (**choice A**) results in a different distribution of symptoms; symptoms would appear in the middle, fourth, and fifth fingers. Entrapment of the radial (**choice C**), sciatic (**choice D**), and peroneal (**choice E**) nerves would cause symptoms along their respective distributions, which do not fit this clinical picture.

6. **The correct answer is A.** Angiotensin-converting enzyme inhibitors (ACEIs) correct both proteinuria and hypertension in patients with Berger disease. Angiotensin receptor blockers can also be used.

   Beta-blockers (**choice B**) may be used to help with extrarenal handling of potassium in end-stage renal disease, but are not indicated for use in Berger's disease. Calcium channel blockers (**choice C**) are not indicated for use in Berger disease. HMG-CoA reductase inhibitors (**choice D**) are indicated for the treatment of hypercholesterolemia. Thiazide diuretics (**choice E**) may cause allergic interstitial nephritis, but are not indicated for use in Berger disease.

7. **The correct answer is D.** Injections are given in the upper, outer quadrant of the buttocks to prevent damage to the sciatic nerve, which is present in the lower quadrant. The other nerves listed are not particularly vulnerable to injections into the buttocks.

   The common peroneal nerve (**choice A**) is a branch of the sciatic nerve that diverges from it in the popliteal fossa. It then divides into the superficial and deep peroneal nerves.

The lateral femoral cutaneous nerve (**choice B**) derives from the lumbar plexus, emerges slightly below the anterior superior iliac spine, and supplies the skin of the anterior thigh down to the knee.

The obturator nerve (**choice C**) derives from the lumbar plexus, diverges from the femoral nerve in the psoas muscle, and passes medially along the lateral pelvic wall to run in the obturator canal, where it divides into anterior and posterior divisions. The anterior division generally supplies the gracilis, adductor brevis, and adductor longus; the posterior division generally supplies the obturator externus and the adductor part of the adductor magnus.

The superior gluteal nerve (**choice E**) is a branch of the sacral plexus. It supplies the gluteus minimus and medius and the tensor fascia lata. Only small branches of this nerve are likely to be encountered in the upper outer quadrant of the buttock, making injection here relatively safe.

8. **The correct answer is B.** This patient has a keloid, which is a benign, hypertrophic scar caused by an excessive deposition of extracellular matrix following trauma. The earlobe is one of the most common sites for a keloid, especially after piercing.

    Blockage of a hair follicle with sebum and keratin (**choice A**) is the initial mechanism for the formation of acne vulgaris. Bacteria, yeast, and inflammation add to the typical lesions called comedones. This patient has acne, but it most likely did not cause the formation of the keloid.

    Nickel exposure from the earrings (**choice C**) may lead to allergic contact dermatitis, which is a type IV delayed hypersensitivity reaction mediated by T cells. The typical lesions are erythematous, vesicular, and pruritic. The treatment involves removing the offending substance and providing antihistamines and possibly corticosteroids.

    Pregnancy (**choice D**) may cause a rash called melasma, which is characterized by tan-to-brown patches on the forehead, cheeks, temples, and upper lip. This does not fit the description of this patient's lesion.

    Sun exposure (**choice E**) is a risk factor for actinic keratosis, basal cell carcinoma, squamous cell carcinoma, and melanoma. These lesions do not typically present in the fashion described by this patient. Also, the histopathology does not correlate with any of these lesions. Nodular melanoma may have a similar presentation; however, the pathology would show a lesion of melanocytes.

9. **The correct answer is D.** The mechanism of action of acarbose, an alpha-glycosidase inhibitor, is that it reduces glucose absorption by decreasing production of the enzyme needed to digest carbohydrates. Increasing sensitivity to insulin (**choice A**) and decreasing hepatic glucose production (**choice E**) are the mechanisms of action of metformin. Increasing insulin receptor activity (**choice B**) is the mechanism of action of thiazolidinediones. Increasing insulin secretion (**choice C**) is the mechanism of action of the sulfonylureas.

10. **The correct answer is D.** Café-au-lait lesions are cutaneous lesions characteristic of neurofibromatosis.

    Ependymomas (**choice A**) are not associated with cutaneous lesions.

    Metastatic tumors (**choice B**) are not associated specifically with café-au-lait lesions, though the patient may have cutaneous manifestations of cancer depending on the cancer's pathology.

    Multiple myeloma (**choice C**) is not associated with cutaneous lesions.

    Staphylococcus aureus infections (**choice E**) are not associated with café-au-lait lesions.

11. **The correct answer is D.** Eczema, or atopic dermatitis, appears to have a hereditary component, and the family history will be positive for atopy (i.e., asthma, allergic rhinitis, atopic dermatitis) in two-thirds of patients.

    Varicella (**choice A**) and mononucleosis (**choice B**) are viral conditions with no association with atopy or eczema. Similarly, neither skin cancer (**choice C**) nor Reye syndrome (**choice E**) is associated with autoimmune phenomena.

12. **The correct answer is A.** Cholera is usually found in endemic areas such as Peru, and history of travel to these countries makes cholera a top differential. Also, this patient has the classic "rice water stools" of cholera—gray and turbid with no fecal odor and no blood or pus. Cholera is also painless, and this patient denies pain. There is also no vomiting or nausea. Because of the high loss of fluid volume in a short period of time, the patient may become dehydrated and go into shock. This patient is already becoming dehydrated, as demonstrated by the tachycardia and poor skin turgor.

    Shigellosis (**choice B**) is characterized by diarrhea with blood and mucus, abdominal cramps, distension, and fever.

Campylobacter dysentery (**choice C**) is also watery diarrhea but is usually grossly bloody. There are also the associated symptoms of abdominal cramping, pain, malaise, and fever.

Giardiasis (**choice D**) is an explosive diarrhea that has associated abdominal cramping, distension, low-grade fever, nausea, and vomiting.

Salmonellosis (**choice E**) usually has associated abdominal cramps, fever, chills, nausea, vomiting, headache, and myalgias. Diarrhea may have pus or blood.

13. **The correct choice is B.** Thiazides are considered first-line monotherapy for African American patients with stage 1 through 3 hypertension. (JNC VII).

    Beta-blockers (**choice C**) and ACE inhibitors (**choice A**) have not been found to be effective in African American patients. Clonidine (**choice D**) is a centrally acting agent and may be used in this patient; however, thiazides and calcium channel blockers are preferred. Prazosin (**choice E**) is an appropriate agent for the concurrent treatment of hypertension and BPH.

14. **The correct answer is D.** Nitrates should be avoided in patients who have taken phosphodiesterase inhibitors (sildenafil, vardenafil, or tadalafil) in the past 24 hours, secondary to the increased risk of myocardial ischemia due to hypotension.

    All patients with a suspected myocardial infarction should receive aspirin (**choice A**). Furthermore, there is no contraindication to the concurrent use of aspirin and sildenafil.

    Metoprolol (**choice B**) is a beta-blocker that can reduce the incidence of ventricular fibrillation. Beta-blockers may be used for the treatment of hypertension, angina pectoris, myocardial infarction, supraventricular tachycardia, and congestive heart failure. Metoprolol is safe to use with sildenafil.

    Morphine (**choice C**) is the drug of choice for relieving pain associated with a myocardial infarction.

    Oxygen at 2 to 5 L/min (**choice E**) is administered, even if blood oxygen levels are normal. This makes oxygen readily available to the tissues of the body and reduces the workload of the heart. It has no effect on sildenafil.

15. **The correct answer is A.** Although the pH is normal, the respiratory rate of 52/min is a very bad prognostic indicator. The patient should have respiratory alkalosis from elimination of CO_2 if he is ventilating properly.

The pCO_2 in a patient with a respiratory rate of 52/min should be *decreased*. This arterial blood gas result indicates that the patient is no longer ventilating and may need mechanical ventilation or other intervention.

16. **The correct answer is C.** The patient has active pilonidal disease. The abscess must be incised and drained.

    Antibiotics alone (**choice A**) are not an effective treatment for pilonidal disease.

    The definitive treatment for pilonidal disease is excision (**choice B**) of the sinus tract. After an incision and drainage is performed, patients who continue to have a draining sinus or fail to heal completely are considered for excision.

    For patients with a recurring pilonidal abscess, shaving of the natal cleft (**choice D**) has been recommended as preventative therapy.

    Warm sitz baths (**choice E**) are not an appropriate treatment for pilonidal disease.

17. **The correct answer is B.** Even uncomplicated grief (**choice A**) usually disrupts a person's ability to carry on daily activities, but a crippling loss in ability to function over an extended period of time is indicative of complicated bereavement and requires therapy.

    Post-traumatic stress disorder (PTSD) (**choice C**) develops after a person experiences a traumatic event. Patients suffer from flashbacks, panic attacks, nightmares, and feelings of isolation, guilt, and paranoia.

    A person with adjustment disorder (**choice D**) often experiences feelings of depression, anxiety, or combined depression and anxiety. As a result, that person may act out to family, work, or society.

    Bipolar disorder (**choice E**) is a condition of extreme highs often followed by debilitating lows. It is also often termed as manic depression.

18. **The correct answer is D.** Sjögren syndrome is a chronic inflammatory disorder of exocrine gland dysfunction. It results in dry eyes, decreased lacrimal and salivary gland production, and rheumatology disorders in its secondary form.

    Schilling test (**choice A**) is used in the diagnosis of pernicious anemia. SPEP (**choice B**) aids in the diagnosis of multiple myeloma. ANA (**choice E**) may be positive in Sjögren but is not used specifically in its diagnosis.

19. **The correct answer is C.** In benign prostatic hyperplasia, the prostate gets larger and there are no malignant or infectious processes occurring. The classic feel of a hyperplastic benign prostate is that it is uniformly enlarged, firm, and nontender without nodules.

A tender and boggy prostate (**choice A**) is common in acute bacterial prostatitis. A prostate with focal nodules and induration (**choice B**) is usually found in prostate cancer. An increase in the tone of the anal sphincter (**choice D**) and periprostatic tenderness (**choice E**) are both found in prostatodynia.

20. **The correct answer is E.** Lesions of the vagus nerve involve nasal speech, nasal regurgitation, dysphagia, palate droop, uvula pointing away from the affected side, hoarseness caused by fixed vocal cords, loss of gag reflex, and loss of cough reflex.

Lesions of the facial nerve (**choice A**) can involve drooping of the corner of the mouth, inability to shut the eye or wrinkle the forehead, loss of blink reflex, hyperacusis, alteration or loss of taste from the tongue, and a dry eye.

Lesions of the glossopharyngeal nerve (**choice B**) involve loss of the gag reflex but do not cause deviation of the uvula.

Lesions of the hypoglossal nerve (**choice C**) result in a deviation of the tongue to the affected side on protrusion.

Lesions of the trigeminal nerve (**choice D**) may involve loss of general sensation in different areas of the face, and if trigeminal motor fibers are involved, a deviation of the mandible toward the affected side.

21. **The correct answer is A.** Cytomegalovirus (CMV) is the most common congenital infection. Pregnant women who have previously been infected with CMV can give birth to children with congenital CMV, but these children generally have no sequelae. However, about 1 to 3% of pregnant women have a primary CMV infection during pregnancy. These women can give birth to infected children who go on to have severe consequences. A small percentage of newborns born to mothers infected with the virus during pregnancy develop the classic cytomegalic inclusion disease with jaundice, petechial rash, pneumonia, and central nervous system disorders. Overall, 30% of those with symptomatic infection die within 2 days to 2 years. Of the survivors, most have mental retardation, microcephaly, hearing and vision loss, and other issues. Infected infants may also be asymptomatic at birth, but subsequently develop varying degrees of hearing loss, chorioretinitis, and mental retardation.

22. **The correct answer is E.** The hypoglossal nerve innervates the tongue and is involved with speech. An abnormality of this cranial nerve can cause the tongue examination to be abnormal, i.e., tongue fibrillations and/or atrophy of the tongue.

During physical examination, cranial nerve II abnormalities (**choice A**) are manifested by visual field deficits and/or abnormal pupillary reaction to light and accommodation.

During physical examination, cranial nerve V abnormalities (**choice B**) are manifested by loss of corneal reflex, atrophy/weakness of the temporalis muscle, and/or abnormal jaw jerk.

During physical examination, cranial nerve VII abnormalities (**choice C**) are manifested by asymmetric elevation of one corner of the mouth and/or flattened nasolabial folds.

Cranial nerves IX and X (**choice D**) are generally considered together. Abnormalities of these nerves are manifested by an absent gag reflex during physical examination.

23. **The correct answer is C.** Striae is a possible side effect of long-term topical steroid use. Hypopigmentation, increased skin infections, skin atrophy, and tachyphylaxis are also side effects of topical steroid use (compare with other choices).

24. **The correct answer is D.** Xanthomas are lesions characterized by accumulations of lipid-laden macrophages. Xanthomas may be due to abnormal lipid metabolism and may be the first sign of a familial dyslipidemia. Diagnosing and treating underlying lipid disorders is necessary to decrease the size of the xanthomas and to prevent the risks of atherosclerosis. Treatment of the hyperlipidemia initially consists of diet followed by lipid-lowering agents, such as statins, fibrates, bile acid–binding resins, or nicotinic acid. In this case, the most appropriate tests in diagnosing an aberration of lipid metabolism would be the HDL, VLDL, and LDL.

The other laboratory studies listed are not relevant to the workup of xanthomas.

25. **The correct answer is E.** Vitamin B_{12} must be combined with intrinsic factor (produced in the parietal cells of the stomach). Once bound, the vitamin B_{12}-intrinsic factor complex is absorbed in the terminal ileum. Gastrectomy and bariatric surgery would reduce the amount of intrinsic factor available to bind vitamin B_{12}. Crohn disease of the terminal ileum would reduce the absorptive ability of the vitamin B_{12}-intrinsic factor complex. Patients should be monitored for vitamin B_{12} deficiency.

Aplastic anemia (**choice A**) is a bone marrow failure syndrome characterized by peripheral pancytopenia and marrow hypoplasia. It is not related to gastrointestinal surgery or vitamin deficiencies.

Folic acid deficiency (**choice B**) is typically a nutritional deficiency commonly found in alcoholic patients.

Glucose-6-phosphate dehydrogenase deficiency (**choice C**) is an acquired enzyme deficiency.

Choice D is incorrect. Iron is absorbed in the duodenum.

26. **The correct answer is A.** The patient is exhibiting classic symptoms of herpesvirus. It usually starts with a prodrome of malaise and low-grade fever, along with paresthesias and burning in the area of infection. There may also be inguinal adenopathy.

A firm, punched-out lesion with rolled borders (**choice B**) is the classic chancre of primary syphilis. Soft, fleshy growths on the vulva that may form "kissing lesions" (**choice C**) are characteristic of venereal warts. Irregularly shaped lesions with red, undermined margins on a yellow or gray base (**choice D**) is characteristic of *Haemophilus ducreyi* (chancroid). Elevated lesions with rolled, elevated margins on a red, rough base (**choice E**) are characteristic of *Calymmatobacterium granulomatis* (granuloma inguinale).

27. **The correct answer is A.** This constellation of symptoms is consistent with atrial fibrillation secondary to mitral stenosis. Patients frequently demonstrate signs of heart failure and pulmonary hypertension. Fifty to 80% of patients with mitral stenosis develop paroxysmal or chronic atrial fibrillation. Patients with significant mitral obstruction who experience atrial fibrillation may abruptly develop marked worsening of congestive heart failure. The enlarged left atrium often beats in an irregular pattern; as a result, cardiovascular efficiency is reduced.

Patients may progress to ventricular tachycardia (**choice B**) if the ventricular rhythm is not controlled, but it is not a common anomaly.

First-degree heart block (**choice C**) is uncommon with mitral stenosis alone. ECG findings in patients with moderate-to-severe mitral stenosis may demonstrate left atrial enlargement, right ventricular hypertrophy, and right atrial enlargement.

Atrial flutter (**choice D**) may be seen in later stages of the disease process. Patients at highest risk for atrial flutter include those with long-standing hypertension, left ventricular hypertrophy, coronary artery disease, or diabetes.

Left ventricular hypertrophy (**choice E**) is more typically seen with mitral regurgitation.

28. **The correct answer is A.** Hepatitis A is usually spread by the fecal-oral route. Spread occurs more commonly in areas of poor sanitation and crowding. Recent travel to an area with high rates of hepatitis A is consistent with the diagnosis. Hepatitis A has an incubation period of 2 to 4 weeks with an acute onset of symptoms.

The route of transmission of hepatitis B (**choice B**) is primarily parenteral or sexual. A history of intravenous drug use or unprotected sexual activity is consistent with hepatitis B. Hepatitis B has an incubation period of 2 to 6 months.

Hepatitis C (**choice C**) is most frequently transmitted via intravenous drug use. Often, patients with hepatitis C are asymptomatic. Hepatitis C has an incubation period of 2 to 22 weeks.

Hepatitis D (**choice D**) is associated with hepatitis B. Hepatitis D is transmitted as a coinfection with hepatitis B in individuals who already have hepatitis B. Hepatitis D has an incubation period of 7 to 26 weeks.

Hepatitis G (**choice E**) is a flavivirus and is transmitted parenterally. It is not associated with any chronic liver disease.

29. **The correct answer is B.** Attention deficit hyperactivity disorder presents with symptoms of hyperactivity and inattention that have lasted for at least 6 months. Onset is usually prior to age 7 and is more common in boys.

Asperger disorder (**choice A**) is found more predominantly in males and is characterized by impaired social interaction and stereotyped behaviors. However, unlike people with autistic disorder, these individuals have normal cognitive function.

It is important to differentiate oppositional defiant disorder (ODD; **choice C**) from ADHD and conduct disorder. ODD is diagnosed after 6 months of negative, hostile, defiant behavior. This behavior is most often directed against authority figures. ODD often results in conduct disorder. In contrast, ADHD is characterized by inattention and hyperactivity.

Autistic disorder (**choice D**) is characterized by problems with social interaction, communication impairment, and stereotyped behaviors. Of patients with autistic disorder, 75% are mentally retarded.

Rett disorder (**choice E**) is seen only in females and is characterized by developmental delay and stereotyped hand movements.

30. **The correct answer is C.** A history of sickle cell disease will cause the patient to be treated differently than he would with any other etiology. The patient with sickle cell usually requires hydration and may need a blood transfusion. In patients with sickle cell disease, priapism usually occurs in males between the ages of 6 and 20.

Obtaining a sexual history (**choice A**) would be helpful because priapism usually occurs in the absence of sexual stimulation. However, if this sustained erection did occur after sexual stimulation, detumescence will still be the goal of treatment. Obtaining a sexual history is also useful in determining a history of sexually transmitted diseases, but these have not been found to be an etiology of priapism.

A history of cryptorchidism (**choice B**) has not been found to be an etiology of priapism inasmuch as it affects the testes, not the penis.

A history of drug (**choice D**) or alcohol (**choice E**) abuse is an etiology of priapism; however, in these cases, the patient would not be treated differently from any other cause outside of sickle cell disease.

31. **The correct answer is A.** This patient presents with gestational hypertension (elevated blood pressure without edema or laboratory abnormalities). Treatment of gestational hypertension consists of labetalol, methyldopa, or hydralazine. Aliskiren (**choice B**) and valsartan (**choice D**) are contraindicated in pregnancy. The use of diltiazem (**choice C**) and nitroprusside (**choice E**) is advised against in pregnancy.

32. **The correct answer is B.** This patient most likely has giant cell arteritis (commonly called temporal arteritis, although many of the larger vessels of the head may be affected). Presentation includes jaw claudication, loss of vision, and elevated sedimentation rate. Diagnosis is made by biopsy of the artery.

Migraine headache (**choice A**) presents with supraorbital pain with associated phonophobia, photophobia, nausea, vomiting, and possible aura. Trigeminal

neuralgia (**choice C**) presents with intense facial pain ("like an electric shock") that lasts minutes to hours. Pain can be aggravated by wind, high-pitched sounds, loud noises, and chewing. Ophthalmic zoster (**choice D**) presents with facial pain in the location of the vesicular face related to varicella zoster infection. Bell's palsy (**choice E**) presents with weakness of the facial muscles that are controlled by the facial nerve.

33. **The correct choice is B.** In the elderly, or in any patients with cardiovascular compromise, thyroid replacement must be done at low doses and titrated up to a therapeutic TSH level. This is the best method of slowly achieving therapeutic levels of Synthroid. In this manner it is possible (and necessary in this case) to give Synthroid to the elderly and to people with heart problems (**choice E is incorrect**)

Full replacement doses of Synthroid (**choices A and C**) may precipitate congestive heart failure in this patient.

Although it is correct to start with the lowest dose (**choice D**), this regimen may take many months to achieve therapeutic Synthroid levels.

34. **The correct answer is A.** Auras are associated with migraine headaches and epilepsy. They usually manifest just prior to the seizure or the headache as flashing lights and/or scintillating scotoma.

In Huntington chorea (**choice B**), there mainly is an increase in involuntary movements (i.e., tremors and/or repetitive and irregular movements). These are not findings or diagnostic indicators for epilepsy and are not manifested by auras.

Parkinson disease (**choice C**) presents with a loss or slowness of voluntary movement and an increase in involuntary movements, but does not manifest with seizures. It is not associated with auras.

Tardive dyskinesia (**choice D**) presents with involuntary movements of the face, mouth, and tongue and is not a symptom of epilepsy. It is not associated with auras.

Transient ischemic attacks (**choice E**) usually involve localized neurologic symptoms, such as *Amaurosis fugax*, numbness/weakness of an extremity, or hemiparesis. Auras are not associated with transient ischemic attacks.

35. **The correct answer is C.** This patient has most likely already tried topical benzoyl peroxide (**choice E**); therefore, clindamycin would be the treatment of choice. Oral contraceptives (**choice A**) are not an appropriate choice due to the age of the patient. The addition of an oral contraceptive may disrupt the menstrual cycle in

a pubertal female. Topical hydrocortisone (**choice B**) is not an appropriate treatment for acne. Isotretinoin (**choice D**) may be employed later if the clindamycin does not result in improvement.

36. **The correct answer is D.** This patient has genital warts, which are caused by human papilloma virus. Genital warts are characterized by the presence of warty growths on the vulva, vaginal walls, cervix, or perianal area. They are described as white, prominent papillae. There is no associated discharge or pain. Human papillomavirus predisposes to cervical and vulva cancers. Human papillomavirus is a DNA virus that belongs to the class Papovaviridae.

    Herpesviridae (**choice A**) is a DNA virus that causes herpes. Poxviridae (**choice B**) is a DNA virus that causes smallpox and molluscum contagiosum. Adenoviridae (**choice C**) is a DNA virus that causes upper respiratory tract infections. Parvoviridae (**choice E**) is a DNA virus whose B19 strain causes erythema infectiosum.

37. **The correct answer is A.** The first DTaP vaccine is administered at age 2 months. The second DTaP is administered at 4 months (**choice B**). The third DTaP is administered at 6 months (**choice C**).

38. **The correct answer is A.** A good way to remember what goes through the superior orbital fissure is that everything that innervates the eye, other than the optic nerve, passes through this fissure. This includes the oculomotor nerve (CN III), the trochlear nerve (CN IV), the ophthalmic nerve (V1), and the abducens nerve (CN VI). The facial nerve (CN VII; **choice B**) passes through the internal auditory meatus. The mandibular nerve (V3; **choice C**) passes through the foramen ovale. The maxillary nerve (V2; **choice D**) passes through the foramen rotundum. The middle meningeal artery (**choice E**) passes through the foramen spinosum.

39. **The correct answer is E.** Attention deficit disorder presents with a 6 month history of inattention to detail, trouble keeping attention, inattention when spoken to, frequent failure to follow directions, trouble organizing activities, avoiding work that takes sustained mental effort, and easy distractibility.

    Depression (**choice A**) in children presents with depressed mood, or at times, irritable mood; loss of interest in activities and decline in academic performance may be noted. Conduct disorder (**choice B**) presents with a prolonged pattern of antisocial behavior, with violations of laws and social norms. Absence seizures (**choice C**) present with abrupt onset of impaired consciousness, interruption of ongoing activities, and a blank stare. Episodes last seconds to minutes and there is no post-ictal period. Intellectual disability (**choice D**) presents with delay in achieving intellectual milestones and developing self-help skills, and lack of social inhibitions.

40. **The correct answer is D.** This patient has symptoms of pulmonary embolism (PE) with probable signs of deep venous thrombosis. Spiral chest CT scan is the usual initial diagnostic test for PE. Normal results virtually exclude the diagnosis.

    Magnetic resonance imaging (**choice A**) has sensitivity and specificity equivalent to contrast venography for the diagnosis of deep venous thrombosis. However, it remains expensive and is not widely available. Further, artifacts introduced by breathing and cardiac motion limit the use of MRI in the diagnosis of PE.

    Pulmonary arteriography (**choice B**) is the gold standard for the diagnosis of PE. The test is appropriate in patients with nondiagnostic $\dot{V}/\dot{Q}$ scans. It is an invasive procedure.

    D-dimer (**choice C**) is not indicated in cases that have a high probability of PE. An echocardiogram (**choice E**) would be helpful to determine pulmonary hypertension or right ventricular dysfunction, but it is not an initial test of choice.

41. **The correct answer is A.** Inhaled albuterol nebulizer is indicated in this patient. Therapy may be repeated three times at 15-minute intervals. Peak flows, pulse oximetry, lung examination, and questioning for symptomatic improvement are done after each nebulizer treatment.

    Prednisone therapy (**choice B**) may be used as an adjunct therapy.

    Theophylline (**choice C**) is rarely used in acute or chronic asthma management anymore because of its narrow therapeutic window and significant toxicity.

    Oxygen therapy (**choice D**) is not indicated in this patient because her pulse oximetry reading is in the 90th percentile.

    Subcutaneous epinephrine (**choice E**) may be used in acute anaphylaxis, but it is typically not used in an acute exacerbation of asthma.

42. **The correct answer is D.** The treatment for phenylketonuria is to restrict the dietary intake of phenylalanine. Foods high in protein, such as fish, meat, eggs, milk, and soy products, should be avoided as they contain high levels of phenylalanine.

Fruits (**choice B**), cereals (**choice A**), vegetables (**choice E**), and grains (**choice C**) typically have lower levels of phenylalanine.

43. **The correct answer is D.** Although all of the answer choices may present with dementia, this clinical picture fits Alzheimer disease (AD). AD begins gradually and affects multiple cognitive functions: memory, orientation, language, visuospatial processing, judgment, and insight.

    Parkinson disease (**choice A**), vitamin B_{12} deficiency (**choice B**), multiple sclerosis (**choice C**), and alcoholism (**choice E**) would also manifest in other clinical findings on exam or in the labs.

44. **The correct answer is A.** Many autoantibodies are found in patients with SLE. Ninety-nine percent will be positive for ANA when a sensitive assay is used.

    Rheumatoid factor (**choice B**), C-reactive protein (**choice C**), and erythrocyte sedimentation rate (**choice E**) all may be elevated or present in SLE, but do not have high sensitivities for the disease. RPR/VRDL (**choice D**) is used to diagnose syphilis.

45. **The correct answer is B.** Attention and concentration can be tested by spelling "world" backward or performing "serial sevens" subtraction.

    Indicating the year, season, month, day, and date (**choice A**) is a test for orientation. Copying intersecting pentagons (**choice C**) assesses visuospatial processing. Repeating the phrase "No ifs, ands, or buts" (**choice D**) tests language repetition. Interpreting a proverb such as "Don't cry over spilled milk" (**choice E**) examines the patient's abstract thought processes.

46. **The correct answer is B.** Antiphospholipid antibody syndrome is a disorder of the immune system characterized by excessive blood clotting and pregnancy complications (miscarriages, unexplained fetal death, or premature birth). Diagnosis is made by combining laboratory findings of antiphospholipid antibodies and clinical presentation.

    Evaluation for in vitro fertilization (**choice A**), progesterone challenge (**choice C**), and laboratory testing of FSH/LH (**choice D**) are incorrect answer choices because the patient should be worked up for an underlying cause of the abortions before an infertility workup is begun.

    Duplex ultrasound (**choice E**) is performed to rule out DVT, which is not of immediate concern in this case.

47. **The correct answer is D.** Bulging anterior fontanel in infants represents an increase in intracranial pressure. This may be secondary to trauma, meningitis, hydrocephalus, tumor, or cerebral hemorrhage.

48. **The correct answer is A.** Orchiopexy, a surgical procedure used to move undescended testes, is the treatment of choice in patients at or older than the age of 2.

    Orchiectomy (**choice B**), the removal of the testicles, is usually performed to remove the primary source of testosterone in the body, as in cases of prostate cancer. Prostate cancer is usually dependent on testosterone to continue growing.

    Testes usually descend spontaneously by the first year of life (**choice C**). If not, then surgery should be performed.

    Human chorionic gonadotropin injections (**choice D**) may stimulate descent but are not the treatment of choice in 2 year olds. Ultrasound (**choice E**) does help in locating the missing testes; however, it is not therapeutic.

49. **The correct answer is B.** Tapeworm infections are best treated with praziquantel. Niclosamide (**choice C**) can be used but is not first-line. Mebendazole (**choice A**) is used to treat roundworms, hookworms, and pinworms. Pyrantel pamoate (**choice D**) is used in the treatment of hookworms and roundworms. Metronidazole (**choice E**) is used in the treatment of *Giardia*, *Entamoeba*, and *Trichomonas*.

50. **The correct answer is A.** Most patients with hyperlipidemia are asymptomatic and the clinician should exclude other risk factors for coronary artery disease. The family history and poor dietary habits warrant a fasting lipid profile.

    Nonfasting total cholesterol level (**choice B**) would be inappropriate. Lipid values would be falsely elevated.

    An oral glucose tolerance test (**choice C**) is indicated for the symptomatic patient with a fasting plasma glucose level less than 140 mg/dL. Finally, all pregnant patients should undergo testing for gestational diabetes with a 50-gram glucose screen at 24 to 28 weeks of pregnancy. A subsequent glucose tolerance test should be performed if the result of that test is abnormal.

    Sigmoidoscopy (**choice D**) is most commonly used in screening for colorectal cancer, but the procedure also can be helpful in evaluating many common complaints that prompt patients to seek medical care (i.e., rectal bleeding, unexplained weight loss, or painful defecation).

Prostate specific antigen (**choice E**) is used to screen for prostate cancer in men age 50 and older; to monitor the effectiveness of antihormonal therapies (LHRH agonists or anti-testosterone agents) in men who are being treated for prostate cancer; and to determine if cancer has relapsed.

51. **The correct answer is D.** The patient is presenting with signs and symptoms of Raynaud's disease: This condition is commonly associated with the development of episodic bilateral digital pallor, cyanosis, and rubor. This condition is precipitated by cold or emotional stressors and is relieved by warmth. Vasodilators are generally used in patients who cannot be controlled with nonpharmacologic methods. Nifedipine is a commonly used calcium channel blocking agent in patients with hypertension, heart failure, and peripheral vascular disorders, such as Raynaud's disease.

Atenolol (**choice A**) is a beta-adrenergic blocking agent indicated for the treatment of hypertension.

Furosemide (**choice B**) is a loop diuretic indicated for the treatment of a variety of edematous states and for treatment of hypertension.

Gabapentin (**choice C**) is an antiepileptic agent used adjunctively in refractory cases of seizure, has efficacy in pain of neuropathic origin, and may be useful in migraine.

Vecuronium (**choice E**) is a nondepolarizing skeletal muscle blocker.

52. **The correct answer is E.** The motor component (special visceral efferent) of the facial nerve (CN VII) exits the skull via the stylomastoid foramen, passes lateral to the styloid process, and then enters the parotid gland. Within the gland, two divisions can usually be identified (upper and lower), which in turn give off five named branches that innervate the muscles of the face. The upper division gives rise to the temporal and zygomatic branches, which collectively innervate the frontalis, corrugator, and orbicularis oculi muscles. The lower division gives off the buccal, mandibular, and cervical branches. The largest, the buccal, innervates the muscles attaching to the upper lip, including the orbicularis oris and the levators, as well as the buccinator and the muscles of the nose. The mandibular branches innervate the muscles of the lower lip and of the chin, whereas the cervical branch innervates the platysma muscle. There are usually communicating

branches between the named terminal nerves so that overlapping innervation of the muscles occurs. If the lower division is injured, there will be weakness (not frank paralysis because of the innervation overlap) of the muscles that attach to the lower lip.

An inability to furrow the brow (**choice A**) would be caused be denervation of the corrugator supercilii and frontalis muscles, which are innervated by the upper division of the facial nerve.

Choice B is wrong because once the facial nerve emerges from the stylomastoid foramen, it is a pure motor nerve (special visceral efferent, or branchiomotor nerve). It carries no sensory nerve fibers.

Ptosis (a drooping of the upper eyelid; **choice C**) is the result of a paralysis of the levator palpebrae muscle, which is innervated by the oculomotor (CN III) nerve.

Choice D is not correct because the orbicularis oculi muscle is innervated by branches from the upper division of the facial nerve.

53. **The correct answer is E.** Glucose-6-phosphate dehydrogenase deficiency is a hemolytic anemia that presents with malaise and jaundice. Hemolysis is triggered by use of sulfa drugs in patients with the disorder. Because this is a hemolytic anemia, the reticulocyte count will be elevated. In patients with beta thalassemia (**choice A**) and vitamin B_{12} deficiency (**choice C**), the reticulocyte count would be decreased, not elevated. Sickle cell anemia (**choice B**) and hereditary spherocytosis (**choice D**) are hemolytic anemias, but neither is triggered by the use of medications.

54. **The correct answer is C.** Cervical cytology screening (i.e., Pap smear) is largely responsible for the tremendous decrease in the incidence and mortality from cervical cancer that occurred in the late 20th century. The issue of when to begin screening is an important one because of the high costs and benefits associated with the screening program. It is difficult to determine the exact, correct time to begin cervical cytology screening in women because large, population-based, randomized-controlled trials are not available and would be difficult, if not impossible, to do. The benefits of earlier screening are the earlier detection of cervical neoplasia and the opportunity to intervene earlier. The disadvantage of earlier screening is the increased anxiety that women would experience from starting the screening earlier. Earlier screening also has the disadvantage of generating increased morbidity and expense from earlier and more frequent intervention. Current recommendations from the American

College of Obstetrics and Gynecology are that screening begins at age 21 or 3 years after the onset of sexual activity.

To recommend that this patient begin having cervical cytology screening at age 12 or with menarche (**choice A**) would be incorrect. Starting screening this early would lead to a significant increase in anxiety for patients and parents. Furthermore, given the natural history of infection with human papillomavirus (the causative organism of cervical neoplasia), screening this early would not be necessary.

To recommend screening at age 18 or with the onset of sexual activity (**choice B**) was the standard of care for screening for many years. However, improved understanding of the human papillomavirus and the impact of cervical cytology screening programs have led to the change in recommendation to age 21 or 3 years after the initiation of sexual intercourse.

To recommend screening at age 30 or 10 years after the onset of sexual activity (**choice D**) would not be correct. Cervical neoplasia can develop within 3 years after initiation of sexual activity, so to wait 10 years would be too long. Furthermore, women from age 20 to 30 are at very high risk, so to wait until age 30 would also be too late.

To state that Pap tests will not be necessary in this patient (**choice E**) is incorrect. As stated above, the Pap test has proven itself over many years to reduce the incidence and mortality from cervical cancer. This patient should begin having cervical cytology screening at age 21 or 3 years after the onset of sexual activity.

55. **The correct answer is A.** Amantadine is an agent used in the treatment of Parkinson disease as an initial agent or in combination with other anti-Parkinson agents. Amantadine is also used for the symptomatic treatment of influenza A infections because of its antiviral properties.

Bromocriptine (**choice B**) is a dopamine agonist used as an adjunctive agent to levodopa in the treatment of Parkinson disease. It is also used in the short-term management of amenorrhea/galactorrhea or female infertility associated with hyperprolactinemia.

Carbidopa (**choice C**) has no pharmacologic action for the treatment of Parkinson disease; however, it does decrease the metabolism of levodopa in the body. Levodopa (**choice D**) is the most effective agent available for the treatment of Parkinson disease. It is decarboxylated to dopamine in the brain. Remember, dopamine deficiency is the etiology for Parkinson's

disease. Selegiline (**choice E**) is effective for the treatment of Parkinson disease because it inhibits the intracerebral metabolic degradation of dopamine by irreversibly inhibiting monoamine oxidase type B.

56. **The correct answer is A.** The patient has a small bowel obstruction. Adhesions are the most common cause of a small bowel obstruction.

Choices B, C, and **E** are less frequent causes of small bowel obstructions.

Neoplasms (**choice D**) are a common cause of large bowel obstructions. Radiographically, a large bowel obstruction shows a dilated large bowel, which can be distinguished from a small bowel by the haustral markings, fluid levels, and peripheral location in the abdomen.

57. **The correct answer is B.** Borderline personality disorder (BPD) is a serious mental illness characterized by pervasive instability in moods, interpersonal relationships, self-image, and behavior. This instability often disrupts family and work life and the individual's sense of self-identity. People with BPD often have highly unstable patterns of social relationships. Although they can develop intense but stormy attachments, their attitudes towards family, friends, and loved ones may suddenly shift from idealization to devaluation.

Patients with narcissistic personality disorder (**choice A**) are grandiose and have a sense of entitlement.

Avoidant personality types (**choice C**) are sensitive to the possibility of social rejection and are reluctant to enter into relationships. Dependent personality disorder overlaps somewhat with avoidant personality disorder. These patients lack self-confidence and self-reliance, passively allowing another person, their codependent, to assume responsibility.

Passive-aggressive personality disorder (**choice D**) consists of people who resist the demands of others in both social and work situations. This resistance is often seen as aggressive behavior.

Obsessive-compulsive personality disorder (**choice E**) is characterized by a pattern of perfectionism, inflexibility, and preoccupation with unimportant details.

58. **The correct answer is C.** The recommended follow-up for early-stage vaginal carcinoma is every 3 months for 2 years, then every 6 months for 3 years, and annually thereafter.

59. **The correct answer is A.** The prostate cancer gene is believed to be passed on in a mendelian fashion. If a Punnett square is established, there will be a 50%

chance of an offspring receiving the dominant allele. However, there is only a 50% probability that the offspring will be male. Therefore, $50\% \times 50\% = 0.50 \times 0.50 = 0.25 = 25\%$.

60. **The correct answer is A.** The left anterior descending artery branches off the left coronary artery and supplies blood to the anterior side of the heart, thus demonstrating changes in leads V1–V4.

The posterior descending branch of the right coronary artery (**choice B**) would be represented by changes noted in the inferior leads (II, III, and aVF).

The pulmonary artery (**choice C**) may demonstrate signs of right ventricular hypertrophy, such as tall right precordial R waves, right axis deviation, and right ventricular strain if pulmonary hypertension is suspected.

The circumflex branch of the LCA (left coronary artery) (**choice D**) would represent the lateral portion of the heart and would be seen in leads I, aVL, V5, or V6.

The aortic artery (**choice E**) most likely shows evidence of left ventricular hypertrophy with or without a strain pattern, conduction defects that include first-degree heart block, or left bundle-branch block.

Block 4

1. **The correct answer is B.** The patient is exhibiting the signs and symptoms of hypertrophic obstructive cardiomyopathy. Syncope is common and is typically postexertional. In cases with outflow obstruction, a loud systolic ejection murmur is present, which increases with upright position or Valsalva maneuver and decreases with squatting.

   The ejection murmur of hypertrophic cardiomyopathy can be altered by maneuvers that decrease venous return, reduce left ventricular diastolic volume, or increase apposition of the anterior mitral valve leaflet with the hypertrophied interventricular septum.

   Inhaling amyl nitrate (**choice A**) should lower aortic pressure and increase the intensity of the murmur.

   Standing up (**choice C**) will increase the intensity of the murmur.

   Digoxin (**choice D**) is not usually used in this type of cardiomyopathy because it can worsen the obstruction of blood flow out of the heart. Treatment for outflow obstruction can include medications such as propranolol and verapamil. These agents are designed to slow the heart rate and decrease the obstruction.

   The Valsalva maneuver (**choice E**) increases the intensity of the murmur by increasing the outflow tract pressure gradient.

2. **The correct answer is C.** This patient has a viral upper respiratory tract infection and requires only symptomatic relief. Her peak expiratory flow rate is within the normal range for her age.

   Albuterol and oral prednisone (**choices A and D**) are indicated in an acute asthma exacerbation.

   Penicillin and amoxicillin (**choices B and E**) are indicated in a bacterial infection.

3. **The correct answer is D.** Diverticulitis most commonly occurs in the descending colon. Symptoms of diverticulitis include nausea, vomiting, and left-sided abdominal pain.

4. **The correct answer is C.** Compulsions are impulses to engage in acts repeatedly. Handwashing is a common action seen in patients suffering from obsessive-compulsive disorder.

   Obsessions (**choice A**) are intrusive and recurring thoughts and images that are uncontrollable.

Delusions (**choice B**) are false beliefs about the self, or about persons or objects outside the self, that persist despite the facts. Delusions occur in some psychotic states.

Hallucinations (**choice D**) are perceptions of something (i.e., visual images or sounds) with no external cause.

A phobia (**choice E**) is a persistent and irrational fear.

5. **The correct answer is C.** Reactive arthritis (formerly called Reiter syndrome) is a triad of urethritis, conjunctivitis, and aseptic arthritis. It commonly follows a dysenteric infection or sexually transmitted infection and is HLA-B27 (+) 50 to 80% of the time.

   Findings in **choices A, B, and D** are not associated with reactive arthritis.

   Rhinorrhea, lacrimation, and diaphoresis (**choice E**) are the symptoms that characterize opioid withdrawal.

6. **The correct answer is D.** The patient has allergic conjunctivitis, and the most appropriate treatment would be with either ocular antihistamines or nonsteroidal anti-inflammatory agents. Allergic conjunctivitis is a benign disease that may be seasonal or perennial, and the clinical signs are usually limited to conjunctival hyperemia and edema. However, other signs may include tearing, redness, and stringy discharge.

   Intranasal saline (**choice A**) and steroids (**choice B**) are both effective treatments of allergic rhinitis that may also produce sneezing, but these would be of little benefit to the ocular symptoms.

   Ocular antibiotics (**choice C**) are appropriate for treating bacterial conjunctivitis, which normally presents with purulent discharge. However, discomfort is minimal and itching is more indicative of atopy.

   Saline drops (**choice E**) would help wash away potential allergens on the conjunctiva but would treat only the ocular symptoms and not the underlying etiology.

7. **The correct answer is C.** Because this patient's hemoglobin is <10 g/dL, she is anemic according to the definition. Her mean corpuscular volume (MCV) is between 80 and 100 fl and thus normocytic. The red cell distribution width (RDW) is also <15. She has anemia caused by volume expansion during pregnancy.

   Even though she has a risk factor for folate deficiency anemia (**choice A**) (phenobarbital), her MCV is 84 fl (normocytic). Folate deficiency anemia is macrocytic (MCV >100 fl).

Iron deficiency anemia (**choice B**) is microcytic (MCV <80 fl) and the RDW is >15.

Even though this patient is of Mediterranean descent, she does not automatically have thalassemia (**choice E**) or sickle cell trait (**choice D**). To diagnose these conditions, you should perform serum electrophoresis. However, this patient most likely has physiologic anemia.

8. **The correct answer is D.** Eighty-five percent of patients are asymptomatic and diagnosed with screening laboratory tests. If symptoms are present, they usually represent the mnemonic "stones (kidney stones), bones (osteopenia), groans (abdominal pain/constipation), and moans (somnolence and lethargy)."

A solitary thyroid nodule (**choice A**) would not cause hypercalcemia. The parathyroid adenoma would not typically be palpable as a "thyroid" nodule.

Hyperactivity and restlessness (**choice B**) are more commonly seen in thyrotoxicosis. Tetany and muscle spasms (**choice C**) are seen in hypocalcemia from hypoparathyroidism.

Weight gain, dry skin, and cold intolerance (**choice E**) are the symptoms of hypothyroidism.

9. **The correct answer is A.** In adults, 78% of spine tumors are located in the extradural space.

Tumors originating in the intradural, extramedullary space (**choice B**) account for approximately 18% of all adult spine tumors. These tumors generally are meningiomas or schwannomas.

Tumors originating in the intradural, intramedullary space (**choice C**) account for approximately 4% of all adult spine tumors. These tumors generally are astrocytomas.

The peripheral nerves distal to the dorsal root ganglia (**choice D**) are not a site of origin for spine tumors.

The spinal column vasculature (**choice E**) is only involved if there is extension of a spine tumor into the vessels. Spine tumors, by themselves, do not originate within the blood vessels.

10. **The correct answer is A.** This is a clinical description of erysipelas—a skin infection typically caused by group A beta-hemolytic streptococci. The infection involves the dermis and lymphatics and is a more superficial subcutaneous infection of the skin than cellulitis. Intense, beefy red erythema, induration, and a sharp border predominate the clinical presentation.

Neisseria gonorrhoeae (**choice B**), varicella-zoster (**choice C**), and *Pseudomonas aeruginosa* (**choice D**) are not common etiologies for erysipelas.

Rickettsia rickettsii (**choice E**) has a characteristic maculopapular rash that appears initially on the wrists and ankles and progresses centrally. The organism is responsible for Rocky Mountain spotted fever.

11. **The correct answer is E.** Sulfonamides, antimalarials, nitrofurantoin, and dapsone can precipitate hemolytic reactions in patients with glucose-6-phosphate dehydrogenase deficiency.

Amiodarone (**choice A**) is a class III antiarrhythmic that when toxic may result in pulmonary fibrosis, hepatotoxicity, and thyroid dysfunction.

Amphotericin B (**choice B**) is an antifungal that can cause fever, chills, hypotension, and nephrotoxicity.

Gentamicin (**choice C**) is an aminoglycoside antibiotic that can result in ototoxicity and nephrotoxicity.

Phenytoin (**choice D**) is an epileptic with the following side effects: nystagmus, lethargy, diplopia, peripheral neuropathy, gingival hyperplasia, hirsutism, ataxia, and megaloblastic anemia.

12. **The correct answer is D.** Based on this patient's clinical presentation, the clinician should suspect *Trichomonas vaginalis*, a sexually transmitted disease that causes a frothy, malodorous yellow-green discharge, pruritus, diffuse vaginal erythema, and red "strawberry" cervix with petechiae. Saline wet mount from vaginal swabs reveal motile, flagellated organisms called trichomonads.

Filaments and spores (**choice A**) that form a "spaghetti and meatballs" (**choice E**) appearance are characteristic of *Candida*. Epithelial cells covered with bacteria (**choice B**) are "clue cells," which are characteristic of bacterial vaginosis. White, prominent papillae (**choice C**) are characteristic of genital warts caused by human papilloma virus.

13. **The correct answer is A.** This patient has symptoms consistent with Prinzmetal/variant angina. It typically occurs at rest and exhibits a circadian pattern, with most episodes occurring in the early hours of the morning. The pain is severe and may be associated with palpitations, presyncope, or syncope secondary to arrhythmia. Transient ST-segment elevation is the characteristic finding in patients with variant angina.

Unstable angina (**choice B**) differs from stable angina in that the discomfort is usually more intense, longer in duration, and easily provoked. ST-segment depression or elevation on ECG may occur. Patients relate prolonged chest pain at rest, which is clinically indistinguishable from an acute myocardial infarction at the time of presentation.

Acute myocardial infarction (**choice C**) has many presentations but typically presents with chest pain, usually across the anterior precordium. The pain is described as a tightness, pressure, or squeezing. The pain may radiate to the jaw, neck, arms, back, and epigastrium. The left arm is affected more frequently than the right arm. Dyspnea, which may accompany chest pain or occur as an isolated complaint, indicates poor ventricular compliance. Nausea and/or abdominal pain often are present in infarcts involving the inferior wall. Anxiety, light-headedness, nausea, vomiting, cough, and syncope may all be present. The pain may be relieved with nitrates or morphine.

Myocardial ischemia (**choice D**) is a condition in which oxygen deprivation to the heart muscle is accompanied by inadequate removal of metabolites because of reduced blood flow or perfusion. It can occur because of increased myocardial oxygen demand and/or reduced myocardial oxygen supply. In the presence of coronary obstruction, an increase of myocardial oxygen requirements caused by exercise, tachycardia, or emotion leads to a transitory imbalance. This condition is frequently termed "demand" ischemia and is responsible for most episodes of chronic stable angina. The patient may report the following signs and symptoms: chest discomfort, dyspnea, fatigue, reduced exertional capacity, palpitations, dizziness, or leg swelling.

Stable angina pectoris (**choice E**) usually only lasts a few minutes. The pain is described as a discomfort, pressure, or squeezing sensation. The pain is most often in the substernal area, precordium, or epigastrium with radiation to the left arm, jaw, or neck. It is often provoked by exertion, emotion, exposure to cold, eating, or smoking. Rest, removal of provoking factors, or sublingual nitrates provide relief.

14. **The correct answer is D.** All inguinal hernias should be treated with surgical intervention, unless there are contraindications to surgery. The risk of developing an incarceration, obstruction, or strangulation is greater than the risk of surgery.

15. **The correct answer is B.** Clozapine is an antipsychotic medication that works by blocking brain receptors for several neurotransmitters. A potentially fatal side effect of clozapine is agranulocytosis, which affects more than 1 in 100 patients. Therefore, the white blood cell count is measured weekly while patients receive this medication, and for 4 weeks after it is stopped.

Liver function tests (**choice A**), urinalysis (**choice C**), renal function tests (**choice D**), and thyroid function tests (**choice E**) are not routinely assessed with clozapine use.

16. **The correct answer is C.** A slipped capital femoral epiphysis is a separation of the ball of the hip joint from the femur at the upper growth plate (epiphysis) of the bone. It presents with limping and pain in the hip and knee.

Osgood-Schlatter disease (**choice A**) and patellofemoral syndrome (**choice D**) both affect the knee, and neither would result in decreased hip range of motion (ROM). Bursitis (**choice B**) is usually a result of overuse and would likely not result in decreased ROM. In this case, the patient has not participated in exercise or sports.

Osteomyelitis (**choice E**) is unlikely because there are no signs of infection.

17. **The correct answer is E.** Of the choices given, prazosin is the only drug approved for use in benign prostatic hyperplasia. Prazosin is an alpha-adrenergic antagonist; as a class of drugs, these are equally effective to the drugs of choice, alpha$_1$-adrenergic antagonists.

Oxybutynin (**choice A**) is used for detrusor instability. Imipramine (**choice B**) is also used for detrusor instability and sphincter incompetence. Pseudoephedrine (**choice C**) is used for sphincter incompetence. Bethanecol (**choice D**) is used for an atonic bladder and overflow incontinence.

18. **The correct answer is B.** Patients with aortic aneurysms greater than 5 cm in width should be referred for surgery.

19. **The correct answer is A.** There are two general categories of twins: dizygotic and monozygotic. Dizygotic twins also are known as fraternal twins, and they develop from two separate fertilized eggs. Monozygotic twins result when a single fertilized egg divides to form two separate embryos. Dizygotic twins are not genetically identical. Monozygotic twins are genetically identical. This patient has a male fetus and a female fetus, which means that her twins are not genetically identical; therefore, she must have dizygotic twins (i.e., two separate eggs fertilized by two separate sperm). Dizygotic twins are dichorionic/diamnionic virtually 100% of the time. This means that each twin has its own chorion and its own amnion.

Dichorionic/monoamnionic (**choice B**) does not exist as a twin classification. Monozygous twins that "split" very early in development become dichorionic/diamnionic. This happens approximately 25% of the time. We know, however, that this wasn't the case with this patient because the twins are of different sexes and, therefore, not genetically identical (monozygous). If the "split" occurs somewhat later, monochorionic/diamnionic (**choice C**) twins are the result. This happens approximately 75% of the time with monozygous twins and is an important occurrence because monochorionic/diamnionic twins can develop the twin-twin transfusion syndrome in which one twin "transfuses" the other, resulting in overgrowth of one twin and undergrowth of the other. If the "split" occurs even later, monochorionic/monoamnionic (**choice D**) twins are the result. This occurs less than 1% of the time. This is an important condition because monochorionic/monoamnionic twins can develop cord entanglement, as there is no membrane separating them.

This is currently no vanishing twin pregnancy (**choice E**), as both twins are fully visualized on the ultrasound. A vanishing twin occurs when one twin from a twin pregnancy is lost early in the pregnancy.

20. **The correct answer is A.** "Mass effect" is the term used to describe the effects of a tumor compressing other structures. Headache and visual field changes (from pressure on the optic chiasm) are the most common mass effects seen with a pituitary macroadenoma. The field deficits can become irreversible if left unchecked.

Significant weight loss (**choice B**) would not typically occur with hyperprolactinemia, and is not a mass effect of a large tumor.

Bilateral nipple discharge (**choice C**) could occur with hyperprolactinemia of any cause and is not dependent on the size of the tumor. It is not a "mass effect."

Elevated blood pressure (**choice D**) is not a result of hyperprolactinemia, nor is it a result of either a micro- or macroadenoma.

An increase in appetite (**choice E**) should not be seen with a pituitary adenoma. Furthermore, it is not an indication for surgery.

21. **The correct answer is C.** Intramuscular or intravenous methylprednisolone is effective in treating or significantly lessening the pain of a prolonged migraine headache in status migrainosus.

Some calcium channel blockers (**choice A**) are used for migraine prophylaxis in resistant cases of recurrent migraine headaches, but they are not indicated for status migrainosus.

Gabapentin (**choice B**) is an anticonvulsant indicated in the treatment of partial seizures. It also is often used off-label for the treatment of nerve pain and paresthesias.

Lithium carbonate (**choice D**) is used mainly for bipolar disorder.

Muscle relaxers (**choice E**) are not beneficial in treating classic migraines. They are most beneficial for tension headaches.

22. **The correct answer is D.** The patient has laryngotracheitis, or croup. This disease is characterized by wheezing, a low-grade fever, a "barking-seal" cough, and hoarseness. Neck radiographs reveal a subglottic narrowing, or the steeple sign. There is an inspiratory and expiratory stridor. Laryngotracheitis usually occurs in children aged 3 months to 3 years and is preceded by an upper respiratory tract infection.

Pharyngitis (**choice A**) usually presents with a sudden-onset sore throat, fever, dysphagia, swollen and erythematous pharynx and tonsils, hypertrophic tonsils, patchy exudates of the tonsils, and tender, enlarged cervical nodes. Pharyngitis may be caused by a virus or bacteria.

Epiglottitis (**choice B**) is supraglottic. It is caused by *Haemophilus influenzae* b and a. There is soft inspiratory stridor, retractions, muffled voice, and drooling. The infected patient usually sits in the tripod position and leans forward. Fever is usually greater than 38.9°C (102.0°F). Neck radiographs reveal a swollen epiglottis, or thumbprint sign. Epiglottitis usually affects children aged 2 to 6 years.

Bronchiolitis (**choice C**) is caused by respiratory syncytial virus. It usually occurs within the first 2 years of life, with a peak at 6 months. Clinical features include fever for 1 to 2 days, rhinorrhea, irritability, decreased appetite, cough, wheezing, tachypnea, intercostal retractions, and nasal flaring. Chest x-ray usually aids in diagnosis and may reveal hyperinflation of the lungs with mild interstitial infiltrates.

Pertussis (**choice E**) is commonly called whooping cough and is caused by *Bordetella pertussis*. It usually affects children younger than age 5. It has three stages: preparoxysmal (1 to 2 weeks), paroxysmal (2 to 4 weeks or longer), and convalescent (1 to 2 weeks). The preparoxysmal stage is when most patients are contagious. The characteristics are rhinorrhea, conjunctival injection, lacrimation, mild cough, and low-grade fever. The characteristics of the paroxysmal stage are forceful coughs during expiration, followed by a sudden, massive inspiration producing the whoop, facial redness and petechiae, cyanosis, and post-tussive vomiting. The convalescent stage consists of a decrease in coughing attacks. Radiographs are not needed for diagnostic purposes.

23. **The correct answer is C.** This patient has a classic history and examination consistent with deep venous thrombosis (DVT). Many patients are asymptomatic. However, the history may include unilateral edema. Leg pain occurs in 50%, but this sign is entirely non-specific. Pain can occur on dorsiflexion of the foot (Homan's sign). Tenderness occurs in 75% of patients. The pain and tenderness associated with DVT does not usually correlate with the size, location, or extent of the thrombus. Warmth or erythema of skin can be present over the area of thrombosis.

Superficial vein thrombophlebitis (**choice A**) may occur spontaneously or as a complication of medical or surgical interventions. Patients with superficial thrombophlebitis often give a history of a gradual onset of localized tenderness, followed by the appearance of an area of erythema along the path of a superficial vein. Normal veins are distended visibly at the foot, ankle, and, occasionally, in the popliteal fossa. Normal veins may be visible as a blue subdermal reticular pattern, but dilated superficial leg veins above the ankle usually are evidence of venous pathology.

Raynaud phenomenon (**choice B**) is a condition in which blood vessels in the fingers and toes (and sometimes in the earlobes, nose, and lips) constrict. It is usually triggered by cold or emotional stress. Episodes are intermittent and may last minutes or hours. Women are affected five times more often than are men. It usually occurs between the ages of 20 and 40 in women and later in life in men.

Multiple sclerosis (**choice D**) is a chronic disease of the central nervous system that predominantly affects young adults during their most productive years. Viral and autoimmune etiologies predominate. Genetic and environmental factors are known to contribute to MS, but the specific cause for this disease has not been identified. Symptoms may include numbness and/or paresthesia, mono- or paraparesis, double vision, optic neuritis, ataxia, and bladder control problems. Subsequent symptoms also include more prominent upper motor neuron symptoms. Vertigo, cerebellar dysfunction, depression, emotional lability, ataxia, dysarthria, fatigue and pain are common.

Varicose veins (**choice E**) are veins that have dilated under the influence of increased venous pressure. They are the visible surface manifestation of an underlying syndrome of venous insufficiency. Venous insufficiency

syndromes allow venous blood to escape from its normal flow path and flow in a retrograde direction down into an already congested leg. Most patients with venous insufficiency have subjective symptoms that may include pain, soreness, burning, aching, throbbing, cramping, muscle fatigue, and "restless legs." Over time, chronic venous insufficiency leads to cutaneous and soft tissue breakdown, which can be extremely debilitating.

24. **The correct answer is B.** This presentation is classic for gout. Gout presents with a painful, red, swollen joint. Examination of the synovial fluid reveals monosodium urate crystals. Gout is triggered by consumption of alcohol, fructose-sweetened drinks, meat, and seafood.

25. **The correct answer is B.** Mannitol is an osmotic diuretic often administered in the setting of acute head trauma with increased intracranial pressure. Mannitol is filtered into the tubule but not reabsorbed. In the tubule, mannitol increases tubular osmolarity and thus draws water into the tubule, increasing urine output.

Agonism of the aldosterone receptors (**choice A**) will result in fluid retention, not diuresis. Patients with hyperaldosteronism display alkalosis, hypokalemia, and hypovolemia.

Ethanol triggers diuresis by inhibiting the release of ADH from the posterior pituitary (**choice C**). Mannitol does not inhibit ADH secretion. Mannitol does not inhibit carbonic anhydrase (**choice D**). Carbonic anhydrase inhibitors prevent $NaHCO_3$ reabsorption from the proximal tubule.

Mannitol does not inhibit the Na/K/2Cl megatransporter (**choice E**) in the thick ascending loop of Henle. Loop diuretics, such as furosemide, potently trigger diuresis through this mechanism.

26. **The correct answer is C.** This patient is demonstrating unstable angina. The accelerating nature of her anginal pattern and the rest angina are characteristic of the condition. Patients with unstable angina, especially those with a prolonged episode, require admission to the hospital for telemetry monitoring and serial measurements of CK-MB and troponin levels.

Emergent cardiac catheterization (**choice A**) in unstable angina is only indicated when angina is refractory to medical therapy or when hemodynamic instability is present.

Administration of thrombolytic therapy (**choice B**) is not indicated for the treatment of unstable angina or non-ST elevation myocardial infarction. In this setting, it is associated with an increased mortality.

Immediate exercise tolerance test (**choice D**) is contraindicated in patients with active unstable angina, but may be performed once the patient is stable.

Transthoracic echocardiogram (**choice E**) can identify regional wall motion abnormalities if active ischemia or prior myocardial infarction is present, but it does not add significant diagnostic information.

27. **The correct answer is A.** The classic symptom of acute pancreatitis is epigastric pain that radiates to the back and is accompanied by nausea and vomiting. Objective findings usually are fever, jaundice, tachycardia, and a soft but tender epigastrium.

    Choice B is incorrect. Patients with alcoholic hepatitis complain of nausea, loss of appetite, and abdominal pain. Physical examination reveals hepatomegaly, splenomegaly, and jaundice.

    Cholecystitis (**choice C**) is characterized by a severe right upper quadrant pain, nausea, and vomiting. A history of a large, fatty meal prior to developing the pain is suggestive of the diagnosis. Objective findings reveal a Murphy's sign, fever, and leukocytosis.

    Retrocecal appendicitis (**choice D**) may have 1) classic symptoms of an appendicitis, such as periumbilical pain that migrates to the right lower quadrant and is associated with nausea and vomiting, 2) symptoms that may be more variable, such as flank pain and abdominal fullness, or 3) no abdominal symptoms at all.

    Small intestinal obstruction (**choice E**) presents with cramping abdominal pain. The pain starts out as mild and intermittent and progresses to severe and constant. Vomiting follows the onset of pain. Distension may or may not be present, depending on the location of the obstruction. Objective findings reveal high-pitched tinkles on abdominal auscultation and visible peristalsis.

28. **The correct answer is B.** Somatization disorder presents with patients complaining of numerous vague physical symptoms that involve multiple organ systems in the absence of organic disease. These patients have histories of concomitant psychiatric illness that may include depression, suicidal tendencies, and anxiety. The diagnostic criteria for somatization disorder according to DSM-IV-TR requires that at some point during the course of illness, the patient must have had all of the following: at least four pain symptoms, two gastrointestinal tract symptoms, one sexual symptom, and one pseudoneurologic symptom.

    Munchausen syndrome by proxy (**choice A**) is when a person (often the parent) provokes symptoms in a child.

Conversion disorder (**choice C**) involves an obvious loss of neurologic function in the absence of organic disease. Phobic disorders (**choice D**) involve irrational fears of specific events or objects. Panic disorder (**choice E**) is characterized by at least 1 month of panic attacks coupled with a persistent fear of recurrent attacks.

29. **The correct answer is B.** de Quervain tenosynovitis of the wrist involves the abductor pollicis longus and extensor pollicis brevis tendons. It is usually due to a repetitive pinching motion (e.g., factory work, weed-picking). The Finkelstein test is used to confirm the diagnosis.

    Gamekeeper's thumb (**choice A**) is a tear of the ulnar collateral ligament and typically presents with pain and swelling directly over the torn ligament at the base of the thumb. Patients will often have a difficult time grasping objects or holding objects firmly in their grip.

    Gonococcal tenosynovitis (**choice C**) presents with erythema, warmth, and swelling, which this patient does not demonstrate. Volar flexor tenosynovitis (trigger finger) (**choice D**) presents with pain in the thumb or ring finger.

    Carpal tunnel syndrome (**choice E**) is a painful, progressive condition caused by compression of the median nerve. Symptoms usually start gradually with pain, weakness, or numbness in the hand and wrist radiating up the arm. This does not fit the present clinical presentation.

30. **The correct answer is B.** Radionucleotide scan is the gold standard for diagnosing blood flow to the testes.

    Doppler ultrasound (**choice A**) is also useful in detecting blood flow to the testes, but it is not the gold standard. Emergency surgical exploration (**choice C**) may be warranted but is not the gold standard for diagnosis. Prehn sign (**choice D**) is useful in differentiating testicular torsion from acute epididymitis, but is not the gold standard. Urinalysis (**choice E**) may be useful in diagnosing infectious processes and hematuria but is not useful in diagnosing testicular torsion.

31. **The correct answer is E.** A PSA level >10 ng/mL requires a radionucleotide scan to rule out bony metastasis.

    A PSA of 2 ng/mL (**choice A**) is considered a normal level. A PSA of 4 ng/mL (**choice B**) is a borderline level. A PSA >4 ng/mL is indicative of prostate carcinoma.

    A PSA level >4 ng/mL but <10 ng/mL is at low probability for bony metastasis. Therefore **choices C** and **D** are incorrect.

32. **The correct answer is C.** The structure described is a staghorn calculus, which is sometimes picked up as an incidental finding on an upper abdominal x-ray. Staghorn calculi are large renal stones that form in the collecting system of the renal pelvis. The stones are composed of radiolucent magnesium ammonium phosphate (struvite), but they often complex with enough calcium salts to become at least partially radiopaque. Infection with urea-splitting bacteria such as *Proteus*, *Klebsiella*, and *Pseudomonas* tends to increase the ammonia content of the urine, predisposing for stone formation. Staghorn calculi are usually treated with percutaneous fragmentation and extraction.

The other organisms listed in the choices do not contain the enzyme urease, and consequently, infection with these organisms is not a specific risk factor for staghorn calculus formation.

33. **The correct answer is B.** The third stage of labor begins with the delivery of the infant and ends with the delivery of the placenta. It is perhaps the most dangerous stage of labor for the mother, as postpartum hemorrhage is a common cause of significant maternal morbidity and mortality worldwide. The placenta usually is delivered 1 to 5 minutes after the birth of the infant. Several studies have demonstrated that active management of the third stage of labor can reduce the incidence of postpartum hemorrhage and the need for transfusion. Active management of the third stage involves immediate clamping and cutting of the umbilical cord, immediate starting of oxytocin after the delivery of the infant, and controlled traction on the cord to deliver the placenta. The third stage is not considered to be prolonged until 30 minutes have elapsed from the delivery of the infant. This is an arbitrary time limit, however, and as long as there is no evidence of active bleeding or maternal compromise, expectant management is reasonable. In this case, 30 minutes have not yet elapsed since the delivery of the infant, and the patient is stable with no evidence of bleeding; therefore, expectant management is appropriate.

Dilation and curettage (**choice A**) would not be necessary at this point. First, dilation would likely not be necessary, as the postpartum cervix is usually open enough to pass instruments without a dilation procedure. Second, curettage of the uterus to remove a placenta after 15 minutes would be overly aggressive.

Exploratory laparotomy (**choice C**) or hysterectomy (**choice D**) would not be necessary in this patient at this point. Only 15 minutes have elapsed since the delivery of the infant. It is reasonable to wait at least

30 minutes (or longer, as long as no bleeding is present). Furthermore, the next step would be an attempt at manual removal of the placenta and not exploratory laparotomy or hysterectomy.

To perform a manual removal of the placenta (**choice E**) at this point would be premature. Manual removal of the placenta carries with it the risk for infection. It is reasonable to wait 30 minutes for the third stage before intervening.

34. **The correct answer is A.** Subacute thyroiditis (typically viral in etiology) frequently presents as fever, malaise, and a tender, painful, diffusely enlarged thyroid gland.

Hashimoto thyroiditis may present as diffuse enlargement of the thyroid (**choice B**), has an insidious onset (**choice C**), and may result in a fullness in the anterior neck (**choice D**). The thyroid is not painful.

Hashimoto thyroiditis is an autoimmune process that results in hypothyroidism. Its symptoms are weight gain, cold intolerance, and dry skin (**choice E**).

35. **The correct answer is D.** Carpal tunnel syndrome involves symptoms related to compression and/or irritation of the median nerve, which innervates the first, second, and third fingers as well as the lateral aspect of the fourth finger. Carpal tunnel syndrome can be manifested by weakness of abduction and apposition of the thumb.

Weakness of the fifth digit (**choice A**) is the result of injury to the ulnar nerve or injury to the digiti minimi muscles of the fifth digit.

Palpable tenderness over the lateral epicondyle (**choice B**) is most often associated with lateral epicondylitis, known as "tennis elbow."

Decreased sensation in the fifth digit (**choice C**) is the result of injury to the ulnar nerve or the distal branches of the ulnar nerve.

Wrist swelling and tenderness with increased warmth and erythema of the wrist (**choice E**) are found in direct trauma to the wrist, inflammatory arthritis of the wrist, or infection in the wrist.

36. **The correct answer is C.** In severe cases of contact dermatitis with blistering, topical steroids are ineffective. Topical lotions, solutions (Sarna lotion [**choice A**] and Domeboro packs [**choice B**]), or steroids (**choice E**) may be used as adjunct therapies but not as primary therapies in severe cases. Antibiotics (such as amoxicillin; **choice D**) should be used only if a secondary cellulitis is a concern.

37. **The correct answer is A.** This patient has epiglottitis that can be caused by *Haemophilus influenzae*. There is a soft inspiratory stridor, as well as retractions, a muffled voice, and drooling. The infected patient usually sits in the tripod position and leans forward. Fever is usually greater than 38.9° C (102.0° F). Neck radiographs reveal a swollen epiglottis, or thumbprint sign. Epiglottitis usually affects children aged 2 to 6 years. Endotracheal intubation is needed in epiglottitis because the swelling of the epiglottis will obstruct the airway.

Cool mist (**choice B**), racemic epinephrine aerosol (**choice C**), systemic steroids (**choice D**), and aerosolized steroids (**choice E**) are all used in the treatment of croup. For this patient, ceftriaxone is recommended to treat the *Haemophilus influenzae* infection.

38. **The correct answer is D.** A CT scan sensitivity for detecting abdominal aortic aneurysm is nearly 100%, and the study offers certain advantages over ultrasound in defining aortic size, rostral-caudal extent, involvement of visceral arteries, and extension into the suprarenal aorta. In addition, CT scanning permits visualization of the retroperitoneum and is not limited by obesity or bowel gas. It also detects leakage and permits concomitant evaluation of the kidneys. A spiral CT scan allows three-dimensional imaging of abdominal contents, enhancing the ability to detect branch vessel and adjacent organ involvement.

Chest x-rays (**choice A**) are obtained on patients with abdominal complaints before the diagnosis of abdominal aortic aneurysm has been entertained. However, the x-ray will not provide an accurate estimation of size.

Abdominal angiography (**choice B**) is useful for the determination of aortic anatomy and has been advocated for preoperative use to rule out aneurysm, renal artery stenosis, or visceral ischemia. The test is limited by its invasiveness, cost, lack of operator availability, time involved, and risk of complications (e.g., bleeding, perforation, and embolization). However, routine use of angiography in evaluation of abdominal aortic aneurysm is not recommended. The technique is not widely available and offers no real advantage over conventional CT scanning.

Abdominal ultrasound (**choice C**) is noninvasive and sensitive, may be performed at the bedside, and can detect free peritoneal blood. Limitations of the study include inability to detect leakage, rupture, branch artery involvement, and suprarenal involvement. Also, the ability to image the aorta is reduced in the presence of bowel gas or obesity. Significant portions of abdominal aorta (at least one third of its length) are not

visualized on bedside emergency ultrasound in 8% of nonfasted patients. This rate is higher than reported for fasted patients receiving elective ultrasound for evaluation of their aortas.

Magnetic resonance imaging (MRI; **choice E**) permits aortic imaging comparable to CT scanning and ultrasound without subjecting the patient to dye load or ionizing radiation. The technique may offer superior imaging of branch vessels compared with CT scan or ultrasound, but it is less valuable in assessing suprarenal extension and is not suitable in patients who are unstable. MRI may have a role in very stable patients with a severe dye allergy. Lack of widespread availability, need for a stable patient, incompatibility with monitoring equipment, and high cost limit its applicability.

39. **The correct answer is C.** Factor V Leiden is the most common inherited coagulation abnormality causing resistance to activated protein C in Caucasians. This trait is present in 20 to 40% of patients with idiopathic deep venous thrombosis.

Both decreased protein C and decreased antithrombin III (**choices A** and **B**) cause hypercoagulability, but they do not present as commonly as factor V Leiden.

Hyperhomocysteinemia (**choice D**) is a genetic or acquired hypercoagulable state associated with a twofold increase in risk for venous thrombosis.

Choice E is incorrect. A decrease, not an increase, in protein S causes hypercoagulability.

40. **The correct answer is E.** Crohn disease is a condition that alternates between recurrent flare-ups and remission. Sulfasalazine is helpful in maintaining remission.

Choice D is incorrect. A low-residue diet, not high-residue diet, is recommended.

Choices A, B, and **C** may be used in the treatment of active disease.

41. **The correct answer is D.** Schizophrenia is a chronic psychotic disorder with onset typically occurring in adolescence or young adulthood. Schizophrenia results in fluctuating, gradually deteriorating disturbances in thinking, behavior, and perception. These disturbances include the presence of "positive" symptoms, such as delusions, hallucinations, and disorganized speech and behavior, and "negative" symptoms, such as poverty of speech (**choice E**), flattened affect, social/emotional withdrawal (**choice A**), and apathy (**choice B**).

42. **The correct answer is B.** Radial head subluxation, or nursemaid's elbow, is a very common injury found in

toddlers. It is often caused by pulling on and twisting the arm. The child may not complain of pain but may simply refuse to use the arm. Unlike the ulnar head (**choice A**), the radial head is subject to dislocation due to the weakness of the annular ligament in childhood.

Olecranon fractures (**choice C**) are uncommon in children and result in swelling and significant pain. Medial epicondylitis (**choice D**) and lateral epicondylitis (**choice E**) are overuse syndromes and do not cause decreased range of motion.

43. **The correct answer is D.** It is recommended that African American men, as well as men with family histories of prostate cancer, start having PSA testing at age 40. Both risk factors are common to this patient. The recommendation for men with no risk factors for prostate cancer is to start screening with PSA at age 50.

44. **The correct answer is A.** Macrosomia is observed in infants of diabetic mothers. Oral glucose tolerance test is preferred because of its high sensitivity.

Fasting blood sugar (FBS) (**choice D**) greater than or equal to 126 mg/dL is diagnostic of diabetes when a repeat FBS confirms this level.

A lipid profile (**choice B**) is not a diagnostic test for diabetes.

Fingerstick blood glucose (**choice C**) should not be used for diagnosis. Plasma glucose levels are the currently accepted method of measuring glucose for diagnosis of diabetes mellitus.

Although a complete blood count (**choice E**) would be useful in the diagnosis of an infectious process, in this scenario the most appropriate test is the fasting blood glucose.

45. **The correct answer is E.** Examine and categorize the patient using the Glasgow coma scale. This assesses the severity of hemorrhage because it is related to the patient's clinical state on initial presentation. This, in turn, is often predictive of overall patient outcome. This coma scale correlates well with the patient's final outcome and provides a prognostic index.

Checking the patient for ataxia (**choice A**) is incorrect. Ataxia is indicative of loss of coordination. It can be tested by watching the patient ambulate or by asking the patient to repeatedly run her heel from the opposite knee down the shin to the big toe. These tests may be abnormal in this patient, but they require an alert patient (unlike this woman) who can follow commands.

Evaluation of cranial nerve VII (facial nerve) (**choice B**) is incorrect. Facial nerve abnormalities are not specific to intracranial bleeds.

Evaluation of deep tendon reflexes (**choice C**) is a part of the coma scale assessment but, by itself, is not specific to cerebral abnormalities. The evaluation can also indicate spinal pathology.

Pronator drift (**choice D**) evaluates pyramidal weakness (i.e., a weakness arising from damage to the motor cortex). Again, this may be abnormal in this patient, but the test requires an awake and cooperative patient.

46. **The correct answer is B.** Angular cheilitis (also called perlèche, cheilosis, or stomatitis) is a condition that presents with deep cracks and fissures at the corners of the mouth. If severe, the splits or cracks may bleed when the mouth is opened and may result in shallow ulcers or crusts. Perlèche is associated with the collection of moisture at the corners of the mouth, which encourages infection by *Candida albicans* (most common), staph, and strep. In rare cases, it may be caused by vitamin B deficiency.

Vitamin C deficiency (**choice A**), squamous cell carcinoma (**choice C**), and lack of moisture in the mouth (**choice D**) are not associated with angular cheilitis. Iron deficiency, not overabundance of iron (**choice E**), is associated with angular cheilitis.

47. **The correct answer is C.** MRI scanning is more sensitive to soft tissue changes than is CT scanning, though it does not necessarily distinguish, for example, a demyelinating process from ischemic changes.

Patients with claustrophobia (**choice A**) often experience exacerbation of their condition due to the closed-in construction of the MRI scanner (termed a *closed scanner*). Light sedation can be beneficial, or an *open MRI scanner* can be used, though such a scanner generally is less sensitive than a closed scanner.

A cardiac pacemaker implanted in a patient (**choice B**) is a relative contraindication to an MRI scanner because the scanner can cause the pacemaker to heat up and possibly burn the skin or it can alter the pacemaker's programming.

Bone imaging is mainly limited to display of bone marrow with MRI scanners (**choice D**). Therefore, for cranial imaging, CT scanning is more sensitive in evaluating osseous lesions of the skull.

Metallic objects in the immediate vicinity of the scanner (**choice E**) pose a problem for MRI scanners due to the large-bore magnets used for producing a radiofrequency pulse.

48. **The correct answer is D.** Centrally acting medications, such as psychotropic drugs, antidepressants, and a variety of antihypertensives, can cause elevated prolactin levels and resulting symptomatology.

A pituitary macroadenoma (**choice A**) would cause much higher levels of prolactin (>100 ng/mL) as well as mass effects of the tumor. A pituitary microadenoma (**choice B**) would likewise cause much higher levels of prolactin but without mass effect.

Hypothyroidism (**choice C**) can cause elevated prolactin levels, and a TSH test would be warranted in this patient; however, in light of the fact that she is taking two medications known to elevate prolactin levels, and in light of the fact that the patient has no complaints relating to symptoms of hypothyroidism, medication-induced prolactinemia is the more likely etiology.

Hyperthyroidism (**choice E**) would not elevate prolactin levels.

49. **The correct answer is A.** This patient has food-ingested botulism, which is caused by *Clostridium botulinum*. Symptoms usually occur within 6 to 8 hours of ingestion; this man's symptoms occurred within 7 hours. Symptoms in food-borne botulinum include dysphagia, dry mouth, diplopia, dysarthria, fatigue, upper extremity weakness, dyspnea, vomiting, and dizziness. Physical exam reveals ophthalmoplegia, ptosis of the eyelids, decreased gag reflex, and facial weakness with normal mentation. Foods that may contain *C. botulinum* are vacuum-packed fish, smoked foods, honey, and any food that was not adequately heated during canning. The patient needs to be intubated and mechanically ventilated because he is already having difficulty breathing, suggesting that his respiratory muscles are becoming paralyzed.

Gastric lavage (**choice B**) can be done but is usually recommended within hours of ingestion. In this case, almost 24 hours have passed.

Antibiotics (**choices C, D, and E**) are not recommended for the treatment of botulism. Botulinal antitoxin should also be given.

50. **The correct answer is A.** Giant cell arteritis (also called temporal arteritis) is a systemic panarteritis affecting medium-sized and large vessels in patients over 50 years. Classic symptoms include headache, scalp tenderness, visual symptoms, jaw claudication, or throat pain. On physical examination, the temporal artery is usually normal but may be nodular, enlarged, tender, or pulseless. This condition accounts for 15% of all cases of fever of unknown origin in patients over the age of

65. The ESR in these patients is often >100 mm/h, and most patients have a mild normochromic, normocytic anemia and thrombocytosis. About half of all patients also have polymyalgia rheumatica symptoms.

Polyarteritis nodosa (**choice B**) usually involves painful extremities (myalgia particularly affecting the calves, arthralgia, and neuropathy) with skin involvement that includes livedo reticularis, subcutaneous nodules, and skin ulcers.

Wegener granulomatosis (**choice C**) usually presents with either upper or lower respiratory tract symptoms. The pathology of this condition is defined by the triad of small vessel vasculitis, granulomatous inflammation, and necrosis of the respiratory tract.

Acute angle glaucoma (**choice D**) presents as severe eye pain and profound visual loss.

Microscopic polyangiitis (**choice E**) is a cutaneous vasculitis of the lungs and kidneys.

51. **The correct answer is A.** NSAIDs are the first-line treatment for osteoarthritis. Corticosteroids (**choice B**) and joint replacement surgery (**choice E**) may play a role in progressed stages.

Colchicine (**choice C**) is used in the treatment of gout. DMARDs (**choice D**) are used as the second-line treatment for rheumatoid arthritis.

52. **The correct answer is D.** Dilated cardiomyopathy clinically presents with symptoms of biventricular heart failure (most commonly dyspnea), a functional murmur consistent with mitral regurgitation, and cardiomegaly on chest x-ray. In this case, the history of a positive toxicology screen points to dilated cardiomyopathy as the cause.

Acute myocardial infarction (**choice A**) would usually be more evident on the EKG, although patients may present with a murmur consistent with mitral regurgitation secondary to papillary muscle rupture and left ventricular dysfunction. Chest/shoulder/jaw pain may be present with diaphoresis and nausea.

Infectious myocarditis (**choice B**) often follows an upper respiratory infection or other febrile illness and presents with either pleuritic or nonspecific chest pain. EKG will show sinus tachycardia and intraventricular conduction abnormalities.

Hypertrophic cardiomyopathy (**choice C**) usually has a history of chronic hypertension or in some cases, another family member with the condition. The EKG will show left ventricular hypertrophy and occasionally septal Q waves in the absence of infarction. Examination will demonstrate a sustained apical impulse and systolic ejection murmur.

Restrictive cardiomyopathy (**choice E**) is relatively uncommon, with the most frequent cause being amyloidosis, radiation, and myocardial fibrosis after open heart surgery.

53. **The correct answer is E.** Vitamin D increases the intestinal absorption of calcium and phosphate. Children who are deficient in vitamin D suffer from rickets, whereas adults who are vitamin D deficient suffer from osteomalacia.

54. **The correct answer is B.** Vitamin B_1 (thiamine) deficiency can lead to both beriberi and Wernicke-Korsakoff syndrome. Thiamine serves as an important cofactor in metabolic pathways. Beriberi clinically presents with dilated cardiomyopathy and polyneuritis.

55. **The correct answer is C.** Pellagra is associated with vitamin B_3 (niacin) deficiency and is characterized by the three "D"s: diarrhea, dermatitis, and dementia.

56. **The correct answer is C.** Primary hyperparathyroidism (due to a parathyroid adenoma) is the most common cause of hypercalcemia. The mnemonic "bones (osteopenia), stones (renal stones), groans (abdominal pain and constipation), and psychic moans (fatigue, depression)" helps to recall the major symptomatology.

Secondary hyperparathyroidism (**choice A**) is less likely. The most common reasons for secondary hyperparathyroidism are low calcium intake and chronic renal failure.

Hypoparathyroidism (**choice B**) most commonly occurs after thyroidectomy, and is manifest by low serum calcium levels and low PTH levels.

Paget's disease of bone (**choice D**) may present as bone pain or fracture. Calcium levels are normal, PTH is normal, and alkaline phosphatase is markedly elevated.

Vitamin D deficiency (**choice E**) would result in a decreased level of calcium because the lack of the vitamin results in decreased calcium reabsorption.

57. **The correct answer is A.** Anytime a fecal occult test is positive, malignancy must be ruled out.

Obtaining a complete blood count (**choice B**) is a good idea but is not the best answer.

Choice C is incorrect. The consumption of large quantities of meats may cause a false-positive result, but to inform the patient of this is not the most appropriate next step.

Choice E is incorrect. The cause for the positive occult test has not been established, so treatment cannot be initiated.

58. **The correct answer is C.** Cauda equina syndrome is a result of a lesion compressing the nerve roots. It presents with low back pain, unilateral or usually bilateral sciatica, saddle sensory disturbances, and bladder and bowel dysfunction.

Scoliosis (**choice A**), spinal stenosis (**choice B**), and spondylolisthesis (**choice D**) may present with low back pain but do not fit this clinical picture.

Disk herniation (**choice E**) can cause pain and paresthesias. The pain often worsens with sitting, but it should not cause bladder dysfunction.

59. **The correct answer is A.** Tardive dyskinesia is a neurologic disorder caused by the long-term use of neuroleptic drugs or antipsychotic medications. The prevalence of tardive dyskinesia in patients taking neuroleptic drugs is estimated to be up to 10 to 20%. Features of the disorder may include grimacing, tongue protrusion, lip-smacking, puckering and pursing, and rapid eye-blinking. Rapid movements of the arms, legs, and trunk may also occur.

Fluoxetine (**choice B**), metoprolol (**choice C**), ibuprofen (**choice D**), and trazodone (**choice E**) do not cause tardive dyskinesia.

60. **The correct answer is C.** *Helicobacter pylori* infections are the main cause of duodenal ulcers. The *H. pylori* infection should be treated along with the ulcer simultaneously. A triple antibiotic regiment is used to eradicate *H. pylori*, and a proton pump inhibitor is used to decrease acid production.

Choice A is incorrect. Antacids will not eradicate *H. pylori*.

A fasting serum gastrin (**choice B**) is usually obtained in patients who are refractory to medical treatment.

Surgical intervention (**choice D**) is used in cases that are refractory to medical treatment.

Because the duodenal ulcer has been diagnosed by endoscopy, there is no need for an upper gastrointestinal series (**choice E**).

Block 5

1. **The correct answer is D.** This patient has gonococcal urethritis. The most common coinfection with gonococcal urethritis is *Chlamydia trachomatis*. *C. trachomatis* is the most common cause of nongonococcal urethritis that usually occurs after treatment of *Neisseria gonorrhoeae*, so it is better to treat prophylactically.

   Treponema pallidum (**choice A**) is the spirochete that causes syphilis. Syphilis usually presents as a painless ulcer that may be found on the penis; it does not occur with dysuria and discharge. Syphilis may occur with *N. gonorrhoeae* but it is not the most common coinfection.

   Gardnerella vaginosis (**choice B**) can be a cause of nongonococcal urethritis; however, it is not the most common coinfection of *N. gonorrhoeae*.

   Ureaplasma urealyticum (**choice C**) is a possible etiologic agent of nongonococcal urethritis but it is not the most common coinfection with *N. gonorrhoeae*.

   Chlamydia psittaci (**choice E**) causes psittacosis from contact with birds and is not sexually transmitted.

2. **The correct choice is A.** Papillary carcinoma of the thyroid makes up 80% of all thyroid cancers. The disease spreads lymphatically and has an excellent prognosis. There is a 98% 10-year survival for stage I or II disease.

   Medullary carcinoma (**choice B**) is a relatively rare thyroid cancer, but is associated with the MEN II syndromes and carries a poor prognosis.

   Follicular carcinoma (**choice C**) is the most aggressive form of thyroid cancer. It spreads hematogenously and can metastasize to the brain, bone, and lungs.

   Anaplastic carcinoma (**choice D**) is an undifferentiated form of thyroid carcinoma with a poor prognosis.

   Adenocarcinoma (**choice E**) is the most common type of esophageal cancer. It usually is found in the lower third of the esophagus.

3. **The correct answer is D.** Peak expiratory flow is the most useful test to perform on a patient with asthma. Nomograms exist for expected performance based on the patient's age, size, and gender. It is also useful in documenting improvement after therapy.

   Arterial blood gases (**choice A**) may be warranted if the patient's condition deteriorates or fails to improve after successive nebulizer treatments, but is not indicated in this patient at this time.

The helical CT of the chest (**choice B**) would be useful in a patient suspected of having a pulmonary embolism.

The posteroanterior and lateral chest x-ray (**choice C**) is warranted only if the patient has signs and symptoms that are suggestive of pneumonia.

Pulmonary angiography (**choice E**) is the most definitive test for pulmonary embolism. Although invasive, it is known as the gold standard in the diagnosis of pulmonary embolism. However, it is not an appropriate diagnostic test for asthma.

4. **The correct choice is B.** The administration of hydrocortisone is the mainstay of treatment for Addison disease. The most common etiology of the disease is autoimmune failure of the adrenal gland.

   The administration of beta-blockers for control of blood pressure (**choice A**) is the appropriate medical therapy for a pheochromocytoma. Surgical management (**choice C**) is also appropriate in the case of a pheochromocytoma. **Choice D** is incorrect because adrenal insufficiency is fatal if left untreated.

   Dextrose IV (**choice E**) usually is given to a patient experiencing Addisonian crisis.

5. **The correct answer is B.** The three key findings in normal pressure hydrocephalus are gait ataxia, memory dysfunction, and urinary incontinence. These are all related to the increased size of the ventricles in the brain, but they are not manifested by measurably increased intracranial pressure. They are not specifically related to central canal stenosis or blockage of cerebrospinal fluid flow by any abnormality, such as tumor or C1 to C2 subluxation due to rheumatoid arthritis or trauma.

   Cranial nerve III (oculomotor) palsy (**choice A**) can be associated with a tremor or hemiparesis in patients with infarction in the oculomotor nerve tract area. It also can be associated with significant complaint of headache (usually severe and rapid in onset) that is, in turn, associated with a subarachnoid hemorrhage.

   Limited extension of neck (**choice C**) is incorrect. Stenosis at the C1 to C2 level of the cervical spine due to spontaneous C1 to C2 subluxation can be seen in a patient with rheumatoid arthritis. The first manifestations of this nontraumatic, insidious-onset C1 to C2 stenosis/subluxation are increasing inability to extend the neck and neck pain. Trauma causing cervical spine subluxation could lead to similar symptoms presented in this patient, but she has no history of trauma.

Loss of sharp/dull discrimination in a nondermatomal distribution in the bilateral lower extremities (**choice D**) is usually associated with peripheral neuropathy, for which this patient is at risk due to her history of diabetes.

Weakness of hand grip in a unilateral distribution (**choice E**) is usually due to cervical spine disease (more specifically from unilateral radiculopathy involving any or all of the C6–C8 nerve roots), such as central cervical spine canal stenosis. It can also be seen with a lesion, such as a tumor or hemorrhage in the left upper cortex of the brain, but complaints of diplopia and dysphagia would be present as well.

6. **The correct answer is A.** Lichen simplex chronicus (also known as neurodermatitis) is a chronic inflammation of the skin (dermatitis) characterized by small, round, itchy spots that thicken and become leathery as a result of scratching.

    Psoriasis (**choice B**) is an inflammatory condition with characteristic plaques with silvery scales. Cellulitis (**choice C**) is an infection that presents with diffuse erythema, swelling, and warmth. Scabies (**choice D**) presents with burrowing and excoriations and is usually not localized to one area.

    Ringworm (choice E) is a contagious fungus infection that presents on the body as a ring-shaped rash.

7. **The correct answer is D.** The most common cause of endocarditis in IV drug users is *Staphylococcus aureus*. The physical examination has many of the classic findings of the condition. Painful nodules of the fingers and toe pads are known as Osler nodes. The red-brown streaks in the proximal nail beds are known as splinter hemorrhages. Also seen are Janeway lesions (nontender hemorrhagic macules of the palms and soles) and Roth spots (retinal hemorrhages).

    Fungal causes and tuberculosis as causes of endocarditis (**choices A, B, and C**) are rare. *Streptococcus viridans* (**choice E**) is a cause of endocarditis in otherwise healthy individuals.

8. **The correct choice is C.** Calcium channel blockers are effective in patients with Raynaud phenomenon and can also be used effectively to control blood pressure.

    Although all of the remaining medications may be used to control blood pressure, calcium channel blockers are preferred in patients with Raynaud phenomenon.

9. **The correct answer is D.** Fitz-Hugh–Curtis syndrome is a complication of pelvic inflammatory disease (PID) that is mostly seen in women. It is a perihepatitis caused by a gonococcal or chlamydial infection. It causes adhesions between the liver and diaphragm. The patient's history of PID, right upper quadrant pain, and a normal ultrasound is indicative of Fitz-Hugh–Curtis syndrome.

Patients with appendicitis (**choice A**) typically have pain in the right lower quadrant. Patients with appendicitis with a high cecum may have symptoms similar to an acute cholecystitis. An ultrasound would show diagnostic evidence of appendicitis.

The ultrasound of cholelithiasis (**choice C**) and cholecystitis (**choice B**) would show gallstones and sludge. Patients can have gallstones (cholelithiasis) and be asymptomatic for years before developing symptoms.

Choice E is incorrect. The pain from a peptic ulcer is located in the epigastrium and may radiate to the back. Food and antacids may provide relief. Endoscopy is diagnostic.

10. **The correct choice is E.** Maintaining an $HgbA_{1c}$ <7 has been found to reduce the risk of *all* complications of diabetes mellitus. The most recent recommendations in the ADA guidelines suggest that tight glycemic control is the most effective means of preventing the chronic complications of diabetes.

    An ACE inhibitor (**choice A**) may delay the progression of diabetic nephropathy but does not affect other micro- or macrovascular complications of DM.

    Frequent eye examinations and testing of the urine for albumin (**choice C**) are appropriate screening exams for detection of the complications of DM; however, these exams do not prevent the complications.

    Checking the feet daily (**choice D**) helps to minimize the complications of diabetic foot infections caused by the insensitivity of the feet in diabetics with peripheral neuropathy. The foot checks, however, do not prevent the neuropathy.

11. **The correct answer is E.** The neonate's respiratory depression is most likely the result of the opioid analgesic given to the mother. The antidote for opioid overdose is to give Narcan (naloxone), a pure opioid antagonist, to reverse the respiratory depression.

    Aminophylline (**choice A**) is an xanthine derivative similar in action to theophylline. This agent potentially would help with the respiratory depression; however, it would not reverse the other untoward effects of the opioids.

Dobutamine (**choice B**) is a cardiostimulant agent indicated for the treatment of heart failure and "shock." This agent increases blood pressure and cardiac output.

Epinephrine (**choice C**) is an agent commonly used in the treatment of anaphylaxis secondary to a food, drug, or toxin allergy. This agent causes immediate bronchodilation.

Flumazenil (**choice D**) is the antidote for benzodiazepine toxicity.

12. **The correct answer is A.** The midbrain, specifically the substantia nigra, is the site of degeneration of dopaminergic neurons in patients with Parkinson disease, such as this patient.

Motor cortex degeneration (**choice B**) may cause a contralateral spastic weakness. Spinal cord lesions (**choice C**) do not result in resting tremors.

Neuronal degeneration in the caudate nucleus (**choice D**) causes Huntington disease, which results in multiple quick, random movements, usually prominent in appendicular muscles instead of the tremor at rest in this patient.

Thalamic degeneration (**choice E**) characteristically results in thalamic pain syndrome. Patients would present with burning or aching pain in contralateral limbs or in the body, not the motor problems evident in a patient with Parkinson disease.

13. **The correct answer is C.** Atenolol is a beta-adrenergic receptor blocking agent used in the treatment of hypertension. Medications in this drug class lower blood pressure by both reducing cardiac output and decreasing renin release from the kidney (to a lesser extent).

Blocking catecholamine release from peripheral sympathetic nerves (**choice A**) is the antihypertensive effect seen with peripherally acting adrenergic neuron blockers (e.g., guanethidine and bretylium). Angiotensin-converting enzyme (ACE) inhibitors block the conversion of angiotensin I to angiotensin II (**choice B**). Diuretics decrease intravascular volume (**choice D**), which ultimately leads to a reduction in blood pressure. Increasing renin release from the kidney (**choice E**) would increase, not decrease, blood pressure.

14. **The correct answer is B.** Esophageal cancer presents with dysphagia to solids, then liquids. Weight loss, chest pain, and hoarse voice may be noted. Barium swallow reveals a polypoid, obstructive lesion.

Achalasia (**choice A**) presents with gradual, progressive dysphagia to solids and liquids. Barium swallow reveals

"bird's beak" dilated esophagus. Lower esophageal web (**choice C**) presents with intermittent dysphagia and barium swallow reveals a thin, diaphragm-like membrane across the esophagus. Plummer-Vinson syndrome (**choice D**) presents with an esophageal web and iron deficiency anemia. Boerhaave syndrome (**choice E**) presents with rupture of the esophagus.

15. **The correct answer is B.** The patient has the classic physical findings of Turner syndrome. The diagnosis can be confirmed by doing a karyotype of her cells.

Biochemical testing (**choice A**) is used to detect the levels of a specific enzyme produced by the patient's cells. It is useful to diagnose disorders such as phenylketonuria.

Linkage analysis (**choice C**) tracks a gene through a family by following the inheritance of a closely linked gene or DNA marker. It is an indirect test for the genetic condition, but it is rapid and cost effective. It is used to test for disorders such as Marfan syndrome and congenital adrenal hyperplasia.

DNA methylation analysis (**choice D**) can reveal whether a promoter for a gene has been shut off by methylation. It is used as part of the workup for such conditions as fragile X syndrome.

PCR multiplex deletion test (**choice E**) is the primary screening test for Duchenne muscular dystrophy. The test evaluates 18 exons for deletions using PCR and will detect approximately 98% of dystrophin deletions.

16. **The correct answer is E.** Mucosal polyps are benign and of no clinical significance. All the other options can give rise to adenocarcinoma of the colon.

17. **The correct answer is A.** Acute pericarditis presents with chest pain and may be noted after a recent viral infection. Viral agents are common etiologies of pericarditis. On physical examination, a pericardial friction rub is pathognomonic for acute pericarditis. Treatment is supportive with NSAIDs.

Pulmonary embolism (**choice B**) presents with tachypnea, tachycardia, shortness of breath, and chest pain. Spontaneous pneumothorax (**choice C**) presents with shortness of breath and chest pain. Physical examination will reveal diminished or absent breath sounds over the pneumothorax. Presentation of pericardial tamponade (**choice D**) may resemble that of acute pericarditis but with the addition of a narrow pulse pressure and pulsus paradoxus. Tietze syndrome (**choice E**) presents with chest pain that is reproduced by local pressure.

18. **The correct answer is C.** The thiazide diuretics (e.g., hydrochlorothiazide, chlorothiazide, benzthiazide) promote diuresis by inhibiting reabsorption of NaCl, primarily in the early distal tubule.

Ethacrynic acid (**choice A**) and furosemide (**choice B**) are loop diuretics. They act by inhibiting electrolyte reabsorption in the thick ascending loop of Henle. If you didn't know where these agents act, but did know that they both belong to the same class of diuretics, you could have eliminated them as possibilities because there can't be more than one correct answer choice.

Mannitol (**choice D**) is an osmotic diuretic. It is freely filtered at the glomerulus and is not reabsorbed. Its primary action occurs at the proximal tubule. Spironolactone (**choice E**) is a potassium-sparing diuretic. It acts on the collecting tubule to inhibit the reabsorption of Na^+ and the secretion of K^+.

19. **The correct answer is D.** Two viruses require reverse transcriptase activity or an RNA-dependent DNA polymerase. HIV is an RNA virus that replicates through a DNA intermediate, thereby requiring a reverse transcriptase. Hepatitis B is a DNA virus that replicates through an RNA intermediate. When the RNA intermediate is copied to make virion DNA, a reverse transcriptase is needed.

20. **The correct answer is E.** Red blood cells (and many other blood cells) contain the enzyme carbonic anhydrase, which catalyzes the intracellular conversion of CO_2 to bicarbonate and H^+ ion. Most of the bicarbonate in the red cell is exchanged across the plasmalemma for chloride ion. This means that although the bulk of the production of bicarbonate occurs in the red cell (**choice D**), the bulk of the actual transport occurs in serum. Carbonic anhydrase is not present in serum. Bicarbonate can also be produced in serum by nonenzymatic means, but the process is slow.

CO_2 is also carried as carbaminohemoglobin (**choice A**), which forms when CO_2 binds to an NH_2 side group of the hemoglobin protein, rather than to the heme iron (Fe^{2+}), as with carbon monoxide and oxygen. CO_2 is not transported in the form of bubbles (**choice B**), which is a good thing because gas bubbles are effectively emboli, which can lead to considerable morbidity or death. Some CO_2 is carried directly dissolved in blood (**choice C**). It is 20 times more soluble in blood than is O_2.

21. **The correct answer is C.** This is a really simple definition question: What is the difference between serum and plasma? Essentially, serum is derived from plasma by the extraction of fibrinogen and coagulation factors II, V, and VIII. This can be achieved by allowing whole blood to clot, then removing the clot.

Albumin (**choice A**) is present in both serum and plasma. Neither erythrocytes (**choice B**) nor granulocytes (**choice D**) are present in either serum or plasma.

Serotonin (**choice E**) levels may be increased in serum because of the platelet breakdown that occurs during the extraction process. Serotonin is normally found in the highest concentration in platelets, as well as in the enterochromaffin cells and mysenteric plexus of the gastrointestinal tract. The brain and the retina contain smaller amounts.

22. **The correct answer is B.** Aortic regurgitation presents with diastolic murmur heard best along the left sternal border. Pulse pressure is wide, and the pulse has a rapid rise and fall ("water-hammer" or Corrigan pulse). Quincke pulse (nail bed capillary pulsations) and Duroziez sign (to-and-fro murmur over a partially compressed artery) are also noted.

Choice A, the cell envelope, is incorrect because both gram-positive and gram-negative microorganisms have this structure, which is defined as all the layers that enclose the cytosol of the bacterium. It is the composition of the envelope that differs between gram-positive and gram-negative microorganisms.

Exotoxin (**choice B**) is not exclusive to gram-negative microorganisms; it is also found in some gram-positives. By contrast, endotoxin (lipopolysaccharide; LPS) is found exclusively in gram-negatives.

Peptidoglycan (**choice C**) is found in the cell walls of both gram-positive and gram-negative microorganisms. Note that there is a larger amount of peptidoglycan in gram-positive microorganisms. Teichoic acids (**choice E**) are found exclusively in gram-positive organisms.

23. **The correct answer is C.** Celiac sprue is a chronic disease of the digestive tract that damages the small intestine and causes malabsorption of most nutrients. Treatment includes removal of gluten from the diet, which results in resolution of symptoms. Rice and corn do not contain gluten.

The remaining answer choices all contain gluten.

24. **The correct answer is A.** This patient has Rocky Mountain spotted fever. The disease is caused by *Rickettsia rickettsii*, which is carried by ticks. The symptoms of Rocky Mountain spotted fever usually appear

2 to 14 days after exposure and include an intractable headache, myalgias, fever, and chills. There is also a characteristic rash that is maculopapular and starts on the wrists and ankles, and then spreads on the extremities toward the trunk. The rash also appears on the palms and soles. In this case, doxycycline is the drug of choice for the treatment of Rocky Mountain spotted fever.

Acyclovir (**choice B**) is an antiviral and is not used for the treatment of *R. rickettsii*. Chloramphenicol (**choice C**) is the drug of choice when tetracycline and doxycycline are contraindicated, as when treating children younger than age 18. Ciprofloxacin (**choice D**) is alternate adult therapy. Sulfonamides (**choice E**) are not used in the treatment of Rocky Mountain spotted fever.

25. **The correct answer is A.** Congestive heart failure may develop secondary to ischemic heart disease, valvular disease, hypertension, and myocarditis. Presenting symptoms include shortness of breath, cough, edema, fatigue, and orthopnea. Chest x-ray reveals increased pulmonary vascularity; if upper lobe veins are dilated it indicates pulmonary venous hypertension.

Coronary artery disease (**choice B**) may presents with fatigue, chest pain, and shortness of breath. Chest x-ray would be normal. Cor pulmonale (**choice D**) is right-sided heart failure noted in patients with a history of chronic bronchitis or emphysema. Symptoms include chronic cough, exertional dyspnea, fatigue, and weakness. Chest x-ray may reveal an enlarged right ventricle. Pneumonia (**choice E**) presents with productive cough and fever. Chest x-ray reveals a pulmonary infiltrate. Pulmonary embolism (**choice C**) presents with tachypnea, tachycardia, shortness of breath, and chest pain.

26. **The correct answer is C.** Paroxysmal supraventricular tachycardia presents with a narrow complex QRS on EKG and is frequently associated with palpitations. If the patient is stable with normal blood pressure and without symptoms, mechanical measures such as vagal maneuvers may convert the patient to normal sinus rhythm. Medications such as adenosine or verapamil can also be used. If the patient is not stable, medications or cardioversion can be used.

27. **The correct answer is D.** Patients with a body mass index (BMI) between 25.0 and 29.9 are considered overweight.

Patients who are muscular (**choice A**) may have higher BMIs. Muscular patients with higher-than-normal BMIs may not have excessive fat, but they are still classified according to the BMI scale.

Patients with a BMI between 18.5 and 24.9 are considered normal (**choice B**).

Patients with a BMI of 30.0 or higher are considered obese (**choice C**).

28. **The correct answer is A.** Neuroleptic malignant syndrome is a life-threatening disorder that consists of muscle rigidity, fever, autonomic instability, and delirium. Laboratory testing reveals an elevated CPK secondary to rhabdomyolysis. Neuroleptic malignant syndrome has been linked to butyrophenones (haloperidol), phenothiazines (chlorpromazine), and metoclopramide (Reglan). Chlordiazepoxide (**choice B**), meperidine (**choice C**), selegiline (**choice D**), and phenelzine (**choice E**) are not commonly linked to neuroleptic malignant syndrome.

29. **The correct answer is A.** This patient has renal vascular hypertension, a disease that usually occurs in females younger than 20 or older than 50. It is suspected if there is an elevated blood pressure, renal artery bruits, and an abrupt deterioration in renal function after administration of an ACE inhibitor.

An abrupt increase of renal function (**choice B**) is incorrect because it is the exact opposite of what is expected to occur and would lead away from the suspected diagnosis.

No change in renal function (**choice C**) would lead away from the suspected diagnosis and a new differential would have to be developed.

An abrupt decrease (**choice D**) and no change (**choice E**) in blood pressure are both incorrect because in this case, the administration of an ACE inhibitor would not have an immediate effect on blood pressure.

30. **The correct answer is C.** Thyroid function tests (TFTs) should be obtained to further evaluate the nodule. If the test indicates that the patient is hypothyroid or euthyroid, then a fine-needle aspirate should be obtained. It should be emphasized that all euthyroid/hypothyroid nodules should be biopsied because the FNA is the definitive test for a solitary thyroid nodule. An ultrasound would be useful to determine whether the mass is solid or cystic, but was not an option in this example.

A repeat exam (**choice A**) is not warranted in this patient. A solitary thyroid nodule has a high risk of being malignant and warrants further investigation. A thyroid scan (**choice B**) provides information on the function of the nodule, but TFTs and an FNA biopsy are necessary for definitive diagnosis.

PTU therapy (**choice D**) is useful in patients with thyrotoxicosis. In this case, there is no evidence to suggest a hyperfunctioning thyroid gland.

Radioablation therapy (**choice E**) is used after thyroidectomy to destroy any remaining malignant cells and lymph nodes. It is useful in the treatment of follicular or papillary thyroid cancer. Nonetheless, a definitive diagnosis should be made before treatment is considered.

31. **The correct answer is A.** Varicella or herpes zoster (shingles) presents with pain followed 48 hours later by grouped, fluid-filled vesicles that distribute unilaterally along a dermatome. Most common dermatomes affected include the trunk or face. Treatment consists of antiviral therapy with acyclovir, famciclovir, or valacyclovir. Fluconazole (**choice B**) is used in the treatment of fungal infections. Beta interferon (**choice C**) is used in the treatment of multiple sclerosis. Tetracycline (**choice D**) is used in the treatment of bacterial infections. Gabapentin (**choice E**) is used in the treatment of seizure disorder and pain control.

32. **The correct answer is D.** Oligoclonal bands are detected via electrophoresis of the cerebrospinal fluid. The bands are found in up to 95% of patients with established multiple sclerosis (MS).

Elevated erythrocyte sedimentation rate (**choice A**) is a nonspecific marker that is found most commonly with vasculitis and inflammatory states, such as arthritis and infection. It is usually normal in MS.

Elevated serum white blood cell count (**choice B**) is found most commonly with infective states. It is usually normal in MS.

Markedly decreased glucose levels in the cerebrospinal fluid (**choice C**) are specific to bacterial meningitis. The condition is not found in MS.

Positive antinuclear antibody titer (**choice E**) is found primarily in systemic lupus erythematosus.

33. **The correct answer is D.** Each of the four cardiac valves can be auscultated at various positions on the chest. The right second intercostal space is the anatomic position for the auscultation of the aortic valve.

The inferior border of the heart (**choice A**) extends from the sixth right costal cartilage to the fifth left intercostal space at the midclavicular line; none of the cardiac valves are auscultated at this anatomic position. The left second intercostal space (**choice B**) is the anatomic position for the auscultation of the pulmonary valve. The left fifth intercostal space (**choice C**) is the anatomic position for the auscultation of the mitral valve. The xiphisternal junction (**choice E**) is the anatomic position for the auscultation of the tricuspid valve.

34. **The correct answer is B.** External hordeolum presents with a localized red, swollen, acutely tender area on the upper or lower eyelid. Warm compresses are first-line therapy. If there is no improvement in 48 hours, then incision and drainage and antibiotics may be needed.

35. **The correct answer is D.** Psyllium is a fiber supplement. An increase in fiber intake may decrease the likelihood of complications, such as diverticulitis.

Antibiotic therapy (**choice A**) is used to treat patients with mild symptoms of diverticulitis.

Patients with diverticulosis are recommended to increase, not decrease (**choice B**), their fluid intake.

Low-residue diets, not high-residue diets (**choice C**), are recommended for diverticular disease.

Surgical intervention (**choice E**) is the treatment of choice for severe disease and patients who fail medical management.

36. **The correct answer is B.** Exophthalmos is pathognomonic for Graves disease. Atrial fibrillation presenting in a previously healthy young woman suggests thyrotoxicosis.

A loud systolic ejection murmur (**choice A**) may be heard in this patient because of the hyperdynamic state, but it would not suggest the diagnosis and may not, in fact, be present at all.

A pericardial friction rub (**choice C**) would present in a patient with pericarditis. A patient with pericarditis may have a tachycardia, but would not necessarily present in atrial fibrillation.

Dry, coarse hair and cool skin (**choice D**) would suggest hypothyroidism and not thyrotoxicosis or Graves disease.

Weight gain (**choice E**) is a hallmark of hypothyroidism.

37. **The correct answer is A.** Otitis media is most commonly noted in infants and develops after upper respiratory tract infections. Patients present with fever, irritability, and tugging at their ears. Physical examination reveals erythematous, bulging tympanic membranes.

Viral rhinitis (**choice B**) and allergic rhinitis (**choice D**) also present with clear nasal drainage and nasal congestion, but the ear examination would be normal and the patient would be afebrile. Otitis externa (**choice C**) presents with purulent ear drainage, and the tympanic membrane is frequently not visualized. Rhinitis medicamentosa (**choice E**) is noted with prolonged use of nasal decongestants and presents with nasal congestion.

38. **The correct answer is B.** Captopril is an angiotensin-converting enzyme (ACE) inhibitor indicated for the treatment of hypertension and congestive heart failure because it has been proven to preserve ventricular function. This agent is commonly used for the treatment of hypertension in diabetic patients because it has been shown to preserve kidney function.

Atenolol (**choice A**) is a beta-receptor blocking agent commonly used in the treatment of hypertension. The usage of beta-adrenergic blocking agents, such as atenolol, may blunt or prevent the appearance of these premonitory signs and symptoms of hypoglycemia in diabetics, and may worsen ventricular function in congestive heart failure patients.

Furosemide (**choice C**) is a potent diuretic commonly used in the treatment of edema associated with congestive heart failure and hypertension. However, the use of this medication in diabetic patients is not recommended because it can cause hyperglycemia and glucose intolerance.

Methyldopa (**choice D**), a centrally acting alpha adrenergic agonist, can be safely used to treat hypertension in diabetic patients. However, due to the severity and frequency of adverse effects associated with this medication, it is not commonly used.

Verapamil (**choice E**) is a calcium channel blocker indicated for the treatment of hypertension, supraventricular tachycardias, and various types of angina. It can be used safely and effectively for the treatment of hypertension in diabetic patients; however, it is not safe for usage in heart failure patients because it has strong negative inotropic effects.

39. **The correct answer is D.** A Rovsing sign is right lower quadrant pain on palpation of the lower left quadrant.

Asterixis (**choice A**) is seen in a metabolic encephalopathy frequently caused by liver disease. Cullen sign (**choice B**) is seen in hemorrhagic pancreatitis. Murphy sign (**choice C**) is seen in an acute cholecystitis.

Shifting dullness (**choice E**) is seen in ascites.

40. **The correct answer is C.** Secondary syphilis presents with a generalized maculopapular rash also noted on the palms of the hands and soles of the feet. The rash typically develops a few weeks after the development of the initial chancre. Generalized nontender lymphadenopathy is also noted. The tests for syphilis—including the screening tests RPR, VDRL, and TP-EIA, and the confirmatory tests FTA-ABS and TP-PA—are all positive.

C-reactive protein (**choice A**) is a test for inflammation and not specific for syphilis. Dark field microscopy and not Gram stain (**choice D**) is used to diagnose syphilis. Lyme titer (**choice B**) is used to diagnose Lyme disease, which does not present with a chancre. Weil-Felix test (**choice E**) is used in the diagnosis of rickettsial infections, which do not present with a chancre.

41. **The correct answer is C.** Specific phobia is an anxiety disorder characterized by intense fear of a particular object (e.g., snakes) or situation (e.g., heights). Many specific phobias remit spontaneously. If treatment is needed, it consists of exposure therapy. There is no role for medications in the treatment of specific phobias.

Lithium (**choice A**) is used in the treatment of bipolar disorder.

Benzodiazepine (**choice B**) is used in the treatment of anxiety disorder but is not considered first line in the treatment of specific phobias.

Insight-oriented therapy (**choice D**) is used in the treatment of mood disorders, anxiety disorders, eating disorders, and sexual dysfunction.

Electroconvulsive therapy (**choice E**) is used in the treatment of major depression, mania, and catatonia.

42. **The correct answer is A.** Phentolamine will reverse the effects of the epinephrine. Unopposed beta activity will cause a decrease in blood pressure.

43. **The correct answer is E.** Methanol (wood alcohol) is found in a number of solvents. Methanol is metabolized to the toxic substance formic acid. Treatment options for patients with methanol poisoning include hemodialysis, ethanol, or fomepizole.

44. **The correct answer is D.** Tuberculosis occurs disproportionately in patients who are malnourished, homeless, or living in crowded conditions. Presenting symptoms include malaise, anorexia, weight loss, fever, cough, night sweats, and hemoptysis. Diagnostic testing

consists of acid-fast smears and cultures. Chest x-ray findings in tuberculosis consist of unilateral infiltrates, hilar adenopathy, pleural effusions, and discrete nodules or cavitary lesions in the upper lobes or superior segments of the lower lobes.

Bilateral interstitial infiltrates (**choice E**) are noted in pneumonia secondary to pneumocystis, viral, and mycoplasma infection. Hyperinflation with a flattened diaphragm (**choice B**) is noted in emphysema. Eggshell calcification of hilar lymph nodes (**choice A**) is noted in silicosis and treated lymphoma. Pleural thickening and hyperinflation (**choice C**) are noted in mesothelioma and asbestosis.

45. **The correct answer is A.** Reye syndrome is associated with aspirin consumption in children with a viral infection. Patients present with rash, vomiting, mental status changes, liver damage, and hypoglycemia. Guillain-Barré syndrome (**choice B**) presents with an ascending weakness and loss of deep tendon reflexes. Phenylketonuria (**choice D**) is an inborn error of metabolism and presents with seizures, mental status changes, and a musty odor to the baby's sweat and urine. Lesch-Nyhan syndrome (**choice E**) is a rare inherited disorder that presents with neurologic dysfunction, cognitive and behavioral disturbances including self-mutilation, and uric acid overproduction. Acute bacterial meningitis (**choice C**) presents with fever, nuchal rigidity, and change in mental status. There would be no abnormality on liver examination.

46. **The correct answer is E.** This patient presents with findings consistent with cerebrovascular accident (CVA). With no evidence of hemorrhage on CT scan, the patient with symptoms less than 34 hours old should be treated acutely with a thrombolytic, such as tissue plasminogen activator.

Anticoagulant medications, such as aspirin (**choice A**) and clopidogrel (**choice C**) are used in the prevention of stroke. Vena cava filter (**choice D**) is also used as a preventive measure for stroke. Warfarin (**choice B**) is used in patients ineligible for thrombolytic therapy and for long-term anticoagulation.

47. **The correct answer is B.** Niacin, or vitamin B_3, is a pharmacologic agent that causes a reduction in LDL cholesterol in around 5 to 7 days with the maximal effect seen in 3 to 5 weeks. Triglycerides and VLDL are reduced by 20 to 40% in 1 to 4 days. Furthermore, HDL levels can increase by 20%. This agent is indicated as adjunctive therapy in patients with elevated choles-

terol and triglycerides when diet and other nondrug therapies are inadequate. The most common adverse effect of this agent is generalized flushing with a sensation of warmth, especially in the facial area. This reaction is noted to be so severe in some patients that they discontinue therapy for this reason alone. Other common adverse effects include hepatotoxicity, tachycardia (**choice A**), hypoalbuminemia (**choice C**) and hyperglycemia (**choice D**), as well as nausea, vomiting, hyperuricemia, glucose intolerance, pruritus, peptic ulcer disease, and dry skin.

48. **The correct answer is E.** The clinical scenario is consistent with adrenal insufficiency (AI). The hyperpigmentation and hypotension are the hallmarks of the disease. The most rapid test that will help rule out AI is the random cortisol level. A random cortisol level of greater than or equal to 18 μg/dL excludes adrenal insufficiency.

A 24-hour urine collection for cortisol (**choice A**) is the most appropriate first test for Cushing's syndrome. Serum cortisol levels rise in the morning (**choice B**); therefore, a single serum cortisol level that is >1.8 μg/dL is diagnostic for Cushing syndrome. A dexamethasone suppression test (**choice C**) that suppresses cortisol to <5 μg/dL at 8 A.M. after a dose of dexamethasone at midnight excludes Cushing syndrome in 98% of patients. A CT scan of the adrenals (**choice D**), although useful as an adjunctive test, is not necessary in the initial diagnosis of adrenal insufficiency.

49. **The correct answer is A.** Most patients do not get enough fiber in their diet, so fiber intake must be increased. The management of constipation may include all of the remaining options.

50. **The correct answer is A.** The loading of O_2 is facilitated when the oxygen dissociation curve shifts to the left, and the unloading of O_2 is facilitated when the oxygen dissociation curve shifts to the right. Carbon monoxide (CO) poisoning is extremely dangerous for several reasons. CO left-shifts the oxygen dissociation curve, which interferes with the unloading of O_2. Also, CO, which has approximately 240 times the affinity for hemoglobin than does O_2, preferentially binds to available sites on hemoglobin.

The remaining answer choices all shift the oxygen-hemoglobin dissociation curve to the right. A good way to remember the conditions that promote dissociation of O_2 is to think of exercising muscle, which has decreased pH (**choice B**) due to lactic acid buildup and increased P_{CO_2} (**choice D**), increased 2,3-DPG

(2,3-diphosphoglycerate; **choice C**) due to increased glycolysis, and increased temperature (**choice E**).

51. **The correct answer is C.** Dopamine agonists are now being used more frequently as a first-line medication for treating Parkinson disease. Levodopa is also used, but it has a lower response rate in improving symptoms, and patients who do respond well tend to develop central side effects secondary to the levodopa later in the treatment.

    Anticonvulsants, such as phenytoin (**choice A**), are used in the treatment and prophylaxis of a variety of seizure types.

    A beta-blocker (e.g., propranolol) (**choice B**) is used primarily for treating benign essential tremors. It is also still used predominantly for migraine headache prophylaxis.

    Lithium carbonate (**choice D**) decreases the severity of symptoms in tardive dyskinesia. It is also primarily used in bipolar disorder.

    Placement of a ventricular shunt (**choice E**) is used exclusively for hydrocephalus, which is not an etiology for Parkinson disease.

52. **The correct answer is B.** Propranolol is the recommended drug for treating the cardiac manifestations of thyrotoxicosis.

    Diltiazem (**choice A**) would slow the heart rate, but would not achieve the other desirable effects of reducing tremor and anxiety.

    Propylthiouracil (**choice C**) is generally used for treatment of Graves disease when ablation is not possible. Because it takes weeks to months, patients often need propranolol additionally during therapy to manage cardiac complaints.

    Iodine (**choice D**) ablation is an excellent method of destroying thyroid tissue in patients with Graves disease. It is contraindicated in pregnancy.

    Radioablation therapy (**choice E**) is not indicated in the treatment of Graves disease.

53. **The correct answer is E.** A boxer's fracture is a fracture of the fifth metacarpal neck, often caused by direct trauma.

    A Colles fracture (**choice A**) is a wrist fracture involving a break of the end of the radius bone of the forearm. Salter-Harris (**choice B**) is a classification system for physeal fractures in children. Rolando fractures (**choice C**) are comminuted thumb metacarpal base fractures. Bennett fractures (**choice D**) are fractures involving the base of the thumb.

54. **The correct answer is B.** Deficiencies of the B complex vitamins and folate in particular can cause large increases in homocysteine levels (exceeding 100 mmol/L). Foods rich in B vitamins, i.e. folate, B_{12} and B_6, help keep homocysteine at safe levels. When B-vitamins are provided, the homocysteine levels may decrease. Conversely, low levels of blood folate are consistently related to high levels of homocysteine. Folate (also known as folic acid) seems to have a greater clearing effect on homocysteine levels than does B_6, B_{12}, or both vitamins combined.

    Decreased lipoprotein A (**choice A**) does not directly affect homocysteine, although concomitant lipoprotein abnormalities may also be mechanisms by which hyperhomocysteinemia promotes atherosclerosis.

    Increased cholesterol levels (**choice C**) is another important modifiable factor that can increase the risk of atherosclerosis, but it does not affect homocysteine levels.

    Decreased fibrinolytic activity (**choice D**) is directly affected by elevated lipoprotein A levels but not homocysteine.

    Hyperinsulinemia (**choice E**) appears to influence homocysteine metabolism, yet the association between the two has not been studied extensively and it does not directly lead to hyperhomocysteinemia.

55. **The correct answer is B.** Surgery is not consistently effective in this scenario, though it is routinely successful if the hemorrhage occurs in the cerebellum.

    Anticoagulant therapy (**choice A**) is relatively contraindicated in the setting of a hemorrhagic stroke. It is indicated in strokes that do not present with hemorrhage.

    Immediate and rapid lowering of blood pressure via intravenous labetalol or intravenous nitroglycerine (**choice C**) is not recommended in the initial treatment of stroke. Blood pressure should not be lowered precipitously due to the risk of decreasing blood and oxygen perfusion to the area surrounding the infarct.

    Placement of a ventricular shunt (**choice D**) would only be used in the setting of hydrocephalus. If the intracranial pressure becomes markedly elevated from hemorrhage or hematoma, it is more appropriate to consider surgical evacuation via a craniotomy.

    Streptokinase thrombolytic therapy (**choice E**) is contraindicated in stroke management because of a demonstrated high risk for intracranial hemorrhage. Other thrombolytics are often used as first-line treatments for stroke, although this patient's present hemorrhage is a contraindication for any thrombolytic therapy.

56. The correct answer is D. The therapy for any patient with type 2 diabetes mellitus and hyperlipidemia is a statin. All patients must be counseled on the importance of exercise and low-cholesterol diet—both of which are imperative to long-term control of hyperlipidemia.

57. The correct answer is C. Prednisone is a corticosteroid indicated for the treatment of primary or secondary adrenal cortical insufficiency (primarily cortisone or hydrocortisone) and rheumatic disorders (treatment of pain associated with inflammation, edema, and nerve compression), as well as a variety of dermatologic and allergic disorders. It is associated with the development of fluid and electrolyte imbalances such as sodium and fluid retention, hypokalemia, and hypocalcemia. It is also associated with endocrine abnormalities, such as hyperglycemia, and the development of a cushingoid state (moon face, buffalo hump, and central obesity). Other side effects include immunosuppression, hypertension, psychosis, and osteoporosis.

58. The correct answer is C. Decompression by gentle insertion of a flexible sigmoidoscope should be tried before surgical intervention.

Elective resection (**choice A**) is recommended for good-risk patients who have been treated successfully by decompression. The risk of recurrence is great.

Emergent surgical intervention (**choice B**) is warranted if decompression is unsuccessful or if strangulation or perforation is suspected.

Choice D is not recommended.

Total abdominal colectomy (**choice E**) is not appropriate in this case.

59. The correct answer is B. The local anesthetics are divided into two groups: esters, which are derivatives of para-aminobenzoic acid, and amides, which are derivatives of aniline. These esters are primarily metabolized by plasma esterases, such as plasma cholinesterase.

Examples of esters include chloroprocaine, procaine, and tetracaine. Bupivacaine (**choice A**), etidocaine (**choice C**), mepivacaine (**choice D**), and prilocaine (**choice E**) are all amides and are metabolized in the liver.

60. The correct answer is C. Cisplatin is an antineoplastic commonly used in the treatment of metastatic ovarian and testicular cancers as well as advanced bladder cancer. This medication, in addition to numerous other toxicities, is associated with the development of profound nausea and vomiting. In fact, it is considered to be one of the most emetogenic agents on the pharmaceutical market. The selective 5-hydroxytryptamine 3 (5-HT3) receptor antagonists are potent antinauseant and antiemetogenic agents indicated for prevention of emesis in cancer therapy, including high-dose cisplatin. Examples of 5-HT3 receptor antagonists include ondansetron, granisetron, and dolasetron.

Diphenhydramine (**choice A**) is an antihistamine with anticholinergic activity; it is indicated in the treatment of allergy signs and symptoms. It can be used in the treatment of nausea and vomiting associated with motion sickness.

Dronabinol (**choice B**) is the principal psychoactive substance present in *Cannabis sativa* (marijuana). The mechanism of its antiemetic action is largely unknown; it is indicated for the treatment of severe nausea and vomiting when conventional therapies are ineffective.

Metoclopramide (**choice D**) is a prokinetic agent indicated for the treatment of GERD and diabetic gastroparesis. Because this agent blocks dopaminergic receptors in the chemotrigger zone, it is also effective in the treatment of severe nausea and vomiting.

Prochlorperazine (**choice E**) is a phenothiazine antiemetic that exerts its action through the blocking of dopaminergic receptors in the chemotrigger zone.

PART V

PANCE/PANRE Resources

Common Medical Abbreviations and Laboratory Values

Abbreviation	Meaning
a	Before
AED	Automated external defibrillator
ac	Before meals
AMA	Against medical advice
AMI	Acute myocardial infarction
ASA	Aspirin
ASHD	Arteriosclerotic heart disease
bid	Twice a day
BP	Blood pressure
BS	Breath sounds, bowel sounds, or blood sugar
BVM	Bag-valve-mask
c/o	Complaining of
ca	Cancer/carcinoma
CC	Chief complaint
CHF	Congestive heart failure
CO	Carbon monoxide
COPD	Chronic obstructive pulmonary disease
CPR	Cardiopulmonary resuscitation
CSF	Cerebrospinal fluid
CVA	Cerebrovascular accident
CXR	Chest x-ray
d/c	Discontinue
DM	Diabetes mellitus
DOA	Dead on arrival
DOB	Date of birth
Dx	Diagnosis
ECG, EKG	Electrocardiogram
e.g.	For example
ETA	Estimated time of arrival
EtOH	Alcohol (ethanol)

Abbreviation	Meaning
Fx	Fracture
GI	Gastrointestinal
GSW	Gunshot wound
gtt	Drop
GU	Genitourinary
GYN	Gynecologic
h, hr	Hour
H/A	Headache
HEENT	Head, ears, eyes, nose, throat
Hg	Mercury
h/o	History of
hs	At bedtime
HTN	Hypertension
Hx	History
ICP	Intracranial pressure
ICU	Intensive care unit
IM	Intramuscular
IO	Intraosseous
JVD	Jugular venous distension
KVO	Keep vein open
L	Left, liter
LAC	Laceration
LOC	Level of consciousness, loss of consciousness
LR	Lactated Ringer's solution
mcg	Micrograms
MS	Morphine sulfate, multiple sclerosis
NAD	No apparent distress
NC	Nasal cannula
NKA	No known allergies
npo	Nothing by mouth
NRB	Non-rebreather mask
NS	Normal saline
NSR	Normal sinus rhythm
NTG	Nitroglycerin
N/V	Nausea/vomiting
O_2	Oxygen
OB	Obstetrics
OD	Overdose
OR	Operating room
PCN	Penicillin

Abbreviation	Meaning
PEA	Pulseless electrical activity
PERRLA	Pupils equal, round, and reactive to light and accommodation
PID	Pelvic inflammatory disease
PND	Paroxysmal nocturnal dyspnea
po	By mouth
PRN	As needed
PSVT	Paroxysmal supraventricular tachycardia
Pt	Patient
PTA	Prior to arrival
PVC	Premature ventricular contraction
qh	Every hour
qid; QID	Four times a day
R	Right
r/o	Rule out
Rx or Tx	Treatment
SIDS	Sudden infant death syndrome
SOB	Shortness of breath
stat	Immediately
SVT	Supraventricular tachycardia
TIA	Transient ischemic attack
tid; TID	Three times a day
TKO	To keep open
VS	Vital signs
x	Times
w/o	Without
WNL	Within normal limits
y/o or yo	Years old
Δ	change
+	Positive
−	Negative

STANDARD REFERENCE LABORATORY VALUES
* Included in the Biochemical Profile

	REFERENCE RANGE	SI REFERENCE INTERVALS

BLOOD, PLASMA, SERUM

	REFERENCE RANGE	SI REFERENCE INTERVALS
* Alanine aminotransferase (ALT), serum	8–20 U/L	8–20 U/L
Amylase, serum	25–125 U/L	25–125 U/L
* Aspartate aminotransferase (AST), serum	8–20 U/L	8–20 U/L
Bilirubin, serum (adult) Total // Direct	0.1–1.0 mg/dL // 0.0–0.3 mg/dL	2–17 µmol/L // 0–5 µmol/L
* Calcium, serum (Ca^{2+})	8.4–10.2 mg/dL	2.1–2.8 mmol/L
* Cholesterol, serum	Rec: <200 mg/dL	<5.2 mmol/L
Cortisol, serum	0800 h: 5–23 µg/dL // 1600 h: 3–15 µg/dL	138–635 nmol/L // 82–413 nmol/L
	2000 h: ≤ 50% of 0800 h	Fraction of 0800 h: ≤ 0.50
Creatine kinase, serum	Male: 25–90 U/L	25–90 U/L
	Female: 10–70 U/L	10–70 U/L
* Creatinine, serum	0.6–1.2 mg/dL	53–106 µmol/L
Electrolytes, serum		
Sodium (Na^+)	136–145 mEq/L	136–145 mmol/L
* Potassium (K^+)	3.5–5.0 mEq/L	3.5–5.0 mmol/L
Chloride (Cl^-)	95–105 mEq/L	95–105 mmol/L
Bicarbonate (HCO_3^-)	22–28 mEq/L	22–28 mmol/L
Magnesium (Mg^{2+})	1.5–2.0 mEq/L	0.75–1.0 mmol/L
Estriol, total, serum (in pregnancy)		
24–28 wks // 32–36 wks	30–170 ng/mL // 60–280 ng/mL	104–590 nmol/L // 208–970 nmol/L
28–32 wks // 36–40 wks	40–220 ng/mL // 80–350 ng/mL	140–760 nmol/L // 280–1210 nmol/L
Ferritin, serum	Male: 15–200 ng/mL	15–200 µg/L
	Female: 12–150 ng/mL	12–150 µg/L
Follicle-stimulating hormone, serum/plasma	Male: 4–25 mIU/mL	4–25 U/L
	Female: premenopause 4–30 mIU/mL	4–30 U/L
	midcycle peak 10–90 mIU/mL	10–90 U/L
	postmenopause 40–250 mIU/mL	40–250 U/L
Gases, arterial blood (room air)		
pH	7.35–7.45	[H^+] 36–44 nmol/L
Pco_2	33–45 mm Hg	4.4–5.9 kPa
Po_2	75–105 mm Hg	10.0–14.0 kPa
* Glucose, serum	Fasting: 70–110 mg/dL	3.8–6.1 mmol/L
	2 h postprandial: < 120 mg/dL	< 6.6 mmol/L
Growth hormone – arginine stimulation	Fasting: < 5 ng/mL	< 5 µg/L
	Provocative stimuli: > 7 ng/mL	> 7 µg/L
Immunoglobulins, serum		
IgA	76–390 mg/dL	0.76–3.90 g/L
IgE	0–380 IU/mL	0–380 kIU/L
IgG	650–1500 mg/dL	6.5–15 g/L
IgM	40–345 mg/dL	0.4–3.45 g/L
Iron	50–170 µg/dL	9–30 µmol/L
Lactate dehydrogenase, serum	45–90 U/L	45–90 U/L
Luteinizing hormone, serum/plasma	Male: 6–23 mIU/mL	6–23 U/L
	Female: follicular phase 5–30 mIU/mL	5–30 U/L
	midcycle 75–150 mIU/mL	75–150 U/L
	postmenopause 30–200 mIU/mL	30–200 U/L
Osmolality, serum	275–295 mOsmol/kg H_2O	275–295 mOsmol/kg H_2O
Parathyroid hormone, serum, N-terminal	230–630 pg/mL	230–630 ng/L
* Phosphatase (alkaline), serum (p-NPP at 30°C)	20–70 U/L	20–70 U/L
* Phosphorus (inorganic), serum	3.0–4.5 mg/dL	1.0–1.5 mmol/L
Prolactin, serum (hPRL)	< 20 ng/mL	< 20 µg/L
* Proteins, serum		
Total (recumbent)	6.0–7.8 g/dL	60–78 g/L
Albumin	3.5–5.5 g/dL	35–55 g/L
Globulin	2.3–3.5 g/dL	23–35 g/L
Thyroid-stimulating hormone, serum or plasma	0.5–5.0 µU/mL	0.5–5.0 mU/L
Thyroidal iodine (^{123}I) uptake	8%–30% of administered dose/24 h	0.08–0.30/24 h
Thyroxine (T_4), serum	5–12 µg/dL	64–155 nmol/L
Triglycerides, serum	35–160 mg/dL	0.4–1.81 mmol/L
Triiodothyronine (T_3), serum (RIA)	115–190 ng/dL	1.8–2.9 nmol/L
Triiodothyronine (T_3) resin uptake	25%–35%	0.25–0.35
* Urea nitrogen, serum	7–18 mg/dL	1.2–3.0 mmol/L
* Uric acid, serum	3.0–8.2 mg/dL	0.18–0.48 mmol/L

	REFERENCE RANGE	SI REFERENCE INTERVALS
BODY MASS INDEX (BMI)		
Body mass index	Adult: 19–25 kg/m^2	
CEREBROSPINAL FLUID		
Cell count	0–5/mm^3	0–5 × 10^6/L
Chloride	118–132 mEq/L	118–132 mmol/L
Gamma globulin	3%–12% total proteins	0.03–0.12
Glucose	40–70 mg/dL	2.2–3.9 mmol/L
Pressure	70–180 mm H$_2$O	70–180 mm H$_2$O
Proteins, total	< 40 mg/dL	< 0.40 g/L
HEMATOLOGIC		
Bleeding time (template)	2–7 minutes	2–7 minutes
Erythrocyte count	Male: 4.3–5.9 million/mm^3	4.3–5.9 × 10^{12}/L
	Female: 3.5–5.5 million/mm^3	3.5–5.5 × 10^{12}/L
Erythrocyte sedimentation rate (Westergren)	Male: 0–15 mm/h	0–15 mm/h
	Female: 0–20 mm/h	0–20 mm/h
Hematocrit	Male: 41%–53%	0.41–0.53
	Female: 36%–46%	0.36–0.46
Hemoglobin A$_{1c}$	≤ 6%	≤ 0.06
Hemoglobin, blood	Male: 13.5–17.5 g/dL	2.09–2.71 mmol/L
	Female: 12.0–16.0 g/dL	1.86–2.48 mmol/L
Hemoglobin, plasma	1–4 mg/dL	0.16–0.62 mmol/L
Leukocyte count and differential		
Leukocyte count	4500–11,000/mm^3	4.5–11.0 × 10^9/L
Segmented neutrophils	54%–62%	0.54–0.62
Bands	3%–5%	0.03–0.05
Eosinophils	1%–3%	0.01–0.03
Basophils	0%–0.75%	0–0.0075
Lymphocytes	25%–33%	0.25–0.33
Monocytes	3%–7%	0.03–0.07
Mean corpuscular hemoglobin	25.4–34.6 pg/cell	0.39–0.54 fmol/cell
Mean corpuscular hemoglobin concentration	31%–36% Hb/cell	4.81–5.58 mmol Hb/L
Mean corpuscular volume	80–100 μm^3	80–100 fL
Partial thromboplastin time (activated)	25–40 seconds	25–40 seconds
Platelet count	150,000–400,000/mm^3	150–400 × 10^9/L
Prothrombin time	11–15 seconds	11–15 seconds
Reticulocyte count	0.5%–1.5%	0.005–0.015
Thrombin time	< 2 seconds deviation from control	< 2 seconds deviation from control
Volume		
Plasma	Male: 25–43 mL/kg	0.025–0.043 L/kg
	Female: 28–45 mL/kg	0.028–0.045 L/kg
Red cell	Male: 20–36 mL/kg	0.020–0.036 L/kg
	Female: 19–31 mL/kg	0.019–0.031 L/kg
SWEAT		
Chloride	0–35 mmol/L	0–35 mmol/L
URINE		
Calcium	100–300 mg/24 h	2.5–7.5 mmol/24 h
Chloride	Varies with intake	Varies with intake
Creatinine clearance	Male: 97–137 mL/min	
	Female: 88–128 mL/min	
Estriol, total (in pregnancy)		
30 wks	6–18 mg/24 h	21–62 μmol/24 h
35 wks	9–28 mg/24 h	31–97 μmol/24 h
40 wks	13–42 mg/24 h	45–146 μmol/24 h
17-Hydroxycorticosteroids	Male: 3.0–10.0 mg/24 h	8.2–27.6 μmol/24 h
	Female: 2.0–8.0 mg/24 h	5.5–22.0 μmol/24 h
17-Ketosteroids, total	Male: 8–20 mg/24 h	28–70 μmol/24 h
	Female: 6–15 mg/24 h	21–52 μmol/24 h
Osmolality	50–1400 mOsmol/kg H$_2$O	
Oxalate	8–40 μg/mL	90–445 μmol/L
Potassium	Varies with diet	Varies with diet
Proteins, total	< 150 mg/24 h	< 0.15 g/24 h
Sodium	Varies with diet	Varies with diet
Uric acid	Varies with diet	Varies with diet

State Statutory and Regulatory Requirements for Licensure

State	Graduation from PA Program	Passage of NCCPA Exam	Current NCCPA Certification	Additional Requirements	Renewal Requirements
Alabama	X	X			CME
Alaska	X	X	X		NCCPA
Arizona	X	X	X^1		CME
Arkansas	X	X		baccalaureate degree	CME
California	X	X			CME
Colorado	X	X	X		
Connecticut	X	X	X	baccalaureate degree	NCCPA
Delaware	X	X		baccalaureate degree	CME
District of Columbia	X	X			CME
Florida	X	X			CME
Osteopathic	*X*	*X*			*CME*
Georgia	X	X			CME
Hawaii	X	X	X		NCCPA
Idaho	X	X		baccalaureate degree[2]	NCCPA and CME
Illinois	X	X	X		NCCPA
Indiana	X	X	X		NCCPA
Iowa	X	X			CME
Kansas	X	X			CME
Kentucky	X	X	X		NCCPA
Louisiana	X	X	X		NCCPA
Maine	X	X	X		CME
Osteopathic	*X*	*X*			*CME*

State	Graduation from PA Program	Passage of NCCPA Exam	Current NCCPA Certification	Additional Requirements	Renewal Requirements
Maryland	X	X		baccalaureate degree	CME
Massachusetts	X	X		baccalaureate degree	CME
Michigan	X	X			
Osteopathic	*X*	*X*			
Minnesota		X	X		CME (NCCPA for Rx)
Mississippi	X	X	X	master's degree[3]	CME
Missouri	X[4]	X	X	master's degree for those graduating after 1/1/08	NCCPA
Montana	X	X	X		NCCPA
Nebraska	X	X			CME
Nevada	X	X	X		CME
Osteopathic	*X*	*X*	*X*		*CME/NCCPA*
New Hampshire	X	X	X		NCCPA
New Jersey	X	X			CME
New Mexico	X	X	X		NCCPA (CME for controlled Rx)
Osteopathic	*X*	*X*	*X*		*NCCPA*
New York	X	X		baccalaureate degree[5]	
North Carolina	X	X			CME
North Dakota		X	X		NCCPA
Ohio	X	X	X	master's degree[6]	NCCPA
Oklahoma	X	X		For graduates after 7/2007, program must meet specific requirements.	CME
Oregon	X	X			NCCPA for Sch. II
Pennsylvania	X	X	X	baccalaureate degree	NCCPA
Osteopathic	*X*	*X*	*X*	*baccalaureate degree*	*NCCPA*

State	Graduation from PA Program	Passage of NCCPA Exam	Current NCCPA Certification	Additional Requirements	Renewal Requirements
Rhode Island	X	X			CME
South Carolina	X	X	X		NCCPA
South Dakota	X	X			CME
Tennessee	X	X			CME
Texas	X	X	X		CME
Utah	X	X		passage of Utah PA Law and Rules Exam	CME
Vermont	X	X			CME
Virginia	X	X	X		NCCPA
Washington	X	X			CME or NCCPA Certification
Osteopathic	*X*	*X*			*CME (NCCPA for Schedule II Rx)*
West Virginia	X	X	X		NCCPA
Osteopathic	*X*	*X*	*X*		*NCCPA*
Wisconsin	X	X	X		
Wyoming	X	X	X		NCCPA

Notes

1 An applicant who presents a certificate issued by the NCCPA that shows the applicant passed either the PANCE or the NCCPA recertification examination within the six-year period preceding presentation of the certificate to the Board shall be deemed to have met the requirement of A.R.S. § 32-2521(A)(2). See Arizona Admin. Code R4-17-202.

2 Graduate PA licensure may also be considered by the board when all requirements have been met with the exception of a baccalaureate degree. Plan for completion of the baccalaureate degree must be submitted and approved by the board. Degree must be completed within 5 years. See Idaho Admin. Code 22.01.03.036.

3 Board may issue temporary license to PAs enrolled in master's program.

4 Program requirement waived for those employed as PAs prior to 1986.

5 New York requires infection control training as a condition before licensure and then every 4 years after initial licensure. See Office of the Professions site for more details, *http://www.op.nysed.gov/training/icmemo.htm*.

6 The master's degree requirement is waived if the PA has a current, valid license or other form of authority to practice that was issued by another jurisdiction prior to January 1, 2008. Effective March 22, 2013, the masters requirement is also waived if the PA can provide evidence of 1) graduating from an accredited program and 2) experience practicing as a PA for at least three consecutive years while on active duty, in any of the armed forces of the United States or a state national guard, including any experience attained while practicing as a PA at a federal VA health facility.

State/U.S. Territory Licensing Authorities

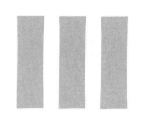

Alabama
Board of Medical Examiners
P.O. Box 946
Montgomery, AL 36101-0946
(334) 242-4116
http://www.albme.org/

Alaska
State Medical Board
Division of Occupational Licensing
550 West 7th Avenue, Suite 1500
Anchorage, AK 99501-3567
(907) 269-8163
http://www.commerce.alaska.gov/dnn/cbpl/ProfessionalLicensing/StateMedicalBoard.aspx

American Samoa
Health Services Regulatory Board
LBJ Tropical Medical Center
Pago Pago, AS 96700
(684) 633-1222
fax (684) 633-1869
https://www.ncsbn.org/American%20Samoa.htm

Arizona
Regulatory Board of Physician Assistants
9545 East Doubletree Ranch Road
Scottsdale, AZ 85258
(480) 551-2700 or (877) 255-2212
http://www.azpa.gov/

Arkansas
State Medical Board
1401 West Capitol Avenue, Suite 340
Little Rock, AR 72201-2936
(501) 296-1802
http://www.armedicalboard.org/

California
Physician Assistant Committee
2005 Evergreen Street, Suite 1100
Sacramento, CA 95815
(916) 561-8780
http://www.pac.ca.gov/

Colorado
Board of Medical Examiners
1560 Broadway, Suite 1350
Denver, CO 80202
(303) 894-7800
http://www.dora.state.co.us/medical/

Connecticut
Division of Medical Quality Assurance
Department of Public Health - PA Licensing
410 Capitol Avenue
PO Box 340308
Hartford, CT 06134
(860) 509-8000
http://www.ct.gov/dph/cwp/view.asp?a=3121&q=389510

Delaware
Board of Medical Practice
Cannon Bldg., Suite 203
861 Silver Lake Boulevard
Dover, DE 19904
(302) 744-4500
http://dpr.delaware.gov/boards/medicalpractice/index.shtml

District of Columbia
Board of Medicine
889 North Capitol Street, NE
Washington, DC 20002
(877) 672-2174
http://doh.dc.gov/node/166752

Florida
Board of Medicine
4052 Bald Cypress Way, Bin #C03
Tallahassee, FL 32399-3253
(850) 488-0595
http://flboardofmedicine.gov/

Board of Osteopathic Medicine
4052 Bald Cypress Way, Bin #C06
Tallahassee, FL 32399-3257
(850) 488-0595
http://floridasosteopathicmedicine.gov/

Georgia
Composite State Medical Board
2 Peachtree Street NW, 36th Floor
Atlanta, GA 30303-3465
(404) 656-3913
http://medicalboard.georgia.gov/portal/site/GCMB/

Guam
Board of Medical Examiners
Health Professionals Licensing Office
651 Legacy Square Commercial Complex
South Route 10, Suite 9
Mangilao, GU 96913
(011) (671) 735-7406
http://www.dphss.guam.gov/content/guam-board-medical-examiners

Hawaii
Board of Medical Examiners
Department of Commerce & Consumer Affairs
Division of Professional Licensing
P.O. Box 3469
Honolulu, HI 96801
(808) 586-3000
http://hawaii.gov/dcca/areas/pvl/boards/medical/

Idaho
Board of Medicine
P.O. Box 83720
Boise, ID 83720-0058
(208) 327-7000
http://www.bom.state.id.us/

Illinois
Division of Professional Regulation
320 West Washington Street, 3rd Floor
Springfield, IL 62786
(217) 785-0820 or (800) 560-6420
http://www.idfpr.com/dpr/WHO/adjmed.asp

Indiana
Professional Licensing Agency
Attn: PA Committee
402 West Washington Street, Suite W072
Indianapolis, IN 46204
(317) 234-2060
http://www.in.gov/pla/pa.htm

Iowa
Board of Physician Assistants
Professional Licensing Division
321 East 12th Street
Des Moines, IA 50319-0075
(515) 281-7689 or (866) 227-9878
http://www.idph.state.ia.us/licensure/PhysicianAssistants.aspx

Kansas
Board of Healing Arts
800 SW Jackson, Lower Level, Suite A
Topeka, KS 66612
(785) 296-7413 or (888) 886-7205
http://www.ksbha.org/

Kentucky
Board of Medical Licensure
310 Whittington Parkway, Suite 1B
Louisville, KY 40222
(502) 429-7150
http://kbml.ky.gov/ah/Pages/Physician-Assistant.aspx

Louisiana
Board of Medical Examiners
630 Camp Street
New Orleans, LA 70130
(504) 568-6820
http://www.lsbme.louisiana.gov/

Maine
Board of Licensure in Medicine
137 State House Station
161 Capitol Street
Augusta, ME 04333-0137
(207) 287-3601
http://www.docboard.org/me/me_home.htm

Board of Osteopathic Examiners
142 State House Station
161 Capitol Street
Augusta, ME 04333-0142
(207) 287-2480
http://www.maine.gov/osteo/

Maryland
Board of Physicians
4201 Patterson Avenue
Baltimore, MD 21215
(410) 764-4777 or (800) 492-6836
http://www.mbp.state.md.us/pages/phys_assi.html

Massachusetts
Board of Physician Assistant Registration
Division of Registration
239 Causeway Street, Suite 500
Boston, MA 02114
(800) 414-0168
http://www.mass.gov/eohhs/gov/departments/dph/programs/hcq/ dhpl/physician-assistants/

Michigan
Physician Assistant Task Force
Bureau of Health Care Services
P.O. Box 30670
Lansing, MI 48909
(517) 335-0918
http://www.michigan.gov/mdch/0,1607,7-132-27417_27529_ 27550---,00.html

Minnesota
Board of Medical Practice
2829 University Avenue SE, Suite 500
Minneapolis, MN 55414-3246
(612) 617-2130
http://www.state.mn.us/portal/mn/jsp/home.do?agency=BMP

Mississippi
Board of Medical Licensure
1867 Crane Ridge Drive, Suite 200B
Jackson, MS 39216
(601) 987-3079
http://www.msbml.state.ms.us/

Missouri
Board of Registration for the Healing Arts
State Advisory Commission for Physician Assistants
P.O. Box 4
Jefferson City, MO 65102
(573) 751-0098 or (866) 289-5753
http://pr.mo.gov/physicianassistants.asp

Montana
Board of Medical Examiners
P.O. Box 200513
Helena, MT 59620-0513
(406) 841-2203
http://bsd.dli.mt.gov/license/bsd_boards/med_board/board_page.asp

Nebraska
Board of Examiners in Medicine and Surgery
P.O. Box 94986
Lincoln, NE 68509-4986
(402) 471-2118
*http://dhhs.ne.gov/publichealth/Pages/crl_medical_medsur_*
pa_pa.aspx

Nevada
Board of Medical Examiners
P.O. Box 7238
Reno, NV 89510
(775) 688-2559 or (888) 890-8210
http://medboard.nv.gov/

State Board of Osteopathic Medicine
901 American Pacific Drive, Unit 180
Henderson, NV 89014
(702) 732-2147 or (877) 325-7828
http://license.k3systems.com/LicensingPublic/
app?page=main&service=page

New Hampshire
Board of Medicine
121 South Fruit Street
Concord, NH 03301-2412
(603) 271-1203
http://www.nh.gov/medicine/assistants/

New Jersey
Physician Assistant Advisory Committee
P.O. Box 183
Trenton, NJ 08625
(609) 826-7100
http://www.njconsumeraffairs.gov/pa/

New Mexico
Medical Board
2055 South Pacheco Street, Bldg. 400
Santa Fe, NM 87505
(505) 476-7220 or (800) 945-5845
http://www.nmmb.state.nm.us/

Board of Osteopathic Medical Examiners
P.O. Box 25101
Santa Fe, NM 87505
(505) 476-4622

New York
State Board for Medicine
Office of the Professions
State Education Bldg., 2nd Floor
Albany, NY 12234
(518) 474-3817
http://www.op.nysed.gov/prof/med/rpa.htm

North Carolina
Medical Board
P.O. Box 20007
Raleigh, NC 27619-0007
(919) 326-1100 or (800) 253-9653
http://www.ncmedboard.org/

North Dakota
Board of Medical Examiners
418 East Broadway Avenue, Suite 12
Bismarck, ND 58501
(701) 328-6500
http://www.ndbomex.com/

Northern Marianas Islands
Medical Professional Licensing Board
P.O. Box 100007, CK
Saipan, MP 96950
(670) 664-4811
http://gov.mp/

Ohio
State Medical Board
30 East Broad Street, 3rd floor
Columbus, OH 43215-6127
(614) 466-3934
http://www.med.ohio.gov/pa_whats_new.htm

Oklahoma
Board of Medical Licensure and Supervision
P.O. Box 18256
Oklahoma City, OK 73154-0256
(405) 962-1400
http://www.okmedicalboard.org/physician_assistants

Oregon
Medical Board
1500 SW First Avenue, Suite 620
Portland, OR 97201-5847
(971) 673-2700 or (877) 254-6263
http://www.oregon.gov/omb/Pages/index.aspx

Pennsylvania
Board of Medicine
P.O. Box 2649
Harrisburg, PA 17105-2649
(717) 783-1400
*http://www.portal.state.pa.us/portal/server.pt/community/state_*
board_of_medicine/12512

Board of Osteopathic Medicine
P.O. Box 2649
Harrisburg, PA 17105-2649
(717) 783-4858
*http://www.recovery.pa.gov/portal/server.pt/community/state_board_*
of_osteopathic_medicine/12517

Rhode Island
Board of Physician Assistants
Division of Health Services Regulation, Health Professionals
3 Capitol Hill
Providence, RI 02908
(401) 222-5960
http://www.health.ri.gov/licensing/#healthcare

South Carolina
Board of Medical Examiners
110 Centerview Drive
Columbia, SC 29210
(803) 896-4500
http://www.llr.state.sc.us/POL/Medical/

South Dakota
Board of Medical and Osteopathic Examiners
101 North Main Avenue, Suite 3-1
Sioux Falls, SD 57104
(605) 367-7781
http://www.sdbmoe.gov/index.php?option=com_content&view=article
&id=16%3Aphysician-assistant-pa&catid=6&Itemid=10

Tennessee
Physician Assistant Committee
Department of Health-Related Boards
665 Mainstream Drive, 2nd Floor
Nashville, TN 37243
(615) 532-3202 or (800) 778-4123
http://health.state.tn.us/Boards/PA/index.htm

Texas
Physician Assistant Board
c/o Texas Medical Board
P.O. Box 2018
Austin, TX 78768-2018
(512) 305-7030
https://www.tmb.state.tx.us/page/licensing-physician-assistants

Utah
Physician Assistant Licensing Board
Division of Occupational and Professional Licensing
160 East 300 South
Salt Lake City, UT 84114
(801) 530-6628
http://www.dopl.utah.gov/licensing/physician_assistant.html

Vermont
Board of Medical Practice
108 Cherry Street
Burlington, VT 05402
(802) 863-7200
http://healthvermont.gov/hc/med_board/bmp.aspx

Virgin Islands
Board of Medical Examiners
Department of Health
48 Sugar Estate
St. Thomas, VI 00802
(340) 774-0117
http://www.fsmb.org/fcvs_paapp.html

Virginia
Board of Medicine
Perimeter Center
9960 Mayland Drive, Suite 300
Henrico, VA 23233-1463
(804) 367-4501
http://www.dhp.virginia.gov/medicine/

Washington
Medical Quality Assurance Commission
P.O. Box 47865
Olympia, WA 98504-7865
(800) 525-0127
http://www.doh.wa.gov/LicensesPermitsandCertificates/
MedicalCommission/MedicalLicensing

Board of Osteopathic Medicine and Surgery
Health Professions Quality Assurance
P.O. Box 47865
Olympia, WA 98504
(360) 236-4700
http://www.doh.wa.gov/LicensesPermitsandCertificates/
ProfessionsNewReneworUpdate/OsteopathicPhysician/
ApplicationsandForms

West Virginia
Board of Medicine
101 Dee Drive, Suite 103
Charleston, WV 25311
(304) 558-2921
http://www.wvdhhr.org/wvbom/

Board of Osteopathy
405 Capitol Street, Suite 402
Charleston, WV 25301
(304) 558-6095
http://www.wvbdosteo.org/

Wisconsin
Medical Examining Board
P.O. Box 8935
Madison, WI 53708-8935
(608) 266-2112
http://dsps.wi.gov/Default.aspx?Page=ee50fe91-099c-49e8-be5d-
a7e23d127c29

Wyoming
Board of Medicine
30 Hobbs Avenue, Suite A
Cheyenne, WY 82002
(307) 778-7053 or (800) 438-5784
http://wyomedboard.state.wy.us/

Authorization for Physician Assistants to Prescribe by State

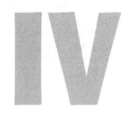

Jurisdiction	Restrictions	Controlled Substances
Alabama		Sch. II-V
Alaska		Sch. II-V
Arizona		Sch. II-III limited to 30-day supply, no refills without written consent from supervising physician; Sch. IV-V not more than 5 times in 6-month period per patient
Arkansas		Sch. III-V
California	PAs may write "drug orders" which, for the purposes of DEA registration, meet the federal definition of a prescription for DEA registration.	Sch. II-V. (Unless the PA has completed a board-approved course on controlled substances, these medications require a patient-specific order from the supervising physician.)
Colorado		Sch. II-V
Connecticut		Sch. II-V
Delaware		Sch. II-V
District of Columbia		Sch. II-V
Florida	Formulary of prohibited drugs	
Georgia	Formulary	Sch. III-V
Hawaii		Sch. III-V
Idaho		Sch. II-V
Illinois		Sch. II-V (Sch. II limited to 30-day supply of oral, transdermal, or topical medication)
Indiana		Sch. II-V (limited to 30-day supply)
Iowa		Sch. II-V (Sch. II excludes depressants)
Kansas		Sch. II-V

Jurisdiction	Restrictions	Controlled Substances
Kentucky		
Louisiana		Sch. III-V
Maine		Sch. III-V (Medical Board may approve Sch. II for individual PAs practicing with MD supervision. No such provision for Osteopathic Board.)
Maryland		Schedule II-V
Massachusetts		Schedule II-V
Michigan		Sch. II-V
Minnesota		Sch. II-V
Mississippi		Sch. II-V
Missouri		Sch. III-V (Sch. III limited to 5-day supply with no refill)
Montana		Sch. II-V (Sch. II limited to 34-day supply)
Nebraska		Sch. II-V
Nevada		Sch. II-V
New Hampshire		Sch. II-V
New Jersey		Sch. II-V (certain conditions apply)
New Mexico	Formulary	Sch. II-V
New York		Sch. II-V
North Carolina		Sch. II-V (Sch. II-III limited to 30-day supply)
North Dakota		Sch. II-V
Ohio	Formulary	Sch. II-V (certain conditions apply to Schedule II Rx)
Oklahoma	Formulary	Sch. III-V (limited to 30-day supply)
Oregon		Sch. II-V
Pennsylvania		Sch. II-V (Sch. II limited to 72 hours for initial therapy; 30 days for ongoing therapy)
Rhode Island		Sch. II-V
South Carolina		Sch. II-V
South Dakota		Sch. II-V (Sch. II limited to 30-day supply)
Tennessee		Sch. II-V
Texas		Sch. II-V (Sch. III-V limited to 90-day supply; certain conditions apply to Schedule II)

Jurisdiction	Restrictions	Controlled Substances
Utah		Sch. II-V
Vermont		Sch. II-V
Virginia		Sch. II-V
Washington		Sch. II-V
West Virginia	Formulary	Sch. III-V (Sch. III limited to 72-hour supply)
Wisconsin		Sch. II-V
Wyoming		Sch. II-V

Adapted from the AAPA.

DEA Registration

The Drug Enforcement Administration (DEA) has a registration category specifically for physician assistants and other so-called midlevel practitioners authorized by state law or regulation to prescribe controlled substances. For more information or to obtain a registration application, contact the DEA Registration Unit at (800) 882-9539.

New PA Graduate Temporary Licensure Availability by State

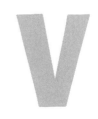

State	Temporary Licensing
Alabama	Yes
Alaska	Yes
Arizona	Yes
Arkansas	Yes
California	No provision
Colorado	No provision
Connecticut	Yes
Delaware	Yes
District of Columbia	Yes
Florida	Yes
Georgia	Yes
Hawaii	Yes
Idaho	Yes
Illinois	Yes
Indiana	Yes
Iowa	Yes
Kansas	Yes
Kentucky	Yes
Louisiana	Yes
Maine	Yes
Maryland	No provision
Massachusetts	Yes
Michigan	Yes

State	Temporary Licensing
Minnesota	Yes
Mississippi	Yes
Missouri	Yes
Montana	No provision
Nebraska	Yes
Nevada	Yes
New Hampshire	No provision
New Jersey	Yes
New Mexico	Yes
New York	Yes
North Carolina	No provision
North Dakota	No provision
Ohio	No provision
Oklahoma	No provision
Oregon	Yes
Pennsylvania	Yes
Rhode Island	No provision
South Carolina	Yes
South Dakota	Yes
Tennessee	Yes
Texas	Yes
Utah	Yes
Vermont	Yes
Virginia	Yes
Washington	Yes
West Virginia	Yes
Wisconsin	Yes
Wyoming	Yes